Comprehensive Book of

MRCPsych CASC

Samir Shah
MBBS, MRCPsych, MSc
Consultant in Liaison Psychiatry (Salford Royal Hospital)
Greater Manchester West Mental Health NHS Foundation Trust
Meadowbrook Unit, Stott Lane, Salford, UK

Madhavan Seshadri
MBBS, DPM, MRCPsych, PGCert ME
Consultant in General Adult Psychiatry
2gether NHS Foundation Trust, Recovery Team South
The Knoll, Ross-on-Wye, Herefordshire, HR9 5NA, UK

Ashok G Patel
MBBS, DPM, FRCPsych
Consultant Psychiatrist
26 Aubreys, Letchworth Garden City
Herts SG6 3TZ, UK

PEEPEE
PUBLISHERS AND DISTRIBUTORS (P) LTD.

Comprehensive Book of MRCPsych CASC

Published by
Pawaninder P. Vij and Anupam Vij
Peepee Publishers and Distributors (P) Ltd.
Head Office: 160, Shakti Vihar, Pitam Pura
Delhi-110034 (India)

***Correspondence Address:* 7/31, First Floor, Ansari Road**
Daryaganj, New Delhi-110002 (India)
Ph: 65195868, 23246245, 9811156083
e-mail: peepee160@yahoo.co.in
e-mail: peepee160@gmail.com
e-mail: pawan_vij@peepeepub.com
www.peepeepub.com

Also Available in United Kingdom at:

Nitika Moore
45 Linden Avenue
Great Barr
Birmingham B43 5JU (UK)
e-mail: nitika_vij@yahoo.com

First Edition : 2017

ISBN: 978-81-8445-211-2

Preface

The MRCPsych examinations (Paper A, Paper B and CASC) are challenging, thought-provoking and essential building block towards higher specialist training in Psychiatry in the United Kingdom. The Clinical Assessment of Skills and Competencies (CASC) is the final examination that demands meticulous preparation and command over clinical and communication skills. To succeed in CASC is every Psychiatry trainee's aspiration that leads to Membership of the Royal College of Psychiatrists. In this book, we have endeavored to provide extensive CASC revision scenarios covering the length and breadth of curriculum essential to pass the examination. We are confident that this book will allow candidates to be thoroughly prepared for CASC and significantly improve their chance of success.

The book is organised in three main sections. The first section aims at providing information and guidance on CASC examination format and structure. The second section includes clinical examination scenarios with sample stations. The third section has extensive coverage of single and linked sample stations from range of sub-specialties in Psychiatry. All sample stations are based on the curriculum and provide clinical scenarios that can be practised with colleagues, seniors and other trainees doing the examination. We strongly recommended practising in groups where one would act as patient, another candidate and third as an examiner.

This is a multi-author book and burden of editorship has been wisely spread to capitalise on breath and depth of expertise, thereby providing trainees the wealth of scenarios and knowledge for CASC. It is our intention that this book will help Psychiatry trainees not only to pass CASC but also to improve their clinical skills, communication and overall patient care. We hope Psychiatry trainees and all involved in Psychiatry education would find this book helpful for the MRCPsych examinations. The authors would like to wish trainees all the best in their endeavor to achieve MRCPsych.

Samir Shah
Madhavan Seshadri
Ashok G Patel

Acknowledgements

We would like to thank our colleagues and friends who have supported us during preparation of this book. They have provided guidance, support, advice and constructive criticism during the planning and preparation this book.

We are most grateful to our publishers Peepee Publishers and Distributors (P) Ltd, New Delhi, India and their staff without whom this book would not have been possible. A special mention and thanks to Dr Dinesh Khanna for his support and encouragement in getting the book published. We would like to thank all the authors who have done an excellent job and ensured that sample stations were compatible with the MRCPsych CASC examination. We would also like to thanks all the trainees, junior doctors and budding Psychiatrists who have encouraged and kept us motivated during this extensive task of preparing this CASC book.

Last but not the least, we would like to thank the families of the authors and our own families who have shown great deal of patience and support. They have been by our side during evenings, weekends and holidays when most of the book has been conceptualized and written.

Samir Shah
Madhavan Seshadri
Ashok G Patel

Contributors

Samir Shah
MBBS, MRCPsych, MSc
Consultant in Liaison Psychiatry (Salford Royal Hospital)
Greater Manchester West Mental Health NHS Foundation Trust
Meadowbrook Unit, Stott Lane
Salford, UK

Madhavan Seshadri
MBBS, DPM, MRCPsych, PGCert ME
Consultant in General Adult Psychiatry
2gether NHS Foundation Trust
Recovery Team South
The Knoll, Ross-on-Wye
Herefordshire, HR9 5NA
UK

Ashok G Patel
MBBS, DPM, FRCPsych
Consultant Psychiatrist
26 Aubreys
Letchworth Garden City
Herts SG6 3TZ
UK

Syed Ashraf
MRCPsych, PGCHM
Specialty Registrar
South Westminster CMHT, 2nd Floor, 190 Vauxhall Bridge Road
London SW1V1DX
UK

Margaret Campbell
MBChB, MSC, FRCPsych
Associate Medical Director and
Director of Medical Education
Greater Manchester West Mental Health NHS Foundation Trust
Trust HQ, Bury New Road
Prestwich
UK

Lalana Dissanayake
MBBS, MRCPsych
Consultant Psychiatrist
East London NHS Foundation Trust
CMHT, Spring House
Potton Road, Biggleswade, SG18 OEL
UK

Sanjith Kamath
MBBS, MRCPsych, MBA
Consultant Psychiatrist
2 Belfry Lane
Collingtree Park, NN4 OPB
UK

Vishelle Kamath
MBBS, MRCPsych
Consultant Psychiatrist
2 Belfry Lane
Collingtree Park, NN4 OPB
UK

Dinesh Khanna
MBBS, MSc, MRCPsych
Child and Adolescent Psychiatrist
Cheadle Royal Hospital, 100, Wilmslow Road
Cheadle SK8 3DG
UK

Juhi Mishra
MBBS
CT-1 Psychiatry, North Essex Partnership Trust
96, Eldon Road, Luton, LU4 0AX
UK

Iqbal Mohiuddin
BSc (Hons), MBBS, HGDip (Human Givens Therapy Diploma)
DipCBT (Diploma in CBT), MRCPsych, FHEA
(Fellow of the Higher Education Academy)
Locum Consultant Psychiatrist
East London NHS Foundation Trust, Luton and Central
Bedfordshire Mental Health Unit, Calnwood Road, Luton
Bedfordshire, LU4 0FB
UK

Laura Pearse
MBChB, BSc (Hons) Phys, MRCPsych, DOccMed
Independent Consultant Psychiatrist
Innovations House, 19 Staple Gardens, Winchester SO23 8SR
UK

Roshelle Ramkisson
MBBS, MRCPsych, MSc (Health and Public Leadership) PGDip
Psychiatry MDCH
Consultant Psychiatrist in Child and Adolescent Psychiatry
Pennine Care NHS Foundation Trust
Royal Oldham Hospital
Oldham, UK

Babu Mani Sandilyan
MBBS, DMH, MRCPsych
Consultant Liaison Psychiatrist
Psychological Medicine Service
Royal Berkshire Hospital
London Road
Reading RG7 1RW
UK

Malarvizhi Babu Sandilyan
MBBS, MRCPsych, DGM
Consultant Psychiatrist
Berkshire Healthcare NHS Foundation Trust
Reading RG30 4EJ
UK

Shazada Hussain Shah
MBBS, MRCPsych, DPM, DCP
Locum Consultant Psychiatrist
NHS Tayside CMHT Arbroath Gowanlea
12-14 Seaton Road
Arbroath DD11 5DX
UK

Ajaya Upadhyaya
MD, FRCPsych
Consultant Psychiatrist
22 West Hayes
Hatfield Heath
Herts CM22 7DH
UK

Nuruz Zaman
MBBS, MRCPsych, PGCert (Medical Education)
Locum Consultant Forensic Psychiatrist
Robin Pinto Unit
Calnwood Road
Luton, Beds LU4 0FB
UK

Contents

List of Stations:

SECTION 1

A Guide to Clinical Assessment of Skills and Competencies (CASC)

1. Format of CASC Examination

Madhavan Seshadri

Introduction

CASC examination follows the principles of objective structured clinical examination (OSCE). A CASC examination consists of a series of stations in which candidates are assessed whilst performing a defined clinical task. These stations comprising a range of clinical scenarios assess competence in a multitude of clinical skills, thus, setting a standard expected of core psychiatric trainees. There are two types of CASC circuits in the MRCPsych examination.

1. **Linked/Paired Stations:** On the day of CASC examination, the morning circuit comprises four linked/paired stations, i.e., eight stations in total. In linked stations, two stations are linked together to form a pair which allows assessment of more 'advanced' clinical skills. Each station lasts 10 minutes with 90 seconds preparation time, i.e., total of 11 minutes and 30 seconds. In the first station, the candidates carry out an assessment, e.g., history from the patient and then carry out a linked task, e.g., communicating their assessment with the patient's carer in the second station.
2. **Stand-alone/Single Stations:** There are eight stand-alone stations in the afternoon circuit. Each stand-alone station lasts 7 minutes with 90 seconds preparation time, i.e., total of 8 minutes and 30 seconds.

In total, CASC examination consists of 16 stations.

Skills and Competencies Assessed

- History taking, either from the patient or from a collateral source.
- Mental state examination.
- Risk assessment.
- Cognitive assessment.
- Physical examination.

- Discussion of diagnosis, treatment options, side-effects, prognosis, consent, etc.
- Difficult communication, e.g., breaking bad news, dealing with angry patient/relative, etc.
- Communications with colleagues from different professions including nurses, social workers as well as doctors from other specialties of medicine.

Each station consists of:

1. Theme.
2. Instructions to the candidates.
3. Instructions to the role player.
4. Construct.
5. Expanded construct.
6. Areas of importance to pass the station.
7. Equipment checklist if applicable.

1. **Theme:**

   Theme indicates the areas of clinical skills and competencies being tested, e.g., history taking, assessment, communication, physical examination, cognitive assessment, etc.

2. **Instructions to the candidates:**

   The candidate instructions should as concisely as possible set the scene for the clinical encounter (i.e., outpatient clinic, A and E, etc.), include circumstances of the presentation as well as inform the candidate of the task or tasks to be completed. The instructions should be set out in bullet points and be limited to as few as possible. The candidates should not be expected to use all the preparation time reading the instructions. It is also not realistic to give them too much information to assimilate before entering the station. Occasionally, negative instructions will be included to allow the candidates to focus on the given tasks.

   Example:

   Elicit the patient's history about:

   - Presenting complaints.
   - Past medical/psychiatric history.
   - Differential diagnosis.
   - You are not required to do mental state examination.

3. **Instructions to role player:**

   The role players are professional actors who are trained to play the roles which could include patients, their relatives/or carers and other professionals, such as, nurses, social workers, psychologists, or indeed consultant psychiatrists. As much as possible, the role should not be gender or race specific unless absolutely required for the construct of the station.

   The information should include:

   - Relevant information about the patient (age, gender, etc.).
   - Information regarding the presentation and circumstances surrounding it.
   - Medical/psychiatric history.

- Social history.
- If the station requires the candidate to perform a particular test or examination (e.g., MMSE), instructions should be given about what the role player should expect as well as any responses that should be given to questions asked by the candidate.
- An opening statement.

4. **Construct:**

It defines the objective to be assessed in the station and makes the examiner aware of what constitutes a competent performance. It requires being concise but precise and unambiguous in setting out the domain to be evaluated.

Examples:

- The candidate is able to establish the content of the patient's delusions and identify the risk to others arising from them in a concise, fluent and focused manner.
- The candidate is able to succinctly communicate with the consultant, over a telephone the assessment of a patient's delusional system and correctly identify the risk arising from this.
- The candidate is able to elicit a history of the mood disorder and related aspects of the patient's past medical/psychiatric and social history.
- The candidate is able to explain the nature, purpose, likely effects, mechanism of action, and practicalities of a proposed treatment. They are required to address the patient's/carer's beliefs, concerns, anxieties, fears and expectations.

It is important that the construct is achievable within the time allowed for the particular CASC format.

5. **Expanded construct:**

The expanded construct defines the objectives to be assessed in the station in more details than the 'Construct'. It needs to be set out in unambiguous language covering the sorts of skills that should be displayed by the candidate.

Example of history taking station:

The candidate is expected to take a history and assess the risk arising from the delusional system.

- They should demonstrate skill in eliciting a history that picks up the relevant information about the onset, duration and progress of the psychotic disorder.
- They should be able to elicit possible aetiological factors.
- Ask a range of questions that demonstrates of the psychopathology.
- They should briefly ask about symptoms of differential diagnosis or comorbid disorders.
- Demonstrates empathy with the patient's experience.
- Need to elicit the patient's fears, anxieties and concerns.
- Show the ability to focus on the specific problem.

In addition to the knowledge, the expanded construct sets out the interview/communication skills expected of the candidate. So a successful candidate would:

- Show an appropriate mixture of open and closed questioning and empathic interview skills.
- Demonstrate advanced listening skills and attending to patients sensitively.

- Ask questions that are structured, focused and fluent.
- Avoid the use of jargon and technical language and false reassurance.

In the explanation stations:

- The candidates are expected to give information in a focused and fluent manner avoiding using jargon and technical language.
- They are expected to demonstrate empathy with the patient's concerns.
- In addition to imparting correct information candidates should be sensitive to the patient's concerns, display an appropriate mix of open-ended and closed questions, transition statements and advanced listening skills.
- They should explain the origin/aetiology (where required) of the patient's symptoms and why they experience the symptoms they do.
- They should explain the practicalities (where appropriate) of the proposed treatment and give information as to how it works. They should discuss the proposed treatment in context with other treatments, physical, psychological and social and be able to explain why this particular treatment is considered most appropriate at this time.
- They should be able to address the patients' relatives or carers' concerns, fears, anxieties, expectations etc. by demonstrating a collaborative approach and not merely offering bland reassurance.

6. **Areas of importance to pass the station:**
   They should be written to cover the basic factual information for examiners, e.g., information for a child and adolescent (CAMH) station that would allow an Old Age Psychiatrist to examine with confidence.
7. **Equipment checklist:**
   Any equipment or material (e.g., examination couch, stethoscope, tendon hammer, etc.) required for the station should be listed.

2. Marking Scheme and Areas of Importance for Unsuccessful Candidates

Madhavan Seshadri

Marking Scheme

Since September 2015, the college has revised the marking scheme. In each station, candidate's overall performance is graded as follows:

1. **Excellent Pass:** Candidate demonstrates excellent knowledge and skills of competence expected of a newly appointed trainee at ST4 grade.
2. **Pass:** Clear level of competence expected of a newly appointed trainee at ST4 grade.
3. **Borderline Pass:** Adequate level of competence expected of a newly appointed trainee at ST4 grade.
4. **Borderline Fail:** Failure to demonstrate an adequate level of competence at ST4 grade.

5. **Fail:** Failure to demonstrate the level of competence by unsystematic, inconsistent and unfocussed approach and omission of many of the essential and desirable components.
6. **Severe Fail:** Failure to demonstrate competence with a clinical approach, i.e., incompatible with good psychiatric practice and accompanied by inadequate reasoning and/or technical competence.

A successful candidate would have passed at least 12 stations. In addition, they should not receive severe fail in two or more marking domains of the station. This would adversely affect the overall score and may lead to failure.

Areas of Importance for Candidates

Unsuccessful candidates receive copies of the marksheets indicating the areas where they have failed. They are broadly divided into five areas:

1. Poor management of interview/discussion, e.g.:
   - Lack of focus on the required task.
   - Lack of fluency.
   - Insensitive interruptions.
   - Lack of systematic and logical line of enquiry.
2. Poor communication skills, e.g.:
   - Lack of flexible approach.
   - Lack of empathy.
   - Excessive use of closed questions.
   - Use of medical jargon and technical language.
   - Failure to listen, identify and respond to concerns of patients and other informants.
3. Significant deviations from the given task, e.g.:
   - Inappropriate avenues of inquiry or discussion.
   - Discussion of inaccurate or misleading information.
   - Poor analysis of problems and synthesis of opinion.
4. Lack of professionalism, e.g.:
   - Harmful interaction.
   - Lack of respect for the patient/informant.
   - Dismissive attitude.
5. Limited depth and/or range to the task, e.g.,
   - Inadequate or superficial risk assessment.
   - Limited range of symptomatology explored.
   - Limited or incomplete address of concerns, anxieties, worries, expectations, etc.

3. Tips for Passing CASC

Lalana Dissanayake

When the CASC exam was introduced in March 2008, it was a major change in the exam practice from the Patient Management Problems (PMPs) and Individual Patient Assessment (long case). It is, therefore, essential to learn the art of the test of Clinical Assessment of Skills and Competencies (CASCs). The candidates must have a good understanding of the Royal College of Psychiatrists' expectations in each station. However, it does not differ from day to day clinical practice except that this is a piecemeal approach. In the CASC examination, even though candidates are interviewing a role player, it is simulating a real life situation; hence, it is important to assume that candidates are examining a real patient.

CASC examination is a highly anxiety-provoking situation as it tests the knowledge and skills in limited time and there is rapid shift from one topic to another. Also in many stations, there is less interaction with the examiner, so, candidates are more prone to be stressed and anxious. On some occasions, this becomes quite obvious to the examiner as well as to the role player. This may create an atmosphere where the candidates are seen as less confident, less competent as well as less professional. Also, role players may not be forthcoming. It is, therefore, important to be calm, confident and professional in the examination. It is important to have a positive attitude that examiners and role players are there to assist the candidates. Generally, what the examiner is looking for is the candidate's knowledge and communication skills, not only verbal, but also non-verbal.

First Impression

When a candidate enters the station, it is better to have some eye contact with examiner and identify with the candidates' number. After that generally one can ignore the examiner's presence until he finishes the interview. Establishing the rapport in the beginning of the interview is a major skill, examiners are looking for. It is better to use first half a minute for this purpose. The patients should be addressed as mentioned in the instructions, as in our view, it is not necessary to be informal with patients during their first appointment. Anybody would respond better if they are called by their name rather addressing 'You'. This is more important for patients who are partially mute, withdrawn, depressed or confused. Some candidates ask patient's name but never use it during the whole interview. It is, therefore, advisable to call the patient by the given names rather than ask "how should I call you".

Good psychiatrists are good observers and good listeners. Examiners look into whether the candidates can pick up the cues given by the role player. So, the candidate should start observing the moment he or she enters the station and demonstrate the same to the examiner. For example, candidates may highlight when the patient is grossly anxious or depressed or distracted by external stimulus. The role players may try to bring the candidate into the task by giving a cue. So, it is important to be vigilant and pick up the cues as the situation evolves. The appearance of the patient may give a cue, e.g., a patient with a cross drawn on his forehead would require the candidate to comment on it politely.

A good candidate would use the information available in the scenario to set the scene. Also, it is useful to remember that a laminated instruction card is always available within the station to refer to the scenario, when necessary. The candidates should not hesitate to look at it if unsure about the task or scenario, as there is a risk of doing something completely out of focus under exam pressure.

Focus on the Task

As it is a time-limited exam, assessment of specific skills in each station is of great importance, so that the candidates remain focused on the task. Generally, in single stations even though the scenarios can be lengthy, the tasks are straight forward. The candidates are expected to demonstrate those skills. In linked/paired stations, the scenarios may be short, but the tasks are more complex. There is a 'question behind the question'. In these situations, candidates should think broadly. The first station is usually geared to information gathering or eliciting psychopathology and the second station is about analysing, interpreting and communicating the findings gathered in the first station as well as explaining the management if needed.

Empathy

The importance of empathy is repeatedly mentioned, as it can often be misunderstood as giving in to patient's every request. For example, in stations where patient is demonstrating personality difficulties or making inappropriate demands, such as asking methadone, the examiner would expect the candidate to maintain boundaries. Showing inappropriate empathy in such situations would be breach of professionalism. The candidates should avoid repeated, unnecessary or premature expressions of empathy.

Communication Skills

Communication skills are the key tool in psychiatric practice. One may use three types of advanced communication skills to approach whatever the scenario.

- **Weaving:** The patient has an agenda in his mind and the candidates should have an agenda to demonstrate to the examiner that he can effectively execute the task. Like in weaving process from one end to another constantly, a good candidate should be able to use advanced listening skills and communication skills to constant move from showing interest to the role players' agenda while focusing on his own agenda.
- **Helicoptering:** There may be situations in during the interview process when the role player would bring a sensitive issue so that one feels 'stuck' and finds it hard to proceed. Here a good candidate uses this technique to smoothly address the issue. It is like police search helicopters 'zoom in and zoom out' appropriately to find something.
- **Clustering:** This is the technique one may use when eliciting complex psychopathology. Once psychotic symptoms are elicited a good candidate would cluster them into hallucinatory experiences and delusional experiences. Within the clustering group, they complete the whole task of establishing all the features of hallucinatory experiences, i.e., type of hallucination (auditory, visual, etc.), pseudo or classic, 2nd or 3rd person, command, etc. Then, he would move to delusion cluster and deal with that separately.

Time Management

CASC exam tests the time management skills of the candidates. This starts the moment candidate starts reading the instructions. The way of managing time is different in single stations compared to paired stations. In single stations, candidates should be clear about the task and how to open the station using available information in hand. It is also important to have a structure in mind to cover the key areas. Each question asked or information given should be relevant to the task. This helps the examiner to score the candidate's performance appropriately. In paired stations, it will be helpful to write down legibly, the information and structure the session so that information can be filled in. This also helps in using the information appropriately in the next station.

When the candidate reads the scenario, he can anticipate what is being tested in particular stations. The candidates should also identify the number of tasks required in each station and allocate time for each task. If there are multiple tasks in a station, candidate should divide the time and try to cover all the tasks, e.g., if there are two tasks, 3 minutes each and 2 minutes to recap or to revisit the tasks. The candidates should try to attend all tasks.

Approach to stations differs depending on the scenario. So, candidates should know how to vary their approach in different scenarios. Having a stereotyped approach can be counterproductive. Many a times candidates practice some stations so much that when they face unexpected scenario they struggle as they assume and expect the station in the examination to be identical to the scenario they have practised. Over-practice and learning the station by heart can limit lateral thinking, which is another skill tested in the exam. So, one should have a structure but still be flexible and open to the exam situation. Generally, you can categorize the scenarios into following areas of testing:

- Eliciting psychopathology and clinical history.
- Mental state examination, cognitive assessment and physical examination.
- Explaining about illness, procedure, situation, side-effects, etc.
- Constructive approach of disturbed patient, breaking bad news, and dealing with demanding relatives.
- Discussing a management plan, psychological treatments.
- Obtaining collateral information and consent.
- Interpreting lab results, ECG, EEG, X-rays, scans, etc.
- Knowledge of practical application of Mental Health Act.

Demonstrating Psychopathology

There are specific stations to assess the candidates' knowledge of psychopathology and how to elicit the signs and symptoms in the patient. In stations, where the main task is to elicit psychopathology, candidates may assume that the examiner has observed the symptoms or signs as patient describes them. However, it is important to emphasize the symptom, sometimes by rephrasing the patient's verbatim. For example, in demonstrating thought echo "so you hear your own thoughts like you hear me now?" Clustering of the symptoms is an easy way to approach such stations as described later. Remember, you need to go into depth of psychopathology by dissecting each experience at this stage rather than touching superficially.

When the task is about explaining something, it is important to assess and make judgments about the level of prior knowledge. One may come across a Professor of Chemistry who is suffering from bipolar affective disorder and the task is to explain about lithium. Of course, then one need not start saying lithium is a type of salt! One should not just try to get answers to a list of questions. Also good interview cannot be monotonous. It should be a conversation, which demonstrates advanced communication skills. Good candidates should be able to respond appropriately to a sudden unanticipated question or comment by the role player.

Finishing the Interview

Certainly, it looks very awkward to finish the interview even before the last minute bell. It may create a negative impression to end the interview before the allocated time, especially if the tasks are not addressed. If one has time left, it is always better to give an opportunity to the role players to raise any questions and clarify anything. Finally, whenever relevant, one should check whether they have understood what you explained. The candidates should be able to continue the conversation to the end of the limited time available. When the last minute bell rings, the candidates should start wrapping up the process. It is not sensible to start a big discussion about something, such as explaining CBT in the last minute. Again finishing the interview abruptly or continuing the interview after the finishing bell would give a negative impression. Thanking the patient for participating in the interview is a good gesture and creates a good impression.

Some candidates who despite their good theoretical knowledge in psychiatry can get lower scores and the reasons are the following:

- Unnecessary anxiety of the candidate, which is obvious and overt to the role player and examiner. It is important for the candidates to remember that they would have the knowledge of all common conditions and situations in the CASC exam. They would have come across most of such situations during day to day clinical practice. The examination is not testing something that they do not know. The candidates sometimes complicate the situation themselves unnecessarily rather than taking a simple approach. So, remember to have a positive attitude and mindset.
- A key to a successful performance is to use the full seven minutes in single stations and 10 minutes in paired stations effectively and constructively without going out of focus. Some candidates waste time by asking unnecessary questions in the beginning and run out of time to ask more relevant information. As the time is limited, one should remember to prioritize symptoms or issues. As an example, if it is about depression, good candidates first cover low mood, lack of interest and lack of energy which are the main criteria in ICD-10, and then move to other symptoms. In the station on eliciting the history of anorexia nervosa in a woman, one would first establish three primary symptoms of body image disturbance, BMI and amenorrhea.

Failure to listen and consequently to pick up relevant cues and not to observe significant body language is a major factor underlying poor performance.

- Due to the nature of the CASC examination, one needs to learn to shift the focus from one station to another within a short period of time. Some scenarios may appear to be difficult and candidates may feel that they have not performed well. It is important to try to push previous stations to the back of one's mind and avoid carrying the negative mindset to the next station. Anxiety can skews the perception about one's performance and it is pointless trying to analyse one's performance when moving from one station to the next. More importantly, it will distract from concentrating on the next station. It is a common observation that some candidates fail in stations which had been perceived to be easy and vice versa.

One should assume that, each station is a clinical encounter, patients are real and do exactly what one would do in their clinical practice. This book gives many of the scenarios that appear in CASC examinations. Practicing the simple techniques described here and following the tips in the exam would help the candidate to deliver a successful performance.

SECTION 2

Clinical Examination with Sample Stations

1. Cognitive Assessment

Madhavan Seshadri and Juhi Mishra

Cognitive functions are basic building blocks of a person's ability to think, feel and act. In every MRCPsych CASC examination, there will be at least one cognitive assessment station (CASC Blueprint www.rcpsych.ac.uk). It will appear as a straightforward task to assess a person's cognitive functions but in these stations examiners expect the candidates to demonstrate a degree of fluency. Also, the candidates should demonstrate the communication skills that are needed in assessing a cognitively impaired patient. Practicing these skills in daily work will help the candidates to shine in the examination situation.

The following set of questions may help the candidate focus on the task:

- Is there a significant cognitive problem?
- Is it a global or focal dysfunction?
- If it is global, what could be the clinical presentation, i.e., delirium or dementia?
- If it is focal, which areas of the brain are involved?
- If possible, ascertain the cause of the cognitive impairment. It is important to rule out depression in old age.
- How does this dysfunction affect patient's life?
- What are the risks the patient is posing due to cognitive impairment?

In the CASC examination, assessment of cognitive dysfunction may involve:

- Taking a focused history from the patient.
- Corroborative/collateral history from a reliable informant.
- Mental state examination.
- Cognitive assessment.
- General medical and neurological examination.

Preliminary steps to follow in all cognitive assessment stations:

- Before entering the station, candidate should read the task carefully. Subtle changes in the task will give a cue to area that needs deeper exploration. For example, if the task mentions cognitive assessment in a person who had a stroke and who has difficulty remembering names, in addition to routine examination naming objects should be explored in depth. Simply asking the name of two objects might not be enough to pass the station.

- It is important to read the CASC vignettes, as they will give some background information to the candidate. Take notes of these points and explore these appropriately.
- Once you see the task of the station as 'cognitive assessment' drawing figures like intersecting pentagon or square triangle and writing down instructions like 'close your eyes' (appropriate to the station) in the 1 minute time (outside the station) can save time.
- Candidate should ensure that the patient is comfortable. They should introduce themselves and explain the process using simple terms.
- Cognitively impaired patients will find it difficult to process information. Using short sentences and simple words are important.
- The older patients may have hearing difficulty or visual problems. These should be clarified sensitively.
- Cognitive functions also depend upon patient's premorbid functioning: educational level, job done etc. Where necessary these should be assessed. Candidate should ask for past history of memory problems.
- Candidate should ask whether they suffer from any medical problems.
- If patient says 'I don't know' one could ask them to guess. If a candidate is stuck in an area for long it is better to move on to complete other tasks. At the same time, it is important not to hurry the patient.
- It is a common mistake that candidates assume that the patient has understood the instructions/tests asked to perform. It is always important to make sure that the patient understands the instructions given to perform a task.
- Mini Mental State Examination (MMSE) is a good screening tool. If patient finds a particular area of MMSE to be difficult then that area needs to be explored in depth.
- In addition to doing the MMSE, candidates should also check for:
    - Personal orientation: Name, age and date of birth. Check whether the patient could remember you and your role (doctor).
    - Long-term memory: For example, Name of the Prime Minister, Year of Second World War or First World War, etc. In early stages of dementia, only short-term memory is impaired. By testing long-term memory candidate can demonstrate to the examiner that he/she screens for all the components of memory.
    - At least one frontal (executive) functions test and one parietal lobe function test.
    - If the candidate has time, he may ask the patient to do 'Clock drawing test'.

Mini Mental State Examination (MMSE)

Orientation:

- Orientation to time: Date, day, month, year and season.

  Better to use standard question, e.g., "Can you also tell me what season it is?" One point for each correct answer.

  Maximum points: 5.

- Orientation to place: Floor number or room number. Ask for the name of the ward, building, town or city and country. If there is no name for the ward you may ask for the name of the hospital. One point for each correct answer.
  Maximum points: 5.

Registration:

- Candidate should explain the patient clearly that memory is being tested. Make it clear that he should repeat the names once you give all three names. Also, he should be clearly told that he will be asked to recall these three names after few minutes.
- Name three unrelated objects (e.g., apple, penny, table) clearly, about 1 second for each. After the completion of all three, patient should be asked to repeat them. This first repetition determines the patient's points. If patient cannot repeat three words, one should keep repeating them until the patient can repeat all three (up to five times). If he/she does not learn all three, the recall cannot be tested.

  Maximum points: 3.

Attention and Concentration:

- One may either do 'serial sevens' or check for spelling 'WORLD' backwards.
- Serial sevens test: Ask the patient to begin with 100 and serially subtract seven. Stop after 5 subtractions (93, 86, 79, 72, 65). Give one mark for each correct answer.
- Spelling 'WORLD' backwards: If the patient cannot perform serial sevens test, ask him/her to spell the word 'WORLD' backwards. Each letter in correct order gives one mark.

  For example, DLROW = 5 marks; DLORW = 3 marks; if patient spells forwards again and again 0 points.

  Maximum points: 5.

Recall:

- Ask the patient if he/she can recall the three words you previously asked him/her to remember. Points one for each correct answer. Apple, penny, table.
  Maximum points: 3.

Language Functions:

- Naming: Show the patient a wristwatch and ask him/her what it is. Repeat for pencil. One point for each correct answer.
  Maximum points: 2.
- Repetition: Ask the patient to repeat the sentence after you.
  'No ifs, ands or buts' allow only one trial. One point if the repetition is completely correct.
  Maximum point: 1.
- Three-stage command: Give a three-stage command first and ask the patient to fulfill the task. Usual command used is "take this paper in your right hand, fold it into half and place it on the floor". Give the patient a blank paper. One point for each step correctly executed.
  Maximum points: 3.

- Reading: Write in big letters 'Close your eyes'. Ask the patient to read and carry out the instruction. Patient may read loudly, but the point is given if the patient closes his/her eyes.
  Maximum point: 1.
- Writing: Give the patient a blank paper and ask him/her to write a sentence. Prompting not allowed. The sentence must contain a subject and verb. Spelling and grammatical errors are accepted. Maximum point: 1.

Construction:

- On a clean piece of paper, draw intersecting pentagons, each side about 1 inch and ask him/her to copy it exactly as it is. The two pentagons must intersect to have the intersected segment with 4 sides. Tremor and rotation are ignored.

  Maximum point: 1

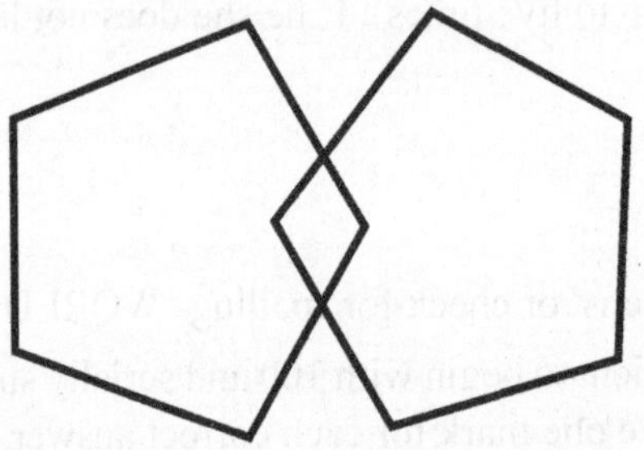

Total score in MMSE = 30. Less than 25 suggests dementia.

Ref: Folstein M, Folstein SE, McHugh PR. "Mini-Mental State" a Practical Method for Grading the Cognitive State of Patients for the Clinician. Journal of Psychiatric Research 1975; 12(3);189–198.

Frontal (Executive) Functions Tests

Impairment of frontal lobe functions typically involves errors of planning, judgment, problem solving, impulse control and abstract reasoning. In the exam situation, it is better to use a standardised scale, e.g., Frontal assessment battery. Components of frontal lobe testing are given below for the benefit of candidates.

Candidates should:

- Introduce themselves, explain the purpose of assessment. Some background questions may be asked for history.
- Check preliminaries that are common to all cognitive examinations.
- **Attention and concentration:** 'Serial seven test' or 'World' Backwards or 'Digit span test'. Normal digit span in humans in up to 7 +/–2 digits.
- **Tests for abstract thinking/concept formation:** Proverb interpretation as well as similarities
  - o Similarities.
- In what way the following are alike?
  - o An apple and a banana.
  - o A table and a chair.
  - o A tulip, a rose and a daisy.

In the CASC exam, eliciting similarities using one of the above pairs is enough.

- Proverb interpretation
  - Ask "What do I mean when I say"
    - A stitch in time saves nine.
    - Make hay while sun shines.
    - Rolling stone gathers no moss.

In the CASC exam, eliciting the abstract meaning using one of the above is enough.

- **Word fluency tests:**
  - *Verbal fluency:* Patients should be asked to tell all the words that start with letter 'A', 'F' or 'S'. One letter is given at a time and the number of words mentioned by the patient in 60 seconds are counted. If the letter is 'A' and if the patient gives no response during the first 5 seconds, candidates may say 'for instance, apple'. If the patient pauses 10 seconds, candidate may repeat the instruction "any word beginning with the letter 'A'." Word repetitions or variations (e.g., attaché, attachment, attached etc.), surnames, or proper nouns are not counted as correct responses.
  - *Category fluency:* Candidates should ask the patient to name all the fruits he can remember in 60 seconds. Alternatively, ask for all the animals or things seen in supermarket aisle.

    Normally, one should be able to tell 15 or more words. Counts less than 9 are significant. Candidates should also observe for verbal perseveration.
- **Motor control**
  - *Luria hand sequence test:* This tests programming ability.

    Ask the patient to closely observe and perform 'fist–edge–palm' sequence. Ask the patient to do it till you say 'stop'.

    Patient should be able to do at least three successful sequences/cycles without error. Observe for motor perseveration.
  - Square triangle test

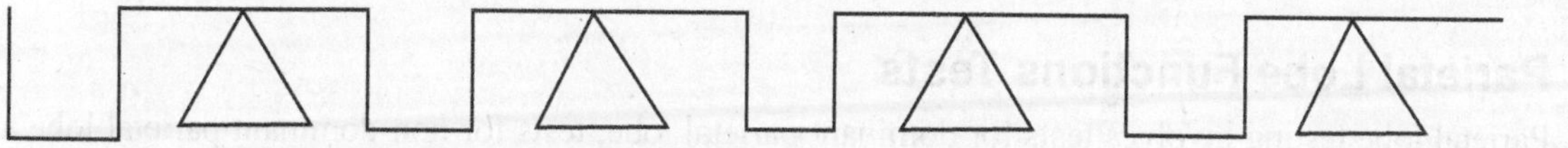

Ask the patient to copy the picture without taking the hand off the paper, i.e., patient should do it continuously with the pen. Observe for perseveration.

- **Conflicting instructions:** They test how a patient can rapidly switch with random changes made by the candidate.

  First instruction "Tap twice when I tap once." To ensure that the patient has understood the instruction, a series of three trials is run. Then give the second instruction. "Tap once when I tap twice." Again do three trials so that you are sure that patient has understood the task. Now combine both steps and perform randomly 1 taps and 2 taps. Observe the patient's response, also observe for motor perseveration.
- **Go-no-go test: Tests the inhibitory control:**

  In this the steps are same as above but the instructions are different.

"Tap once when I tap once." And "Do not tap when I tap twice."

- **Prehension test:** Tests environmental autonomy, i.e., how much control patient has on his behaviour over the environment.

  The examiner is seated in front of the patient. Place the patient's hands palm up on his knees. Clearly tell him not to shake hands with you or take your hands. Now without saying anything or looking at the patient, bring your hands close to the patient's hands and touch the palms of both the patient's hands. If the patient takes or shakes the hands, try again after asking the patient not to take your hands.
- **Cognitive estimates tests:** Cognitive estimates tests test how much a person can guess. The questions asked have no clear-cut or straightforward answers.

  For example,

  What is the height of the 'Tower Bridge'?

  How many elephants are in England?

  How tall is the average Irish woman?

  The responses are documented.
- **Look for released reflexes** like palmomental, glabellar tap or snout.
  - Testing for released reflexes is relevant if the task says 'assess frontal lobe functions' without specifying cognitive functions.
  - In the examination situation, where time is limited it is better to do one test from each domain.
  - Also better to do the word fluency towards the end as the candidates need to wait for one full minute for the responses from the patient.

Clock Drawing Test

In clock drawing test, the patient is asked to draw the face of a clock (circle), mark the numbers so that it resembles a clock. Ask the patient to show a time (e.g., 10 minutes past 6) by drawing the arms of the clock. By giving this task in the examination situation, you can demonstrate the examiner that you are checking for patient's comprehension, visuospatial and constructional abilities.

Parietal Lobe Functions Tests

Parietal lobe testing involves tests for dominant parietal lobe, tests for non-dominant parietal lobe and tests that are common to both the lobes. In fact many books present these differently.

Tests for Dominant Parietal Lobe

- **Calculations:** Ask the patient do simple addition and subtraction. Inability to do calculations is called acalculia.
- **Right–left orientation:** Ask the patient identify right and left body parts. Ask the patient to close the eyes and then touch the right ear with left hand. Inability to perform this is called right left disorientation.
- **Finger agnosia:** Ask the patient to name and identify each digit with eyes closed. Alternatively, you can instruct the patient to close the eyes and ask him to show a specific finger, e.g., right hand ring finger.

- **Agraphia:** Inability to write is called agraphia.
- Some patients also present with aphasia: Tests from the language function component of MMSE, i.e., naming, reading, writing, repetition, comprehension will help to identify these difficulties.
- The syndrome comprising acalculia, agraphia, finger agnosia and right-left disorientation is called Gerstmann syndrome.

Tests for Non-dominant Parietal Lobe

- **Asomatognosia:** Inability to recognise parts of the body. With the eyes closed patient is asked to show his hand, ask him to point to his eyes with fingers, etc.
- **Constructional apraxia:** Tested by asking the patient to do intersecting pentagons or performing clock drawing test.
- **Ideomotor apraxia:** Simple definition of the term 'praxis' would be "to perform a function". The term 'Apraxia' gives a clear understanding, "the inability to perform a complex motor act in the absence of a gross motor deficit". There are various types of apraxias. In the CASC exam, it is enough for the candidate demonstrates one or two tests. Asking the patient to show with his hands "how he would brush the teeth with a toothbrush", "how he would blow a whistle" or "how he would comb his hair". These are the tests for ideomotor apraxia.
- **Hemi-neglect:** Patient with hemi-neglect will present with one side of the body not dressed/not shaven. This will also be seen in clock drawing test where the patient draws only on one side.
- **Prosopagnosia:** Inability to recognise the familiar faces. Show Queen's face on banknote and ask the patient to identify.
- **Anosognosia:** Inability to acknowledge a disabled body part or inability.

Tests Common for Both Parietal Lobes

- **Visual field testing:** As optic tracts pass through the parietal lobes patient might present with hemianopia. So, confrontation technique may be used to assess visual fields in the exam setting.
- **Agraphesthesia:** Parietal lobes are important for perception of sensory information. These are called cortical sensations, e.g., graphesthesia: ability to perceive the letters are numbers written on the hands without looking at them. Ask the patient to close the eyes. Draw 'H' on his hands and ask him to identify the letter.
- **Astereognosis:** Ability to identify the objects placed in hands without looking at them is called stereognosis. Ask the patient to close his eyes and give a pound coin on one hand. He should be able to identify it without opening the eyes or using both the hands. The difficulty is called agraphesthesia and astereognosis.

CASC Stations that Assess Cognitive Functions

Station 1: Cognitive assessment following head injury

Theme: Cognitive assessment of a patient who had forehead injury

1. **Instructions to candidates:**
   You are a CT3 on call in Psychiatry. You received a call from the A and E liaison nurse to assess Henry Malcom, a 32 years old man, who was hit on his forehead with a hammer about 6 months

ago. He was unconscious for 2–3 hours. He suffered a depressed skull fracture and hemorrhagic contusion of the frontal lobes. Mr Malcolm had urinated a few times recently in the security office; hence, his manager brought him to the A and E. The liaison nurse could not find any psychotic or depressive symptoms. Mr Malcolm was over friendly with her and shook hands repeatedly. So, she called you to assess him before he goes home.

- **Assess his cognitive functions focusing mainly on the frontal lobe functions.**
- **Do not take a history.**
- **Do not carry out a mental state examination.**

2. Instructions to the role player:

- You are Henry Malcom. You are 32 years old. You do not see anything wrong with yourself. You work as a security guard in a private company. About 6 months ago you had sustained forehead injury and were hospitalised. You recovered and started going to work. Today, your manager called to ask you why you had urinated in the security office. You do not find anything wrong with this. The manager brought you to the A and E. You think, he is unnecessarily worried about you. You are not depressed or anxious. You don't understand why you should be seeing a psychiatrist.
- If the candidate talks in simple language answer his questions. Otherwise appear confused. Talk less and on-and-off appear as if you are at a loss for words.
- When the candidate asks you to do some actions start doing properly for once, but later repeat a single action. If he tries to explain again, tell him that you understood the task well and you are not a child.
- For example: Fist-palm-side test keep making fist and palm.
- In go-no-go test do the opposite of what you are asked to do.
- If the candidate asks you to draw/çopy a square and triangle keep drawing the triangles.
- If you are asked for a proverb, tell the candidate that you do not know any proverb. If he comes out with a proverb, repeat the proverb and say that is the meaning.
- If candidate ask you to tell the similarity between two objects tell the differences.
- When the candidate asks you to tell all the words starting with a particular alphabet. You can remember tell three or four words, slowly and appear to be at loss. If he hurries tell the names and surnames starting with the alphabet. Repeat this pattern with naming animals, etc. Do not name more than 5–6.
- When the candidate asks you some questions such as "how many camels are in the UK", tell you don't know.
- The candidate may ask you not to shake hands. But shake hands with him readily if he offers the hands.
- If he asks you to spell the word 'WORLD' you say that you can't spell. Repeat up to 3 numbers correctly, beyond which you start making mistakes.
- Rest of the tests perform correctly.

3. Construct:

The candidate fluently demonstrates the cognitive assessment of a patient with frontal lobe dysfunction.

4. Expanded construct:

- Candidate should be able to establish a rapport with the patient who has short attention span.
- Candidate should use jargon-free language.
- Candidate should not hurry the patient to move from one test to other, without giving adequate time.
- Candidate should be able to assess the components of frontal lobe function fluently.
  - Attention and concentration
  - Look for motor or verbal perseveration
  - Test abstract thinking–proverb interpretation as well as similarities
  - Test cognitive estimates
  - Verbal fluency
  - Category fluency
  - Some candidates may do tests to look for release reflexes like palmomental, glabellar or snout. These are signs of frontal lobe dysfunction.

5. Areas of importance to pass the station:

- Communication skills 30%.
- Frontal lobe functions 70%.

6. Equipment checklist if applicable:

- Pens/Pencils
- Paper
- Clipboard.

Station 2: Korsakoff Syndrome

Theme: Patient not willing to stay on the ward

1. Instructions to candidates:

Patient's name: Richard Taylor Age 52 years.

You are a CT3 in Psychiatry. You are called to the surgical ward to assess this patient who was admitted 5 days ago with stomach pain. He was diagnosed as having pancreatitis and was treated by surgeons. The patient received alcohol detoxification treatment for 4 days. Initially he was confused, but this is settling now. He seems to be talking well. But staff on the ward could not follow him. He refused to stay on the ward. His consultant surgeon is worried about this patient's mental state. His serum amylase levels are very high. Hence, he called you to assess the patient.

- **Assess the cognitive functions.**
- **Decide whether this patient could leave the ward.**

2. Instruction to the role player:

- You are Mr Taylor. You live alone in Southend-On-Sea. You were working as a mechanic in a private company. You cannot remember much about your life in the past 3–4 years. You do not recognise your memory problem. You remember being a mechanic and wanted to go to work and report to supervisor. You believe that the current year is 2006. You don't remember anything about recession or you losing the job. But you give stories to candidates about these. You change the story each time the candidate asks the question, or with different professionals.

- You don't know how you reached hospital. Today when you woke up in the morning you were surprised with your hospital dress. You asked the staff and they told that you were in hospital. You changed into your dress and got ready to go home. You don't think that you have any memory problems.
- You don't remember your conversations with the staff nurse on the ward or with your consultant. When the candidate asks about this, you give your own stories. For example, you are in the hospital to visit a friend, who had piles.
- When the candidate asks about drinking pattern you describe yourself as a social drinker. All you say is that you drink in the evening to relax and sleep well.
- If the candidate asks you to copy a diagram do it without problem. You do not know the day, date, month, etc., but you will answer readily to the doctor with a day, date, month, etc. When asked about the year you say it is 2006. You have no problem in telling the place. But you don't think that you are an inpatient.
- If the candidate is empathic and explains what he is doing, in understandable terms cooperate and complete other tasks. Otherwise say that you are in a hurry and pretend as if you are going to call for a taxi.

3. **Construct:**

The candidate is able to assess the cognitive functions in a patient who has alcohol related cognitive dysfunction.

4. **Expanded construct:**

Candidate should be able to:

- Establish rapport with a patient who is eager to leave the ward.
- Use simple jargon-free language to explain.
- Assess cognitive functions focusing on memory.
- Demonstrate that the immediate memory (working memory) is intact.
- Demonstrate short-term memory loss.
- Assess retrograde and anterograde memory loss.
- Pick up inconsistencies in history and demonstrate confabulation.
- Think and formulate about the risks of him leaving the ward.

5. **Areas of importance to pass the station:**

- Advanced communication skills 20%.
- Cognitive assessment 70%.
- Decision making skills 10%.

6. **Equipment checklist:**

- Pen
- Paper
- Paper holder/clipboard.

Station 3: Assess cognitive functions in a patient who suffered a stroke

Theme: Assessment of parietal lobe functions

1. **Instructions to the candidates:**

   Mr George Washington is a 55-year-old accountant. He suffered a stroke 5 months ago. Since then he has difficulty in doing simple calculations and writing.

   Assess parietal lobe functions in this gentleman.

2. **Instructions to the role player:**
   - You are Mr Washington. You worked as a successful accountant. About 5 months ago, you suffered a stroke. Since then, you could not do even simple calculations. You are very upset about this.
   - You do not have memory problems. You answer correctly to all the questions except the following:
     - You can't do calculations. You can't even write simple sentences.
     - You can't name or identify the correct finger when the examiner asks you to do so. Appear perplexed and show a wrong finger.
     - When the examiner asks you to identify right or left side do the opposite.

3. **Construct:**

   The candidate is able to assess the cognitive functions in a patient who had stroke involving left parietal lobe.

4. **Expanded construct:**
   - Candidate should be able to use simple and jargon-free language to explain.
   - Candidate should be able to assess the cognitive functions focusing on parietal lobes.
   - Candidate should be able to demonstrate the signs of acalculia, agraphia, right-left disorientation and finger agnosia.

5. **Areas of importance to pass the station:**
   - Advanced communication skills 20%.
   - Cognitive assessment 80%.

6. **Equipment checklist:**
   - Pen
   - Paper
   - Paper holder/clipboard
   - Coins
   - Key
   - Pictures of HM Queen Elizabeth, Mr Tony Blair, Mr David Cameroon.

2. Physical Examination

Juhi Mishra and Madhavan Seshadri

Introduction

Physical examination is an essential component of psychiatric practice. In fact, patients with mental illnesses are at higher risk for physical morbidity. However, many a times, psychiatrists focus only on mental state examination. According to the Royal College of Psychiatrists CASC blueprint, there will be at least one physical examination station in every circuit.

There are certain basic steps one should follow in physical examination stations.

(i) Read the task carefully and divide the time to complete it.
There is usually more than one task, e.g., examine the patient and address their concerns.

(ii) **Use of alcohol gel:** College is very particular about the use of alcohol gel. In stations involving physical examination candidates are expected to clean the hands with alcohol gel, before and after the examination.

(iii) **Consent:** Explain the purpose of examination and the procedure briefly, and get a verbal consent.

(iv) **Chaperone:** Ask for a chaperone if appropriate.

(v) **Brief focused history:** Rather than straightaway jumping into the exam ask a couple of system specific questions. Ask for past medical history and medication history.

(vi) **General physical examination:** In any given station do a general physical examination.

(vii) **System specific examination:** As you examine comment on the findings. For example, During inspection of neck in thyroid examination the candidate may say, "There are no obvious swellings, trachea appears to be in midline etc."

(viii) Explain the findings and thank the patient.

1. Thyroid Examination

Introduce yourself to the patient and explain the purpose of the examination. Obtain verbal consent.

Ask for a chaperone if appropriate.

Explain that you will be asking a few questions and do a physical examination. Ask a few questions that are relevant to the history.

General Physical Examination:

- Hands: Examine nails, thyroid acropachy, fine tremors and sweating.
- Check the pulse rate and rhythm.
- Eyes: Loss of hair in the eyebrows and xanthelasma.
- Eye signs of hyperthyroidism – exophthalmos and lid lag.
- Examine extra-ocular movements.
- Coarse dry skin, thinning of hair.
- Obesity.
- Examine the legs for pretibial myxoedema.

Examination of Thyroid (Neck) Gland

Patient will need to expose neck and upper chest area.

- **Inspection:**
  - Look from front for scars, swellings or sinuses.
  - Ask the patient to swallow (water) and observe for movement of any swelling in the neck area.
  - Ask the patient to protrude the tongue and observe for the movement of any swelling.
  - Thyroglossal cyst moves up with protrusion of the tongue.
- **Palpation:**
  - Enquire for any pain.
  - Stand behind the patient.
  - Gently palpate the neck looking for any abnormality, observe for tenderness.
  - Have the patient swallow (water) and feel the gland move under your fingers.
  - If you feel a swelling, examine whether it is uniformly enlarged or nodular, consistency, tenderness and mobility.
  - Palpate lymph nodes of the neck.
- **Percussion:**
  - Percussion is useful when there is retrosternal goitre.
- **Auscultation:**
  - Auscultate for thyroid bruit.
- **Focused central nervous system examination:**
  - Examine for pseudomyotonic reflex.
  - Examine for proximal myopathy.

If there is time:

- Examine for signs of cardiac failure.
- Examine abdomen for ascites.

2. Cardiovascular Examination

Ask for permission and a chaperone if appropriate.

- **Take a brief focused history:**
  - Explain to the patient and get permission to expose chest area for examination.
- **General physical examination:**
  - Observe the patient: Is he/she comfortable at rest?
  - Breathing: Look for distress, accessory muscles in action.
  - Examination of the hands
    - Pallor
    - Clubbing
    - Cyanosis

- Osler's nodes (red, nodular painful lesions found on the hands and feet).
- Janeway lesions (non-tender nodular or macular lesions in the hands or legs).
- Splinter haemorrhages (small blood clots seen under the nails).
- Polydactyly or Arachnodactyly (Marfan's syndrome).
- Pulse:
  - Rate, rhythm, character, radio-femoral delay and radio-radial delay.
  - Collapsing pulse, assessed by holding patient's wrist with the palm on the radial artery area. Raising patient's hand above his head leads to examiner feeling the pulse more like tapping on the palm.
  - Feel all peripheral pulses: radial, brachial, carotid, femoral, popliteal, posterior tibial and dorsalis pedis arteries (both sides).
- Take blood pressure.
- Legs for oedema.

- Examination of the eyes.
  - Pallor
  - Jaundice: Ask the patient to look down, look for yellowish sclera.
  - Xanthelasma: Lipid deposits seen as plaques around the eyelids.
  - Corneal arcos (seen in severe hypercholesterolemia).
- Mouth
  - Cyanosis of lips indicates central cyanosis.
  - High arched palate is seen in Marfan's syndrome.
- Examination of the back and legs
  - Sacral oedema.
  - Pedal oedema.

- **Examination of the neck** (Ask the patient to lie at 45% on the couch)
  - Carotid: Look and feel for carotid pulsations one carotid at a time.
  - Check for carotid bruit with bell of stethoscope.
  - JVP: Inspect height with patient at 45 degrees.
- **Chest Inspection:**
  - Scars of cardiac surgery.
  - Deformities of the chest wall.
  - Visible pulsations and heaves.
  - Apex beat.
- **Chest palpation:**
  - Palpate apex beat for character and location.
  - Parasternal heave (checked by placing heel of hand to left side of sternum).
  - Thrills.
- **Chest auscultation:**
  - Heart sounds and murmurs (in all four areas).
  - Specific manoeuvres for various murmurs especially mitral regurgitation.

- **Examination of the abdomen:**
  - Palpate for lower border of liver; Percuss to measure the size.
  - Examine for spleen.
  - Examine for ascites.
  - Aortic pulsations, aneurysm.
  - Auscultate for renal bruit, aortic bruit and femoral bruit.
- **Listen to lung bases for crepitations.**

3. Examination of Respiratory System

Introduce yourself and explain the procedure. Obtain verbal consent. Ask for a chaperone if appropriate. Ensure that the patient is comfortable.

Take a Brief History.

While taking the history, observe whether the patient can talk without becoming breathless.

- **General examination:**
  - General appearance: Thin, obese, etc.
  - Is the patient comfortable at rest?
  - Fingers: Clubbing and cyanosis.
  - Wrists: Pulmonary osteoarthropathy.
  - Pulse rate, temperature.
  - Look at the mouth/lips for central cyanosis, pursed lips.
  - Check for lymph nodes: Cervical and axillary.
  - Examine the throat for tonsillitis/inflammation.

  Ask the patient to remove his shirt.
- **Inspection:**
  - Ask the patient to look straight and observe from front, sides and behind.
  - Look for tracheal deviation.
  - Shape: Any deformity in the chest wall.
  - Scars, swellings or sinuses.
  - Movement of the chest with breathing: Do all quadrants expand equally?
  - Difficulties in breathing.
  - Accessory muscles of breathing in action.
  - If the wheezing is severe, it could be heard.
  - Count breath rate.
- **Palpation:**
  - Feel for any local tenderness.
  - Feel for position of trachea in suprasternal notch.
  - Apex beat.
  - Chest expansion: Using hands in all the quadrants. Assess whether the movement is equal on both sides.

  - Vocal fremitus: In assessing vocal fremitus, the patient is asked to repeat '99' whilst the examiner places the palm of his hand on the patient's chest and feels for the vibrations. All areas of chest are tested.
- **Percussion:**
  All the areas of chest are percussed. Start with percussion of clavicle using middle finger directly. Compare notes on both the sides of the chest including axillae.
- **Auscultation:**
  - Listen to all the areas of the chest using the stethoscope. Compare both the sides.
  - Tactile Vocal Fremitus (TVF): Ask the patient to say '99', whilst listening over the chest. Sounds are louder over areas of consolidation. Compare both the sides.
  - At the end of the examination request the patient to give a sample of sputum for testing.

4. Cranial Nerves Examination

1. Olfactory nerve (I)
   - Ask whether patient could smell coffee, perfume, etc.
2. Optic nerve (II)
   - Check one eye at a time.
   - Examine vision: Acuity of vision using Snellen's chart and reading a newspaper for near vision.
   - Colour vision: Check whether patient could clearly identify green, red, blue and yellow colours.
   - Field of vision: Peripheral field using confrontation technique, central field using red pin.
   - Pupillary reflexes: Light reflex (direct as well as consensual) accommodation reflex.
   - Fundus examination.
3. Oculomotor (III), trochlear (IV) and abducent nerves (VI): Extra-ocular movements.
   - Ask the patient to tell you if he gets diplopia.
   - Also observe for nystagmus.
4. Trigeminal nerve (V)
   - Sensory: Sensations of the face.
   - Motor: Muscles of mastication (temporalis and masseter–clenching of teeth).
   - Lateral and medial pterygoids: Ask the patient to open the mouth and look for deviation of the jaw.
   - Jaw jerk.
   - Mention about corneal reflex.
5. Facial (VII)
   - Test muscles of the upper and lower face.
   - Taste sensation of front part of tongue.
6. Vestibulo cochlear (VIII) (one ear at a time)
   - Hearing whispers or finger clicks.
   - Rinne's test and Weber's test.

- Balance.
- Also do Romberg's test.

7. Glossopharyngeal (IX) and Vagus (X)
   - Look at the position of uvula. Ask the patient to say 'ah' and see the movement of uvula.
8. Accessory nerve (XI)
   - Shrugging of shoulders.
   - Test for sternomastoids.
9. Hypoglossal nerve (XII)
   - Tongue wasting, movements.
   - Ask to press their tongue against the cheek and feel the muscle bulk.

5. Cerebellar Examination

- Focused history.
- Mnemonic for cerebellar signs: DANISH.
- Dysdiadokokinesia.
- Ataxia.
- Nystagmus.
- Intention tremor.
- Slurred speech.
- Hypotonia.
- Examine the eyes: Nystagmus.
- Observe the speech: Staccato speech or scanning in speech. Ask the patient to repeat the word 'British Constitution'.
- Look for intention tremors.
- Finger nose test: Look for past pointing.
- Dysdiadokokinesia.
- Heel shin test.
- Ataxic gait (wide based).
- Tandem walking: Patient can't perform well.
- Examine the tone of muscles for hypotonia.
- Pendular knee jerk.

6. Extrapyramidal System Examination

Take a focused history and establish the link between increase in dose of risperidone or other antipsychotics and restlessness.

- **General examination**
  - Is the patient able to relax?
  - Facial expression/mask like face.
  - Slurring of speech and drooling of saliva.

- Specific examination:
  Observe the patient for restlessness. If the patient is walking it is better to observe the gait first.
- Examine for triad of rigidity, tremor and hypokinesia or akinesia
- Examine with patient sitting and standing.

Sitting:

- Observe the patient at rest.
- Ask the patient to sit on a chair without arms.
- Observe for posturing for longer periods (patient maintaining odd positions for long periods).
- Observe for any abnormal movements unmasked by examination or movement elsewhere, e.g., face, mouth, arms, hands, feet, legs. Are they present at rest or during activity? Do they interfere with activities?
- Observe for oculogyric crisis or dystonia (mainly neck).
- If patient has something in the mouth remove it and inspect for pooling of saliva.
- Observe the patient with tongue resting inside the mouth as well as tongue protruding outside.
- Observe for tremors with outstretched hands.
- Ask the patient to leave the arms hanging and observe for any movement.
- Ask the patient to touch each finger with thumb as rapidly as possible first with right hand and then with left hand (15 seconds each hand).
- Perform glabellar tap.
- Examine rigidity
  - Upper limbs: At wrist, elbow and shoulders.
  - Lower limbs: Ankles and knees.
  - Get permission, rule out cervical pain and then examine neck for rigidity.

Standing:

- Ask the patient to outstretch the arms at shoulder level on either side of the body. Allow it to fall and observe for slowness.
- Observe for drooping of shoulder on one side.
- Engage in conversation and observe for restlessness and movement of legs. Clarify by asking for subjective restlessness.
- Ask the patient to turn around in four stages and observe for truncal unsteadiness.
- Ask the patient to walk fast and observe the gait (e.g., festinant gait).

7. Neurological Examination of Upper Limbs

- Ask for relevant history.
- Explain the process, get verbal consent. Ask for chaperone if appropriate.
- Get patient to remove clothes from top half of the body.
- **General Examination:** Anaemia, clubbing, cyanosis, jaundice, any neck pathology.
- **Inspection:** Observe for any abnormal posturing, asymmetry of sides, fasciculation, tremor or other movement disorder. Muscle wasting especially for muscles of the hand and pronator drift.

- **Palpation:** Before doing this ask for pain and discomfort. Examine muscle bulk and tone. If tone is increased verify whether it is spasticity or hypertonia. Measuring tape may be used to measure the mid arm circumference on both arms and compare.
- **Power of muscles around major joints:** Shoulder, elbow, wrist, fingers.
- **Reflexes:** Biceps, triceps and supinator.
- **Coordination:** Finger nose test, dysdiadokokinesia.
- **Sensation:** Light touch with cotton wool. Look for any dermatomal distribution. Vibration and joint position sense.

8. Neurological Examination of Lower Limbs

- Explain the process, get verbal consent. Ask for chaperone, if appropriate.
- Ask for relevant history.
- Ask patient to expose legs from thighs.
- **General examination:** Anaemia, clubbing, cyanosis, jaundice, any spine pathology.
- **Inspection:** Observe for any abnormal posturing, asymmetry of sides, fasciculation, tremor or other movement disorder.
- Muscle wasting especially for muscles of the foot and pronator drift.
- **Palpation:** Before doing this ask for pain and discomfort. Examine muscle bulk and tone. If tone is increased verify whether it is spasticity or hypertonia.

  Measuring tape may be used to measure the mid-thigh circumference on both arms and compare. Try to elicit ankle clonus.
- **Power of muscles around major joints:** Hip, knee, ankle, subtalar joints, toes.
- **Reflexes:** Knee jerk, ankle jerk, plantar (Babinski sign).
- **Coordination:** Heel shin test, dysdiadokokinesia.
- **Sensation:** Light touch with cotton wool. Look for any dermatomal distribution. Vibration and joint position sense.
- If the patient can stand well ask him to squat and stand. This helps to elicit proximal myopathy.
- **Gait:** Ask the patient to walk and observe.
- **Tandem** walking: Walk on toes, walk on heels.
- **Romberg's test.**

9. Patient with Alcohol Dependence

- Important: In the exam, it is a 7 minutes station so one has to be brief but thorough. Skip unnecessary steps.
- Once you ensure privacy and chaperone, start the general examination and relevant system first.
- For example, if the vignette gives history of hematemesis and melena, conduct abdominal examination first.
- But make sure you show the examiner that you also examine central nervous system.
- Take a brief focused history.

General Physical Examination

Anemia, clubbing, jaundice.

Hands: Clubbing, palmar erythema, hepatic flap, Dupuytren's contracture. Brittle white nails.

Pulse: Rate rhythm and volume, blood pressure.

Face: Eyes for pallor, jaundice, nystagmus and ophthalmoplegia. Enlargement of parotid glands.

Mouth: Foeter hepaticus.

Neck: Lymph nodes, abnormal pulsations.

Chest: Spider naevi, gynaecomastia in males.

Examination of Abdomen

Inspection: Ideally patient should undress from nipples to mid-thigh, cover the private parts.

Look for abdominal distension, caput medusae, if there are distended veins in the abdomen look for the direction of flow.

Any scars or swellings. Movement of the abdomen all quadrants with respiration.

Ask the patient to raise the head off the pillow and observe for divarication of recti.

Palpation: Superficial palpation: Feel for tenderness, warmth, etc. in all quadrants.

Deep palpation of all quadrants. Examine for hepatomegaly and splenomegaly. Palpate kidneys by what is called bimanual palpation, palpate for aortic pulsations.

Percussion: Upper border of liver and liver dullness. Shifting dullness and fluid thrill.

Auscultation: For bowel sounds, renal bruit.

Complete the examination by examining the inguinal area for swelling, impulse on coughing.

Tell the examiner that ideally you would like to examine external genitalia and perform a rectal examination.

Central Nervous System

Motor system: Inspect for wasting of muscles and muscle weakness.

Power, tone and reflexes around major joints.

Cerebellar examination.

Use the mnemonic DANISH.

Observe for tremors.

Finger nose test.

Heel-shin test.

Dysdiadokokinesia.

Sensory System

Enquire about pins and needles.

Fine touch: Cotton wool.

Joint position and vibration sense: Use a tuning fork.

Pinprick and temperature: Just mention.

Rhomberg's test.

Gait: Observe gait ataxia.

Tandem walking.

These are the possible scenarios that can come in the examination. Candidates are advised to practice the examination and more importantly how to explain the patient about the examination as well as findings.

9 Single Stations on Physical Examination

Station 1: Examine the patient who is on lithium carbonate

Theme: Patient on lithium and complaining of weight gain. Examination of thyroid gland

Instruction to candidates:

Mrs Fiona Matthews is a 41-year-old woman suffering from bipolar affective disorder. She is stable on lithium carbonate 800 mg nocte. For the past 6–7 months, she has lost appetite. She has put on one stone in weight. She went to her GP who did thyroid function tests. The results were faxed to you last week.

Thyroid function tests:

1. TSH: 17.5 mU/L (Normal 0.5–5.0 mU/L)
2. T3: 0.4 nmol/L (Normal 1.1–2.8 nmol/L)
3. T4: 40 nmol/L (Normal 50–150 nmol/L)
    - **Perform a thyroid examination.**
    - **Address her concerns.**

Station 2: Examination of cardiovascular system

Theme: Examine the patient who complains of chest pain

Instructions to candidates:

Mr Derek Hunt is a 65-year-old man admitted to the psychiatric ward. He had chest pain and the ward staff asked you to assess him.

- **Examine the cardiovascular system.**
- **Explain the findings to the patient.**

Station 3: Respiratory system examination

Theme: Examine the patient who complained of blood in the sputum

Instructions to Candidates:

Mr Mark Thompson is a 50-year-old patient who has been smoking excessively. He was complaining of blood in the sputum. The staff called you to assess him.

- **Perform a respiratory system examination.**
- **Explain the findings to the patient.**

Station 4: Examine the patient who complained of chronic headache

Theme: Cranial nerves examination

Instructions to the candidates:

Mrs Betty Benjamin is a 40-year-old woman who has been complaining of headache for the past few months.

- **Examine the cranial nerves.**

Station 5: Examine the patient who is unsteady on walking

Theme: Cerebellar examination

Instructions to candidates:

Mr Stanley Wine was admitted to your ward last week for alcohol detoxification. The staff on the ward noticed him to be unsteady on his feet.

- **Perform cerebellar examination.**
- **Explain the findings to the patient.**

Station 6: Examination of a restless and agitated patient

Theme: Examination of extrapyramidal system

Instructions to candidates:

You received a call from A and E that a psychiatric patient is agitated and restless. You were busy on the ward and by the time you reached A and E you found the patient pacing up and down.

Patient's name: Gabriel Agassi, age 23 years.

- **Take a focused history.**
- **Perform relevant neurological examination.**

Station 7: Neurological examination

Theme: Neurological examination of upper limbs

Instructions to the candidates:

You received a call from the A and E that a patient came to the A&E with difficulty moving both arms. She was found to be tearful. Family gave a history of development of symptoms following bereavement. Your liaison nurse told that this patient was not physically assessed.

Patient's name: Charmaine Dollar, 23 years old.

- **Perform upper limb neurological examination.**

Station 8: Neurological examination

Theme: Neurological examination of lower limbs

Instructions to the candidates:

You received a call from the medical ward about a patient who had difficulty walking. She had a breakdown in relationship yesterday. Since then she was found to be tearful. Family gave a history of sudden development of symptoms since this morning. Nurses told that this patient could move her legs in sleep.

Patient's name: Manisha Kaur, 26 years old.

- **Perform lower limb neurological examination.**

Station 9: Physical examination

Theme: Physical examination of patient with alcohol dependence

Instructions to the candidates:

Mr David Eastham is a 38-year-old man with history of heavy drinking. He vomited blood today. His family were worried and took him to the hospital. A and E doctors referred him to Psychiatry unit. On the ward, he passed black coloured stools. He also complained of shaking and sweating. Staff gave him lorazepam and he calmed down. You have been called to examine this patient.

- **Perform a physical examination.**
- **Explain the findings to the patient.**

Fundoscopic Examination

Introduction: In fundoscopy or ophthalmoscopy, the clinician examines the retina by using ophthalmoscope. It is a clinical procedure which is useful in neuropsychiatric practice as retina can give plenty of information about the brain. It is important for the candidates to familiarise with ophthalmoscope. In the CASC exam situation, one will get only 3–4 minutes to perform fundoscopy. Usually there are few other tasks like eliciting appropriate history, examination of eyes and explanation of findings to the patient/relative added to this station. So candidate should know the parts of ophthalmoscope, how to switch it on and off, how to use it practically.

Steps in Fundoscopy/Ophthalmoscopy:

- **Explanation and consent:** Since one will be using hands to fix the patient's head, approaching the patient very closely and more importantly the room light will be switched off; one should explain the procedure and get consent. If needed eye drops may be used to dilate the pupils, after obtaining verbal consent.

- Tell the patient that you will be throwing bright light into the eyes, to look at the back of the eyes. You will be fixing the patient's head with one hand and coming close to the patient.
- Ask for a chaperone if necessary.
- Obtain brief background history.
- Check ophthalmoscope.
- If patient wears spectacles ask him to remove it.
- Ask the patient to look straight at a distant point and not to look at the light.
- **Rule: Patient's right eye:** Examine from right side of the patient, with ophthalmoscope in right hand and with your right eye.
- **Patients' left eye:** Examine from the left side of the patient with ophthalmoscope in left hand and your left eye.
- **First step: Eliciting red reflex:** View the patient's eye at a distance of 30 cms through the ophthalmo-scope with light thrown on the pupils. You will be able to see the red reflex.
- **Examination of retina:** Once you see the red reflex move close to that eye and continue the examination. Look for:

  (a) Optic disc

  (b) Blood vessels

  (c) All the quadrants of retina; and

  (d) Macula.

Optic disc is situated on the nasal side of the fundus. It is slightly pink, has a central cup. A bright candidate can describe the optic disc's colour, margins and the cup-to-disc ratio. Optic disc can become pale in optic neuritis. The margins can become blurred/oedematous in papilloedema. Normal cup to disc ratio is 0.3. It increases in glaucoma.

The arteries emerge from the optic disc into four quadrants (upper nasal, lower nasal, upper temporal and lower temporal). The veins run close to them. One should be able to describe any abnormality like new vessel formation.

While describing the background of retina, candidate should be able to describe the background colour, any haemorrhages or exudates.

Macula is 2 disc spaces away from the optic disc. Macula is seen as a dark spot, well seen when the patient looks at the ophthalmoscope light. So the candidate, after examining the disc, blood vessels and background may ask the patient to look at the light and examine the macula.

1. Normal Fundus:

In a normal fundus, one should be able to see the well-formed optic disc on the nasal side, blood vessels emerging from it to all the four quadrants. Retinal background is seen as clear without exudates, haemorrhages or neovascularisation and finally a clear macula.

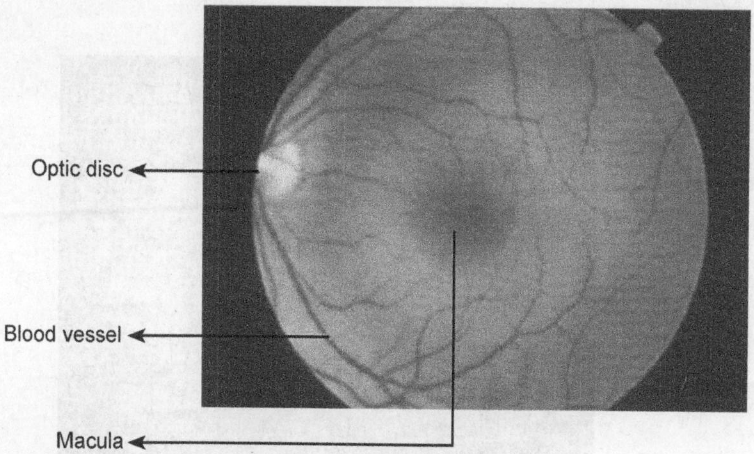

2. Fundus in Glaucoma:

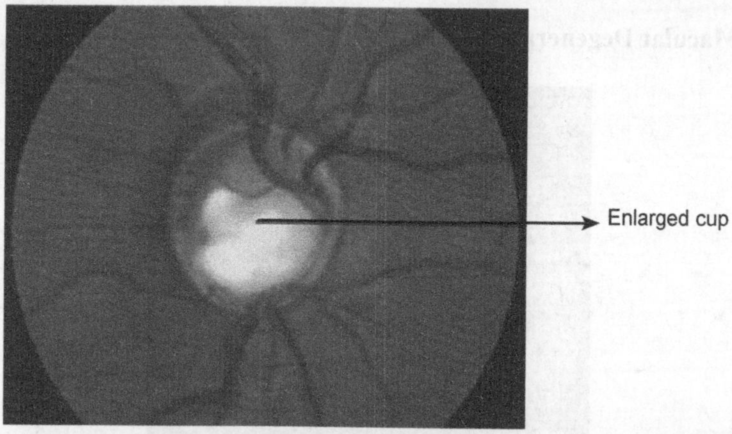

In glaucoma, there will be enlargement of the optic cup. In the above image the cup is occupying almost the whole of optic disc.

3. Fundus in Papilloedema:

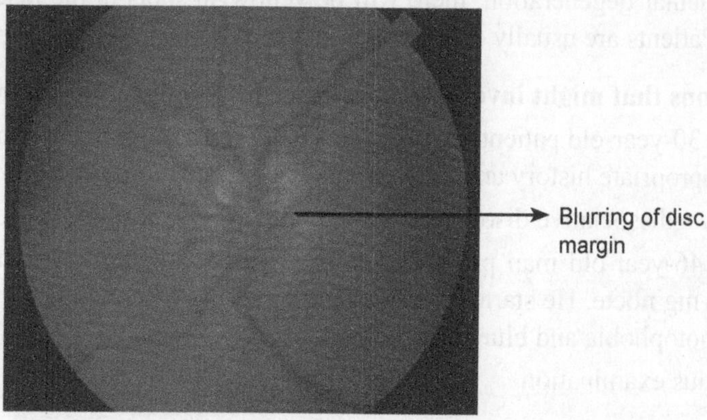

In papilloedema, the disc margins will be blurred because of the swelling of optic disc margins.

4. Diabetic Retinopathy:

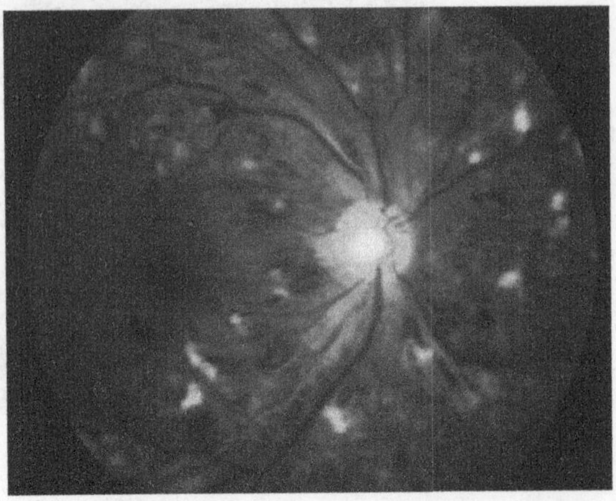

In this image, one can see multiple haemorrhages, exudates as well as neovascularisation.

5. Age Related Macular Degeneration:

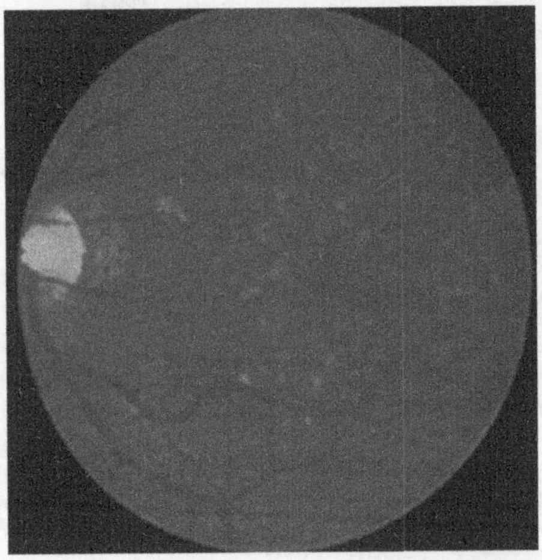

In age related macular degeneration, there will be yellowish spots in the macular area. These are called 'drusen'. Patients are usually elderly with loss of vision.

5 Single CASC stations that might involve ophthalmoscopy/fundus examination

1. Mrs Becham is a 30-year-old patient who has sudden loss of vision. She lost her son recently in an accident. Take appropriate history and perform fundus examination.

   Finding: Usually a dissociative disorder and the fundus will be normal.

2. Mr Saddler is a 46-year-old man presenting with depression and back pain. He was started on Amitriptyline 75 mg nocte. He started complaining of seeing colours in front of the eyes. He also complained of photophobia and blurring of vision.

   - Perform fundus examination.

Finding: Tricyclic drugs are anticholinergic and they can increase intraocular pressure/precipitate glaucoma. Therefore, the fundus will show findings consistent with glaucoma.

3. Mr Rooney is a 54-year-old man complaining of pulsating headache.
   - Perform a fundus examination.

   Finding: Papilloedema.
4. Mrs Melanie Baker suffers from insulin dependent diabetes mellitus. Her blood sugar levels are uncontrolled. She has depression and is on medication.
   - Perform fundus examination.

   Finding: Diabetic retinopathy.
5. Mrs Venessa Butler is a 64-year-old patient with depression. Recently, she started complaining of difficulty in recognising familiar faces and difficulty in reading.
   - Perform a fundus examination.

   Finding: Age related macular degeneration.

   Candidates should remember that occasionally fundus examination could be a stand-alone station with manikin and slides. In this situation, candidate should explain the procedure and describe the findings to the examiner.

3. Physical Investigations

Madhavan Seshadri

ECG Interpretation

Electrocardiogram (ECG) is the tracing of the electrical activity of the heart on the surface of the body. This can give us wealth of information about the cardiac status of the patient.

How to Read the ECG?

- Always check the identity of the patient: Make sure that you are reading the ECG of the person in front of you. Check the date of ECG.
- **Rate:**
  - The standard ECG paper speed is 25 mm/second. One small square in the ECG paper is 0.04 second and one large square is 0.2 second.
  - To calculate the heart rate, first you need to check the R-R interval. This is the distance between two R waves in an ECG. Once you count the number of big squares in one R-R interval use the formula:

    Heart rate = 300/number of big squares in one R-R interval.

    Example: If the R-R interval has four big squares then heart rate would be 300/4 = 75. This gives the approximate heart rate.
  - If one wants to be more accurate with heart rate then the following formula will help.

    1500/number of small squares in one R-R interval.

- For the purpose of CASC exam, it is enough for the candidate to tell the approximate rate by using the first formula.
- Normal heart rate is 60–100 per minute. A heart rate of less than 60 is bradycardia and more than 100 is tachycardia.
- Psychiatrists should at least be aware of few conditions commonly associated with tachycardia: hyperthyroidism, anxiety states, drug induced states like excess of caffeine or nicotine and medication induced tachyarrhythmias.
- Thyrotoxicosis is a common cause of atrial fibrillation.
- Sinus bradycardia can be seen in hypothyroidism, hypothermia and raised intracranial pressure. Beta blockers can cause it.

• **Rhythm:**
  - Normally the heart is in sinus rhythm. In the ECG, this is seen as QRS complexes preceded by P wave.
  - If P waves are completely absent, QRS complexes are present and are followed by T wave, this indicates ventricular rhythm. This is usually seen in atrial fibrillation.
  - In atrial flutter, typical P waves are not seen. These are replaced by 'saw tooth' waves or flutter waves.
  - In nodal rhythm, the electrical activity starts from AV node and spreads to both atria and ventricles. So 'P' waves are absent or they come immediately before or after QRS complex. Occasionally, it may superimpose on QRS complex.
  - In ventricular rhythm, electrical activity of the heart generates from ventricles and then spreads to atria. Hence, QRC complex is followed by P wave. Also the QRS complex will be more than 3 small squares in width or 0.12 seconds.
  - If there is a suspicion that the heart rhythm is irregular, then a **'card method'** will be very useful. In this method, a card is laid alongside the ECG and three successive R waves are marked. The card can be moved to and fro to check that all R-R intervals are equal. If they are not equal then the rhythm is irregular. This irregularity is usually secondary to the block in the cardiac conduction pathway.

• **Electrical Axis of Heart:**

Axis refers to sum of all electrical forces of ventricles during ventricular depolarisation.

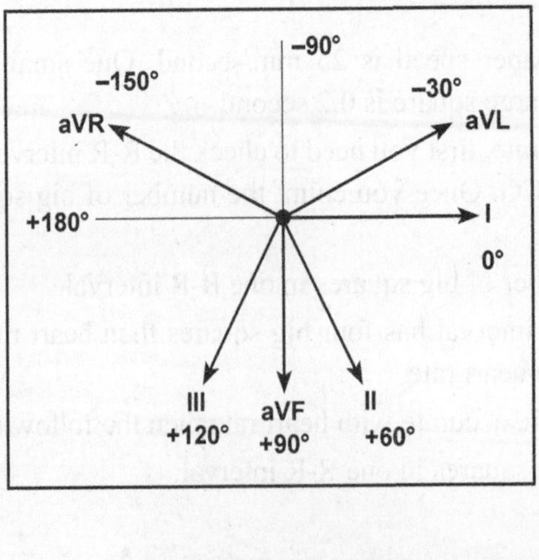

Normal axis is between –30° and +90°.

- Left axis deviation (LAD) means the axis is between –30 and 90°.
  Causes of LAD: Left anterior hemi-block, inferior myocardial infarction, ventricular tachycardia from LV focus and WPW syndrome.
- Right axis deviation (RAD) means the axis is between +90 and +180°.
  Causes of RAD: Right axis deviation could be a normal finding in children and tall thin adults. Right ventricular hypertrophy, pulmonary embolism, anterolateral myocardial infarction, WPW syndrome and left posterior hemi-block.
- Easy way of remembering by reading the deflection of QRS complex:
  - **Deflection of QRS complex in both I and aVF are +ve = normal axis.**
  - **Deflection of QRS complex in lead I is +ve and aVF is –ve but lead II is +ve = normal axis.**
  - **Deflection of QRS complex in lead I is +ve , aVF is –ve and lead II is –ve = left axis deviation.**
  - **Deflection of QRS complex lead I is –ve and aVF is +ve = right axis deviation.**

  Important: Left ventricular hypertrophy is not a cause left axis deviation.
  (Ref: http://www.ecglibrary.com/axis.html)

- **ECG waves and intervals:**

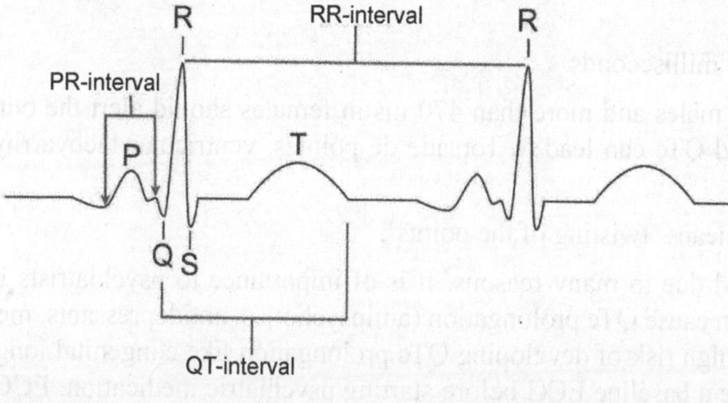

- **P wave:** In a normal sinus rhythm, P waves precede QRS complex. If P waves and QRS complexes have no association then P wave can be seen in the ECG either preceding QRS, on QRS or following QRS complex. In these situations, usually the heart rate is slow and this indicates complete heart block.
  - Absent P wave: Atrial fibrillation, AV nodal rhythm or sinoatrial block.
  - When P waves are tall (more than 2 and ½ small squares) they are called P Pulmonale. Indicates right atrial hypertrophy. It can also be seen in hypokalemia (known as pseudo-P-Pulmonale).
  - P Mitrale is bifid P waves (more than 2 and ½ small squares in width). This indicates left atrial hypertrophy and is usually seen in mitral stenosis.
- **Q wave** is the negative/downward deflection that precedes 'R' wave in the ECG. It might not be seen in some leads. Normal Q wave is less than 0.04 seconds wide and less than 2 mm in depth. They can be seen on LI, aVL, V5 and V6. Pathological Q waves are seen within few hours after myocardial infarction.

- **R wave** is the first positive or upward deflection in the QRS complex.
- **S wave** is the first downward deflection occurring after the R wave.
- **QRS complex** is normally <0.12 seconds in width (3 small squares). A broad QRS complex (>0.12 sec) suggests ventricular conduction defects. Tall QRS complex suggests ventricular hypertrophy.
- **T waves** follow QRS complexes. They are seen as positive deflections except on aVR, V1 and occasionally V2. If T wave inversion is seen in LI, LII and V4–V6 then they are abnormal. Tall T waves are seen in hyperkalemia and flat or inverted T wave is seen in hypokalemia.
- **ST segment** is usually isolelectric. It is abnormal if the elevation is > 1 mm baseline or depression is >0.5 mm baseline. ST elevation is usually seen in ischaemia or infarction. ST depression could be seen in ischaemia or strain pattern (uncontrolled hypertension) can cause strain pattern.

Intervals

PR interval: It is measured as the distance from the start of P wave to the start of QRS complex. Usually it is 3–5 small squares (0.12–0.20 seconds). Short PR interval is seen as the beginning of R wave immediately after P wave. It is also called 'Delta' Wave and is seen in WPW syndrome. These patients are prone for arrhythmias.

QT interval: Distance from the beginning of Q wave to the end of T wave. In patients with tachycardia QT will be shorter. Hence it is corrected and is known as (QTc). QTc is calculated using Bassett's formula:

$$QTc = QT/\sqrt{R\text{-}R}$$

Normal QTc 380–420 milliseconds.

More than 440 ms in males and more than 470 ms in females should alert the clinician to review the medication. Prolonged QTc can lead to Torsade de pointes, ventricular tachyarrhythmias and sudden cardiac death.

Torsade de pointes means 'twisting of the points'.

QTc can be prolonged due to many reasons. It is of importance to psychiatrists because most of the psychiatric medication cause QTc prolongation (antipsychotics, antidepressants, methodone and so on). Some patients are at high risk of developing QTc prolongation like congenital long QT syndromes. So it is important to have a baseline ECG before starting psychiatric medication. ECG can be repeated as per guidelines for individual drugs.

Heart Blocks

1. Heart block is usually classified into first degree heart block, second degree heart block and complete heart block.
   (a) First degree heart block is the prolongation of the PR interval on an electrocardiogram (ECG). In first degree AV block, conduction is slowed, there are no missed beats. Prolonged PR interval is seen in patients who take beta blockers.
   (b) Second degree heart block is characterised by disturbance in conduction of atrial impulse to the ventricles through the atrioventricular node (AVN). Electrocardiographically, some P waves are not followed by a QRS complex. Second degree AV block is further classified as either Mobitz I (Wenckebach) or Mobitz II AV block.

(i) Mobitz I second degree AV block is characterised by a progressive prolongation of the PR interval and at after few beats there will be a missed beat as the atrial impulse is not conducted to the ventricles.

(ii) Mobitz II second degree AV block is characterised by a few P waves not followed by QRS complexes, i.e., missed beats. The PR intervals remain constant. This is classified into 2:1 block, 3:1 block, etc. depending on, after how many beats the QRS complex is missed.

(c) Third degree heart block or complete heart block is characterised by complete dissociation of the atrial and ventricular activity. Commonly seen following myocardial infarction. The P waves can be seen preceding, superimposed or following QRS complexes. It is a medical emergency and the patient will need a pacemaker.

ECG Changes in Myocardial Infarction

Within hours, T waves become taller associated with ST elevation. Gradually over 24 hours period T waves get inverted and as the infarction becomes complete the ST segment comes to baseline. ST segment may remain elevated if injury continues or left ventricular aneurysm develops. After few days Q waves develop and persist. The site of myocardial infarction is described based on the leads where the ECG changes happen.

Changes in Lead I, II and aVF show ischaemia and infarction on the inferior wall of the heart. Changes in V1–V4 show anteroseptal ischaemia or infarction and V4–V6 show lateral wall ischaemia or infarction. Posterior wall myocardial infarction is characterised by reciprocal changes in the anterior leads (V1–V3), i.e., ST depression and tall R waves.

In summary, a systematic reading of ECG is more than identifying cardiac ischaemia and acute myocardial infarction. Psychiatrist should be able to read the ECG systematically and report about rate, rhythm, axis of the ventricular electrical activity, describe the waves and any abnormality in them. The intervals, i.e., PR interval and QT interval as well as heart blocks should be identified.

Common Scenarios in the CASC Exam

1. **Panic disorder with ECG (usually normal ECG)**

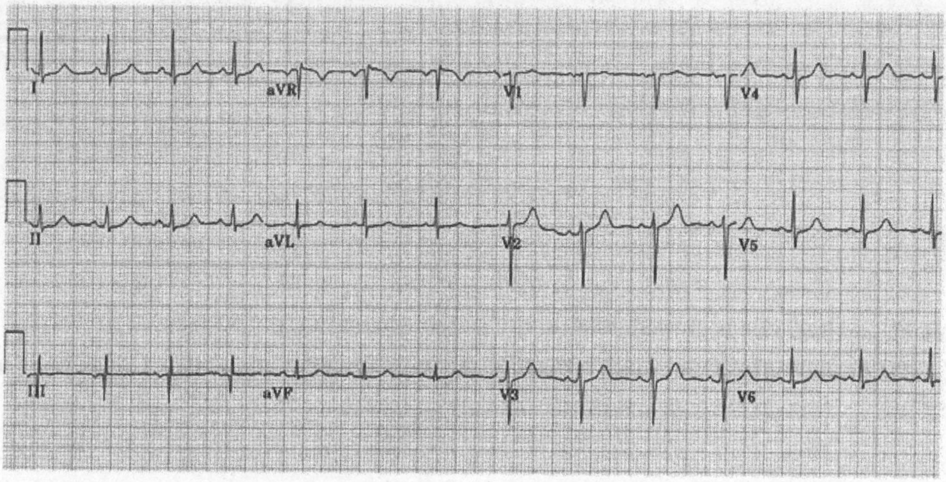

In this ECG, rhythm is sinus rhythm. Heart rate is around 90–100/min. PR interval is around 0.16 sec. No ST/T changes of Myocardial infarction. T waves are normal.

2. **Old age patient complaining of chest pain and is profusely sweating–MI**

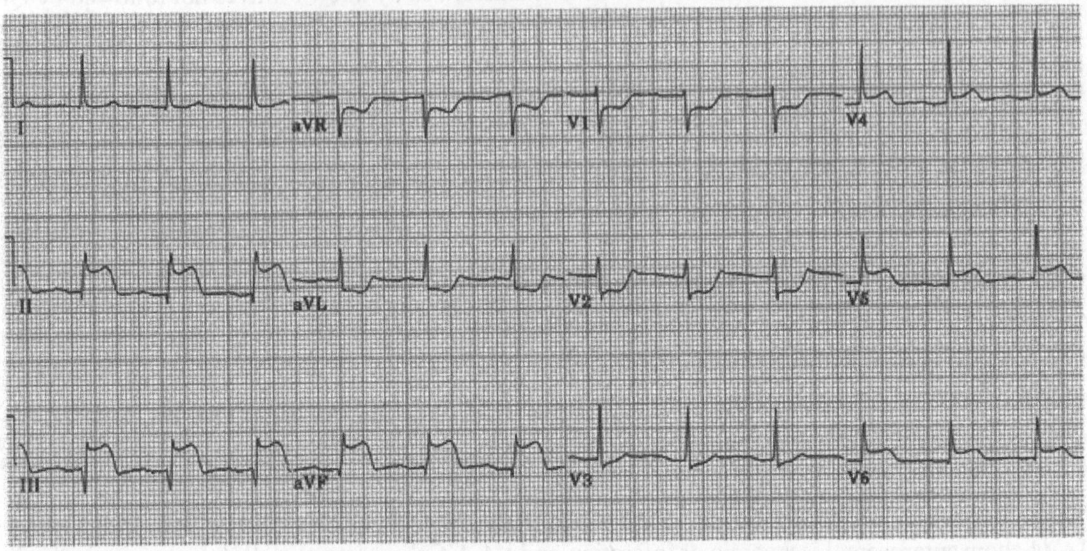

In this ECG, there is ST elevation and T wave inversion in Lead II, III, aVF, V5 and V6. This is suggestive of inferior wall MI. The ST depression in aVR, V1 and V2 is known as reciprocal changes.

3. **Patient on medication read ECG-QTc prolongation**

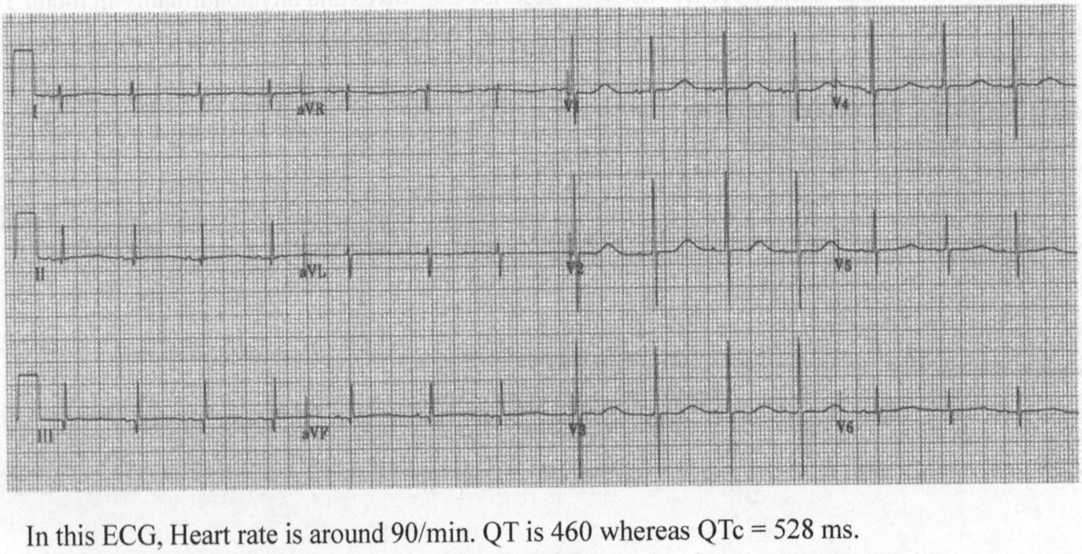

In this ECG, Heart rate is around 90/min. QT is 460 whereas QTc = 528 ms.

ECG station may also come with "Discuss the management plan with Consultant or Ward nurse".

4. **First degree Heart Block (Prolonged PR interval)**

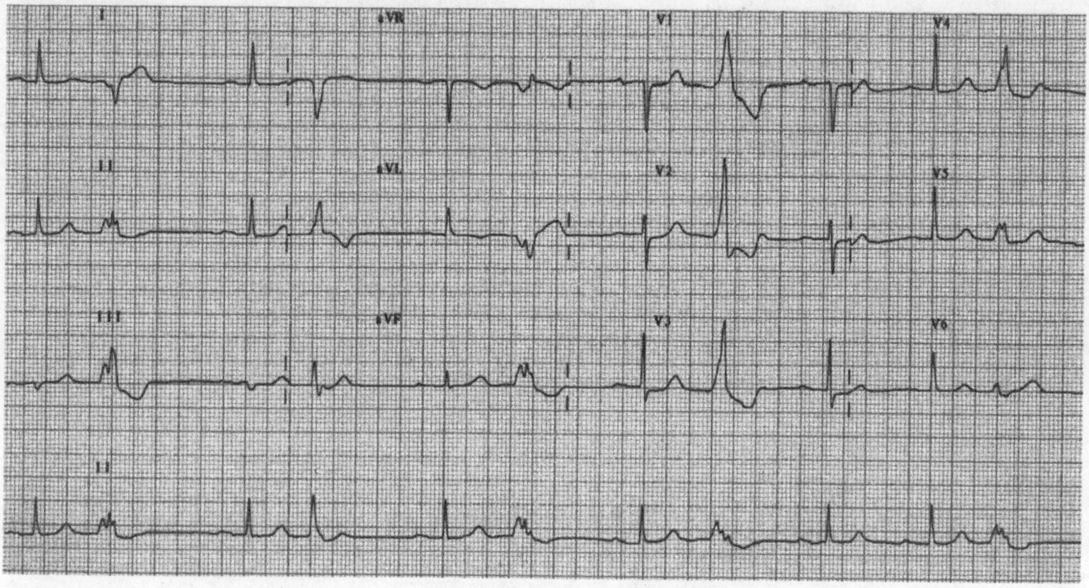

Here the PR interval is about 7–8 small squares, i.e., 0.28–0.32 sec.

5. **Complete Heart Block**

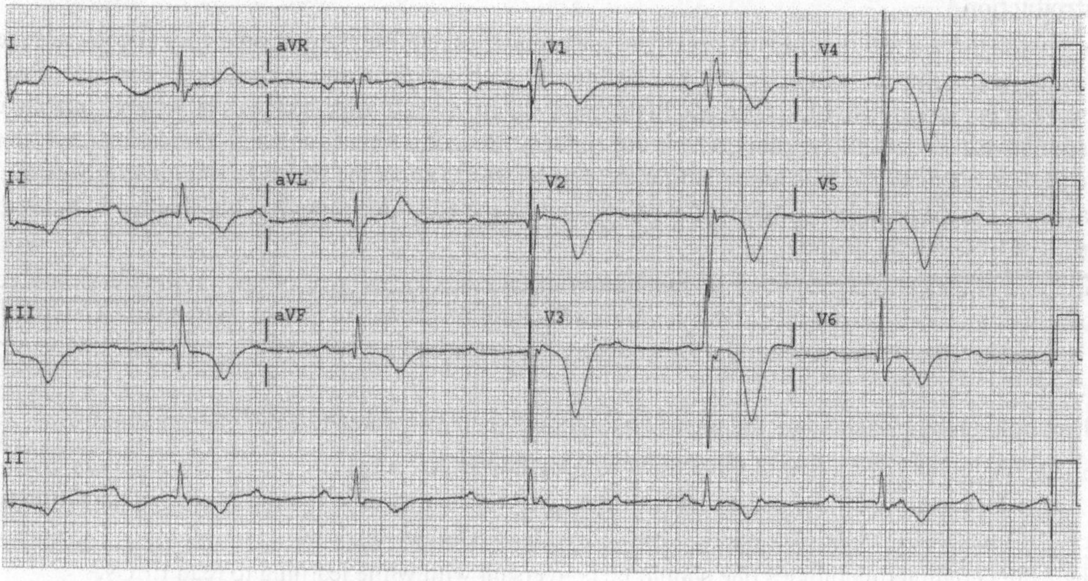

In this ECG, the P waves and QRS complexes have dissociated. P waves vary in position.

6. ECG showing 'Torsade de pointes'

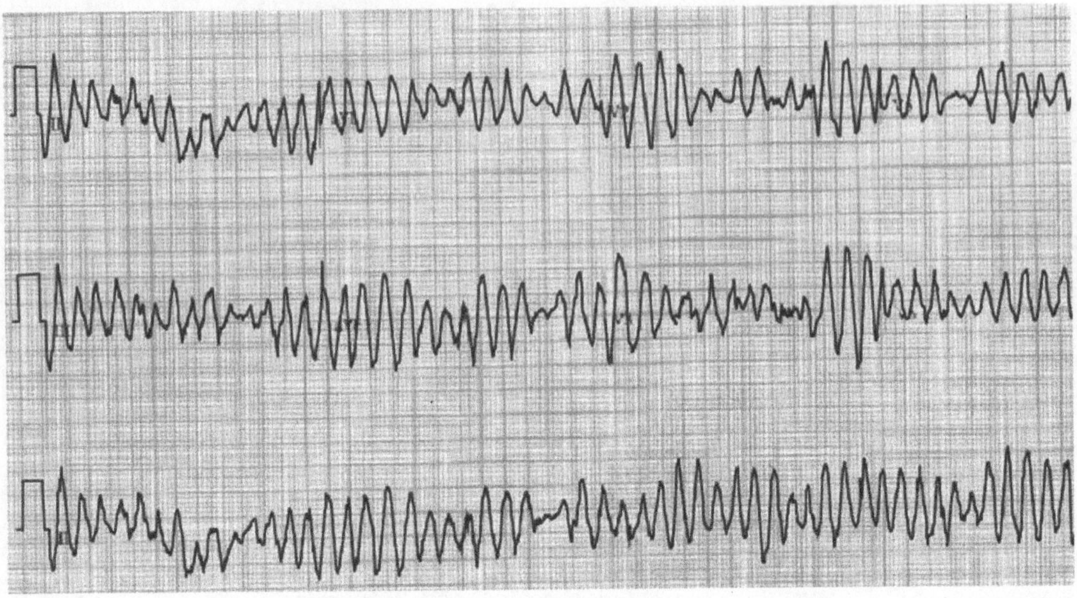

Interpretation of EEG

Introduction

As a psychiatrist one will deal with psychiatric aspects of generalised tonic clonic convulsions, absence seizures and complex partial seizures. Conditions, such as, dementia including Creutzfeldt–Jakob disease may present with EEG changes. In many psychiatric conditions, such as, conversion disorder or dissociative disorders, EEG is done to rule out epilepsy. Benzodiazepines and anti-depressants can affect the EEG frequencies. So, it is important for the psychiatrist to know the basics of EEG interpretation. At least they should be able to interpret the report sent by the EEG department. This chapter includes the basics of EEG interpretation.

EEG is a graphical representation of summation of electrical activity of all the brain cells at a given point in time. Electrical activity of deeper brain structures might not be picked up by the EEG. Usually, it is done for 20–30 minutes period. But in some cases it can be carried out for up to 24–72 hours using an ambulatory EEG device.

Most importantly one should remember two important dictums related to EEG interpretation.

(a) A normal EEG does not rule out underlying pathology.

(b) Treatment is for the person and not the EEG. Once a specific finding is seen clinician should think of the range of possible clinical correlates associated with it.

There are certain terminologies one should be conversant with while learning to read EEGs:

- EED leads and montages.
- 10–20 system of electrode placement.
- Intrinsic rhythm: Denotes normal brain activity.
- Amplitude and frequency of EEG waveforms.
- Phase reversal.

How Electrodes are Designated?

- Capital letters show us the area where electrode is placed, i.e., F = Frontal, T = Temporal, O = Occipital, P = Parietal. C denotes centrally placed electrodes.
- Odd numbers: Electrodes placed on the left side of midline on the scalp.
- Even numbers: Electrodes placed on the right side of midline on the scalp.
- Z denotes midline electrodes.

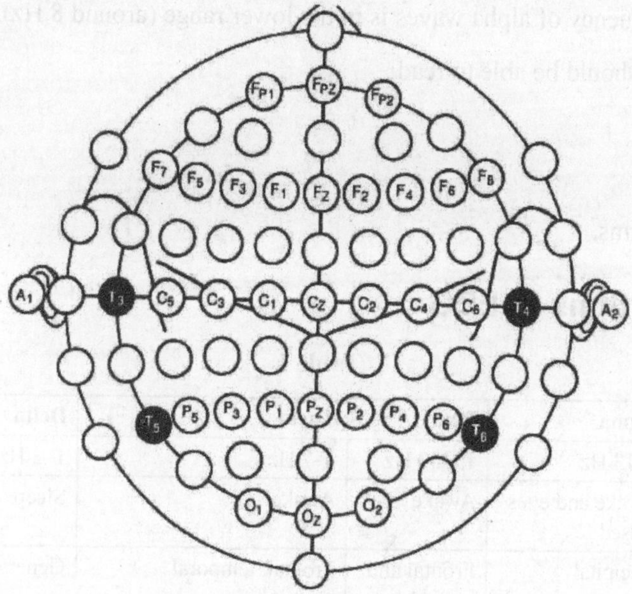

10–20 system of electrode placement

EEG waveforms change with:

- Age
- Position of electrodes
- Sleep
- Activity
- State of the person: Drowsy
- Drugs.

Sometimes certain procedures can unmask underlying abnormality. Then EEG can easily pick up these. These are called activation procedures. These include:

- Hyperventilation
- Medication activation
- Photic stimulation
- Sleep
- Sleep deprivation.

So, it is important to know these details before interpreting the EEG.

EEG Changes with Age

- Infants have irregular, slower and high voltage delta activity.
- Mature rhythms develop between 2 and 6 years – theta to lower alpha range (around 8 Hz).
- By mid-adolescence EEG becomes adult type.
- Normal adult EEGs show predominant alpha rhythm in the background, seen in the occipital region with eyes closed and awake state. Beta activity is seen in the frontal and parietal regions.
- When subject is drowsy, alpha becomes intermittent and theta appears.
- In old age, the frequency of alpha waves is in the lower range (around 8 Hz).

To interpret EEG, one should be able to read:

- Normal rhythm
- Normal variations
- Artefacts
- Abnormal waveforms.

Waveforms/Rhythms in EEG

Table 1

Characteristics	**Alpha**	**Beta**	**Theta**	**Delta**	**Gamma**
Frequency	8–13 Hz	13–30 Hz	4–7 Hz	1–3 Hz	>30 Hz
State of person	Awake and eyes closed	Awake	Awake	Sleep	Awake
Region of brain	Occipital	Frontal and central	Frontal, temporal	Generalised	Generalised
Normal/Abnormal	Normal. Absence of alpha rhythm in the background could be pathological	Normal	Sporadic and Isolated theta in frontotemporal regions could be normal. Excessive generalised or focal theta in a wake state indicates focal pathology. Patients on Benzodiazepines can have fast beta activity in EEG	Delta waves could be normal in a person who is in deep sleep. In awake state, focal or general delta is suggestive of pathology	Some people call it high beta. Indicative of abnormal brain function

Generalised slowing (delta or low theta waves) is seen in:

- Metabolic encephalopathy.
- Endocrine disorders like hypothyroidism.
- Vitamin deficiencies; and
- Toxic encephalopathies.

Focal slowing (delta or low theta) in a wake person is suggestive of:

- Structural lesion like a tumour or abscess.
- They can also be seen in closed head injuries.

EEG Changes with Sleep

As a person becomes progressively drowsy waveforms can get slower and slower, i.e., theta and delta waves. These are also associated with sharp waves and sleep spindles.

Artefacts in EEG

Artefacts are wave patterns detected by scalp electrodes in an EEG that are not due to brain's electrical activity. These may mimic real brain waves. Common causes are:

- Eye blinks.
- Eye movements.
- Contraction of frontalis muscle.
- Clenching of jaw.
- Tongue movements.
- Movement of head.
- Sweating–gives rise to what is called galvanic skin response.

Waves Those are Suggestive of Epileptic Activity

These are also called 'epileptiform pattern'[1]: These are distinctive waves or complexes, distinguished from background activity, and resembling those recorded in a proportion of human subjects suffering from epileptic disorders. These are also seen interictally. They could be focal, hemispherical or generalised. If these waveforms are seen continuously, for longer period they represent underlying seizure activity.

- **Spike:** Same as sharp wave, but with duration of 20 to less than 70 ms.
- **Sharp wave:** Transient, clearly distinguishable from background activity, with pointed peak at conventional paper speeds and a duration of 70–200 ms.
- **Spike and slow wave complex:** Pattern consisting of a spike followed by a slow wave.
- **Multiple spike and slow wave complex:** Same as spike-and-slow-wave complex, but with two or more spikes associated with one or more slow waves.

Many a times the slow waveforms in the background can be associated with spikes or sharp waves in pathological condition, e.g., Brain abscess can irritate surrounding regions and cause spikes along with slowing.

Hepatic encephalopathy can give rise to 'triphasic waves' in EEG. These are also called liver waves. These are characterized by 1–3 Hz (Delta waves) with each slow wave initiated by spike waves.

In this chapter, we did not go into the details of EEG patterns in various psychiatric conditions as well as controversial EEGs. Another topic, i.e., not covered is evoked potential studies.

Ref: 1. International Federation of Societies for Clinical Neurophysiology. A glossary of terms most commonly used by clinical electroencephalographers. *Electroencephalogr Clin Neurophysiol*, Nov 1974;37(5):538–48.

Further Reading: Kaplan and Saddock's Comprehensive textbook of psychiatry, 9th edn., Lippincott Williams and Wilkins; Chapter on Applied Electrophysiology 2009; 211–248.

4 Single Stations

Station 1: EEG and ECT

Theme: EEG in a patient undergoing ECT

1. **Instructions to candidates:**
You are a ST3 psychiatry trainee administering 5th ECT to this patient in the ECT suite. The patient is depressed and receives bilateral ECT at the dose of 256 mc. After the ECT session, the consultant asked you to discuss the findings with him.

Discuss the findings with the consultant.

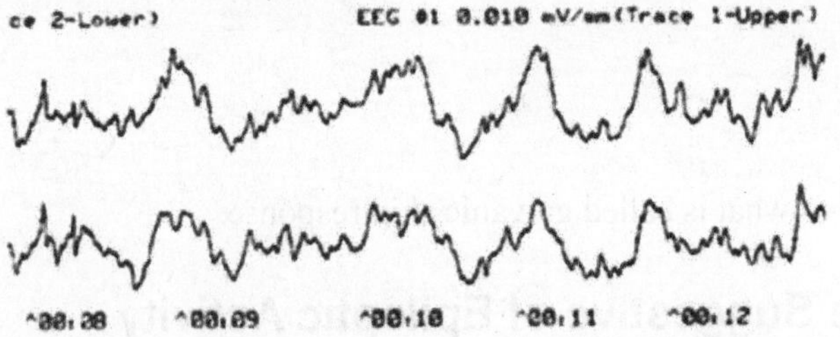

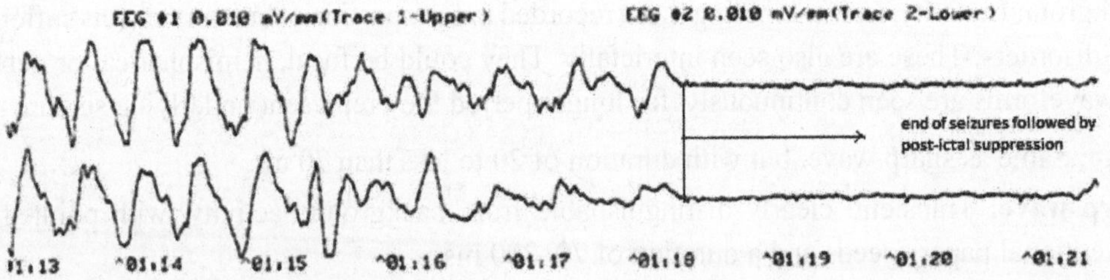

2. **Instructions to consultant (Role player):**
Unless the candidate describes, ask the following questions.
   - **Describe what you see in the upper EEG strip?**
   - **Is it bilaterally symmetrical?**
   - **What is the duration of seizures?**
   - **Is the seizure duration adequate?**
   - **Is there post-ictal suppression?**
   - **What is the importance of post-ictal suppression?**
   - **When do you say a seizure as prolonged one?**
   - **What can be done if the seizure duration is prolonged?**
   - **What is your recommendation regarding the charge setting for next ECT?**

3. **Construct:**
Candidate should be able to interpret the EEG and discuss the findings with the consultant.

4. **Expanded construct:**
   - Candidate should be able to describe the upper strip and lower strip.
   - Candidate should be able tell the duration of seizures.
   - Candidate should be able to discuss the symmetry of EEG waves bilaterally.
   - Candidate should know about the normal duration of seizures during ECT.
   - Candidate should know about prolonged seizures and what to do when the seizures are prolonged.
   - Candidate should be able to decide about the voltage setting for the next ECT based on this EEG.

5. **Areas of importance to pass the station:**
   - Ability to interpret EEG (80%).
   - Demonstrating background theoretical knowledge regarding ECT (20%).

6. **Equipment checklist:**
   Not applicable.

Station 2: EEG in a 65-year-old patient

Theme: Interpretation of EEG in a 65-year-old man with staring spells

1. **Instructions to the candidates:**

   You are a CT3 trainee in General Adult Psychiatry. You are asked to interpret the EEG of Mr Anthony Harper. Mr Harper has been found to be staring vacantly on and off at workplace. He is due to retire in 2 months' time. Hence, colleagues thought he might be depressed. GP referred Mr Harper to you for further advice.

   Interpret the EEG and discuss the findings with the consultant.

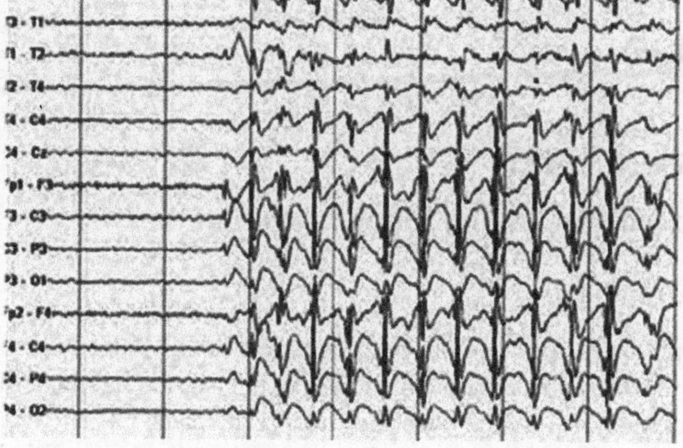

2. **Instructions to the consultant (Role player):**

   Ask the following questions to the candidate:

- **Describe the EEG.**
- **What is the pattern?**
- **What is the likely diagnosis?**
- **How would you assess this patient further?**
- **What further investigations would you do?**
- **How will you manage?**

3. **Construct:**

   Candidate should fluently describe the EEG and discuss the management plan.

4. **Expanded construct:**

   - Candidate should be able to describe the spike waveforms and their frequency.
   - Candidate should be able to tell the diagnosis from the EEG.
   - Candidate should be able to discuss the significance of absence seizures in old age.
   - Candidate should be able to talk about further clinical assessment and neurological assessment.
   - Candidate should be able to talk about investigations including Imaging and Neurology referral.

   This EEG is suggestive of absence seizures. EEG in absence seizures shows spike-waveforms of 3 Hz (i.e., there will be 3 spike-waves/second) which is symmetrical in all the EEG montages. It is common in children and old age. In old age underlying pathology should be ruled out, e.g., degenerative diseases.

5. **Areas of importance to pass the station:**

   - Interpreting EEG (75%).
   - Discussing about the management of the patient 25%.

6. **Equipment checklist:**
   Not applicable.

Station 3: Interpretation of the EEG

Theme: 30-year-old woman having funny turns

1. **Instructions to the candidates:**

   You are assessing a 30-year-old woman with depression. GP started her on Dosulepine 75 mg at night. Her depressive symptoms improved. However, she started having strange episodes where she was found to be picking her skin and vacantly starring at space. On one occasion, she was found to be smacking her lips and muttering. The patient cannot recollect any of these. Your Consultant had requested EEG.

   Interpret the EEG and discuss the findings and management plan with the Consultant.

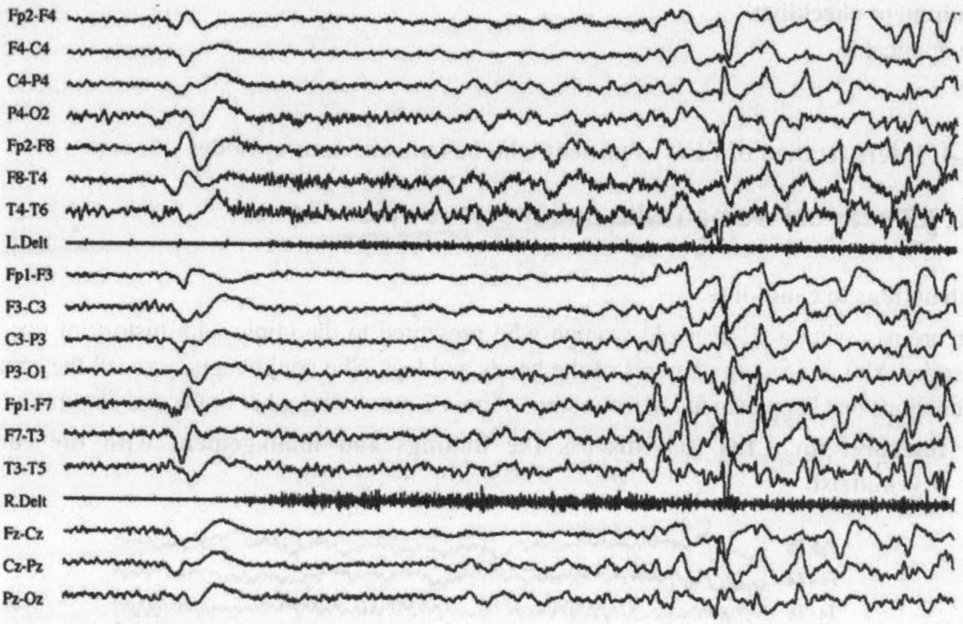

2. **Instructions to the role player:**

You are a consultant psychiatrist.

Ask the following questions to the candidate:

- **Describe the EEG.**
- **What is the likely diagnosis?**
- **How would you manage this patient further?**

3. **Construct:**

Candidate demonstrates knowledge in interpreting EEG and discusses the management plan.

4. **Expanded construct:**

- Candidate should be able to discuss the findings of the EEG.
- Able to discuss the diagnosis of complex partial seizures.
- Able to discuss the management plan including change of anti-depressant, dosulepine if indicated.
- Able to discuss about neurology referral.
- In this EEG, the spikes originate initially from right frontotemporal areas (F8–T4 and T4–T6 montages) but get generalised soon. This is an EEG of complex partial seizure/temporal lobe epilepsy.

5. **Areas of importance to pass the station:**

- Interpretation of EEG (70%).
- Discussion of management including management of depression as well as epilepsy (30%).

6. **Equipment checklist:**
   Not applicable.

Station 4: Interpretation of EEG of patient who has unconscious episodes

Theme: 22-year-old woman with unconscious episodes

1. **Instructions to candidate.**
   You are assessing a 22-year-old woman who presented to the clinic with history of unconscious episodes. You noticed movements of the hands and legs. She could vaguely recall the episode and discussions that happen in her surroundings. About 2 months ago, her boyfriend committed suicide.
   - **Interpret the EEG and discuss the findings and management with the consultant psychiatrist.**

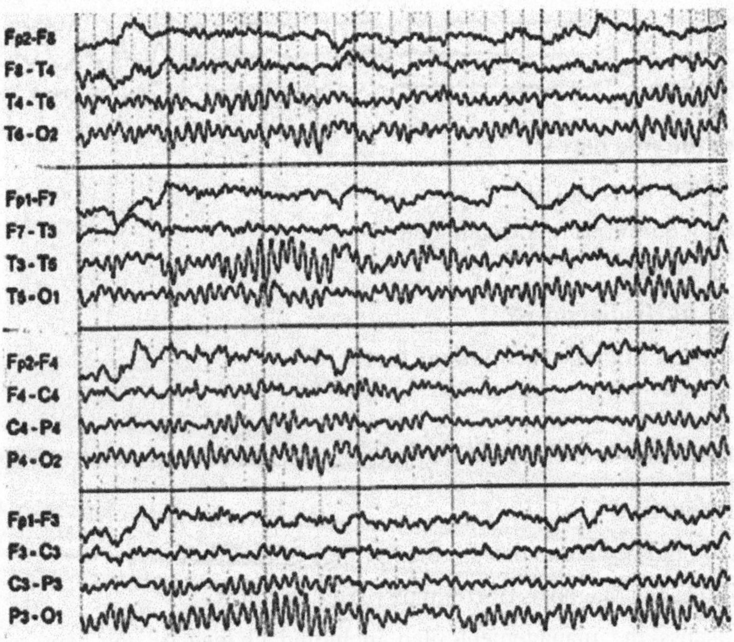

2. **Instructions to the role player:**
   You are a Consultant Psychiatrist. Ask the following questions:
   - **Describe the EEG.**
   - **What is your conclusion?**
   - **What are the normal waveforms in EEG?**
   - **How would you assess this patient further?**
   - **How would you manage this patient further?**
3. **Construct:**
   Candidate demonstrates knowledge in interpreting EEG and discusses the management plan.

4. **Expanded construct:**
   - Candidate should be able to discuss the findings on the EEG.
   - Able to discuss about normal waveforms in the EEG.
   - Able to discuss about the assessment of conversion disorder.
   - Able to discuss the management plan including psychotherapy.
   - This is a normal EEG. There is well-formed alpha activity in the background (8–9 Hz). No spikes, sharp waves or spike-waveforms seen. A normal EEG does not rule out epilepsy. Appropriate history for the seizure pattern along with EEG finding is of diagnostic value.
5. **Areas of importance to pass the station:**
   Interpretation of EEG (60%).
   Discussion of management including management of conversion disorder (40%).
6. **Equipment checklist:**
   Not applicable.

3 Single CASC stations on physical investigations

Station 1: Blood test results in clozapine therapy

Station 2: Anorexia ECG + electrolytes: Interpret

Station 3: Blood test results lithium therapy: Interpret

Station 1: Clozapine induced neutropenia

Theme: Discuss with the consultant psychiatrist about the management of clozapine-induced neutropenia

1. **Instruction to candidates:**
   You are a CT3 trainee in Psychiatry. You received a phone call from Haematology clinic regarding Mr George Gregory a 35-year-old man of Afro-Caribbean origin. He suffers from treatment-resistant schizophrenia with a high risk of violence. He was started on clozapine 3 months ago. He is compliant with medication and his symptoms have been well-controlled over the past few years. The blood tests results are as follows:
   WBC count is 2.9×10^9 ($4.0 - 11.0 \times 10^9$); and
   Neutrophil count is 1.4×10^9 ($2.0 - 7.5 \times 10^9$).
   - **Talk to the consultant and explain about your management plan.**
2. **Instructions to the role player:**
   You are a consultant psychiatrist.
   You should ask the candidate the following questions:
   1. **What do you infer from the results?**
   2. **What assessments will you do with this patient?**

3. **What is the management plan?**
4. **Will you stop clozapine now?**

Option A. If the candidate mentions about continuing clozapine, ask:

5. **How will you monitor the patient if you are going to continue clozapine?**
6. **Will you consider adding medication? Explain.**
7. **If white cell counts continue to fall, what will you do?**
8. **If patient develops infection, what will you do?**

Option B: If candidate mentions about stopping clozapine, ask:

9. **How will you monitor this patient further?**
10. **How would you control his psychotic symptoms?**
11. **Explain about clozapine re-challenge.**
12. **Role of inpatient care.**

3. **Construct:**

   Candidate fluently and confidently explains the management of clozapine induced neutropenia.

4. **Expanded construct:**
   - Candidate should be able to discuss about the normal and abnormal neutrophil and white cell counts.
   - Candidate should be able to discuss about the entity benign ethnic neutropenia.
   - Candidate should be able to explain the management of patient whose neutrophil counts are amber (according to clozapine monitoring services).
   - Candidate should be able to explain about contacting clozapine monitoring service as appropriate.
   - Candidate should be able to explain about assessment of the patient for past history of neutropenia, current infections, etc.
   - Candidate should be able to discuss about twice weekly blood tests, adding lithium etc.
   - Candidate should be able to tell clearly the indications for clozapine in neutropenia and agranulocytosis.
   - Candidate should be able to explain the role of physician and hematologist in the management of clozapine-induced neutropenia.
   - Candidate should be able to discuss about using alternative medication for the management of psychosis.
   - Candidate should be able to talk about clozapine re-challenge and chances of developing agranulocytosis again.

5. **Areas of importance to pass the station:**
   - Demonstrating knowledge of benign ethnic neutropenia and management of a patient with falling neutrophil levels (40%).
   - Involving clozapine monitoring services, physician and haematologist (20%).
   - Discussing about treatment of psychosis (30%).
   - Discussing about clozapine re-challenge (10%).

6. Equipment checklist:

Not applicable.

Ref: 1. Rajagopal S: Clozapine, agranulocytosis, and benign ethnic neutropenia: Current knowledge and clinical implications. *Postgrad Med J* 2005;81:545–546.

2. Taylor D, Paton C, Kapur S: The Maudsley Prescribing Guidelines in Psychiatry, 11th edn.; Wiley-Blackwell. Clozapine, Neutropenia and Lithium 2012;84–87.

Station 2: Anorexia nervosa: Investigations

Theme: Interpretation of ECG and blood results of a patient with anorexia nervosa

1. Instructions to candidates:

Catherine Bennet is a 14-year-old girl admitted with BMI of 13. She had fainted in her dance session and her family and teachers were concerned. She had her blood tests and ECG and the findings are as below:

- **Interpret the results.**
- **Discuss with the nurse in charge about the management plan.**

Blood investigations:

Blood Urea 8 mmol/L (2.5–6.7 mmol/L)

S Creatinine: 120 micromol/L (70–150 micromol/L)

Na+ = 120 mmol/L (135–145 mmol/L)

K+ = 3 mmol/L (3.5–5.0 mmol/L)

T4 = 60 mmol/L (70–140 mmol/L)

ECG:

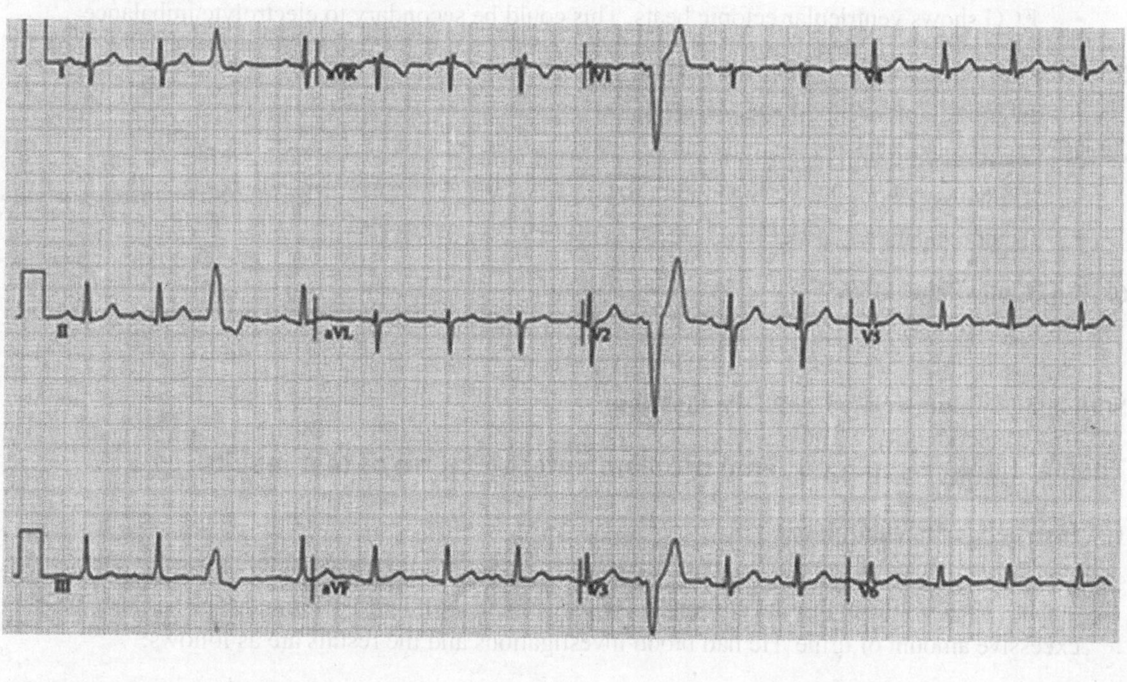

2. **Instructions to the role player:**

   You are the charge nurse of the inpatient psychiatric unit. You and your colleagues are worried about Catherine. Ask the following questions to the doctor.

   1. **What are the blood investigation findings?**
   2. **Does she have kidney failure?**
   3. **Thyroid levels are low, but she is so thin. Could the lab results be wrong?**
   4. **What are the ECG findings?**
   5. **Should we transfer her to medical unit?**
   6. **How to manage her in the psychiatry unit?**

3. **Construct:**

   Candidate fluently explains the findings and management of the patient suffering from anorexia.

4. **Expanded construct:**

   - Candidate should be able to interpret the blood results appropriately.
   - Candidate should be able to interpret the ECG appropriately.
   - Candidate should be able to explain the management of patient suffering from anorexia with very low BMI and abnormal blood results and ECG results.
   - Blood tests show raised urea and normal creatinine. This shows patient is dehydrated. She does not suffer from kidney failure.
   - Sodium and potassium values are low. This could be because of vomiting.
   - T4 levels are low: In patients with anorexia, T3 and T4 levels can be low and rT3 levels can be raised. This is known as sick euthyroid syndrome. No need for thyroid replacement. Treating anorexia will lead to correction of thyroid levels.
   - ECG shows ventricular ectopic beats. This could be secondary to electrolyte imbalance.

5. **Areas of importance to pass the station:**

   - Interpretation of blood results (30%).
   - Interpretation of ECG (30%).
   - Explaining about the management (30%).
   - Communication skills (10%).

6. **Equipment checklist:**

   None listed.

Station 3: Lithium-related renal dysfunction

Theme: Lithium-induced renal problem: Interpretation of test results

1. **Instructions to candidates:**

   You are reviewing Andy Bottoms, a 45-year-old patient. He suffers from bipolar affective disorder and has been stable on lithium carbonate 1000 mg nocte. For the past 2 months, he has been passing excessive amount of urine. He had blood investigations and the results are as follows:

24 hours urine output: 6 liters.

Urine osmolality: 340 mOsmol/L (400–800 mOsmol/L).

Plasma osmolality: 305 mOsmol/kg (285–295 mOsmol/kg).

Serum Na+: 150 mmol/L (135–145 mmol/L).

Serum K+: 3.0 mmol/L (3.5–5 mmol/L).

Blood Urea: 18 mmol/L (2.5–6.7 mmol/L).

S Creatinine: 150 micromol/L (70–150 micromol/L).

- **Interpret the findings to arrive at a diagnosis.**
- **Explain the management plan to the patient.**

2. **Instructions to the role player:**

You are Andy Bottoms and you are 45 years old. You have been stable on lithium 1000 mg at night which you have been taking for 20 years now. For the past 6 months, you have been passing excess of water and GP has done some blood tests.

You are worried about the test results.

You are also worried about what would happen if lithium were to be stopped.

About 10 years ago, you had stopped lithium but your condition had relapsed.

Ask the following questions:

- **What do the results show?**
- **Am I having a kidney problem?**
- **What is the problem–Is there any name?**
- **What is the treatment plan for this problem?**
- **What would be the treatment for bipolar disorder now?**

3. **Construct:**

Candidate should be able to interpret the results and explain the management plan to the patient.

4. **Expanded construct:**

- Candidate should be able to demonstrate advanced listening skills.
- Candidate should be able to interpret the blood results appropriately.
- Candidate should be able to explain the management of diabetes insipidus.
- Candidate should be able to explain the management of bipolar disorder.

5. **Areas of importance to pass the station:**

- Interpretation of results, i.e., diabetes insipidus (50%).
- Explaining the management of bipolar disorder (30%).
- Explaining the management of diabetes insipidus (20%).

6. **Equipment checklist:**

None listed.

SECTION 3

Practice CASC Stations

1. General Adult Psychiatry

Linked Stations: 1–20

Linked Stations 1 and 2

Station 1: Link 1: Suicide risk: Assess

Station 2: Link 2: Suicide risk: Discussion

Station 1: Link 1: Suicide risk: Assess

Theme: Assessment of suicide risk

1. **Instructions to candidates:**

   Patient's name: Hilary Brown

   Mrs Brown is a 60-year-old lady. She was admitted to medical assessment unit following an overdose and she is ready for discharge from medical side.

   Talk to her and assess the risks and suitability for home treatment.

   In the next station, you are going to speak to your consultant about further management.

2. **Instructions to the role player:**

   Mrs Brown is 60-years-old married female who lives with her husband. She doesn't have any dependents.

   - She is a housewife and there is a gradual decline in her activities of daily living. She was able to do household chores till 6 weeks ago.
   - She was worried about her physical health and about her husband who suffers from physical health problem. She had a fall on two occasions but she didn't sustain any head injuries.
   - She suffers from paranoid schizophrenia for the last 20 years. She also suffers from arthritis and hypertension and type 2 diabetes. Her clozapine was stopped due to low neutrophil count. She was commenced on quetiapine and she had been compliant with her medication.

- The signs of her relapses are poor motivation, poor sleep and social isolation. She had two voluntary admissions in the psychiatric ward due to relapses. The common cause of her relapses are non-compliance with her medications.
- She has been hearing three voices for a long time. These voices talk about her and they are derogatory in nature. They do not give any commanding instructions. Gradually, they have been becoming louder. It became so distressing for her that she was not able to cope with it. When she becomes unwell she becomes paranoid as well.
- Her mood has been low for the last 2 months and she is in constant pain. She is not able to sleep well and feels tired all the time. She has lost her appetite. She has been feeling hopeless, helpless and worthless. She feels like she is a burden on her husband. She has been having fleeting thoughts of self-harm for a long time but she never acted on these thoughts. She doesn't have any interference with her thinking or any abnormal perceptions. She knows she has some mental health problem but she doesn't want to be locked away in the ward and see other people with mental health difficulties. There is no history of alcohol dependence.
- Two days earlier she was feeling so miserable that she was not able to rationalise things. In late evening when she was on her own at home, she impulsively took an overdose of 30 tablets of tramadol and 30 tablets of quetiapine after drinking half a bottle of vodka. She was found by chance by her husband in an unconscious state. She doesn't drink alcohol regularly. These medications belong to her. She had access to more medications but she did not take it because she started feeling sick. She has not left any suicidal notes. There was no planning but she took the overdose before going to bed. She has no regret about the overdose.
- She doesn't want to take another overdose but she may try other methods to harm herself. She is not sure about these things and she doesn't have any active plans. She sees her husband as a protective factor, but she believes there is no point in living like this.

3. **Construct:**

Candidates should assess the risk to self, patient's safety as well as the risk to others.

4. **Expanded construct:**

- Introduction
- Background
- Reason for admission
- Deliberate self-harm: Environment, methods, planning, preparation, precaution, intent, suicidal notes, recovery (past, present and future plans).
- Aetiological factors
- Affective symptoms
- Thoughts
- Perception
- Insight
- Past psychiatry history of deliberate self-harm, contact with mental health services, compliance with medication, engagement, care plan and inpatient admissions.
- Past medical history
- Impact
- Coping skills

- Risk of self-harm
- Risk of suicide
- Risk to others.

5. **Areas of importance to pass the station:**
   - Communication (20%).
   - History and mental state examination (40%).
   - Risk assessment (40%).
6. **Equipment checklist if applicable:**
   None.

Station 2: Link 2: Suicide risk: Discussion

Theme: Suicide risk management: Explain the management to the consultant

1. **Instructions to candidates:**
   Patient's name: Hilary Brown
   You have done a risk assessment of a 60-year-old lady was admitted to medical assessment unit who is ready for discharge from medical side.
   Discuss your finding and discuss the management of this patient with your consultant.
2. **Instruction to the role player:**
   You are the consultant and ask your junior the following questions:
   - Summarise the case.
   - Give your provisional diagnosis.
   - Explain the risks.
   - Explain the management plan.
   - Appropriate use of Mental Health Act.
   - Use of Mental Capacity Act.
3. **Construct:**
   Candidate has to demonstrate his ability to summarise the case, formulate the risks and make a management plan using biopsychosocial model. He should communicate these to the consultant appropriately.
4. **Expanded construct:**
   - Introduce yourself.
   - Take the permission from your consultant.
   - Tell the background, i.e., why and where you have seen the patient including background of the patient.
   - Reason of admission to the medical unit.
   - Deliberate self-harm: Environment, methods, planning, preparation, precaution, intent, suicidal notes, recovery (past, present and future plans).

- Affective symptoms.
- Thoughts.
- Perception.
- Insight.
- Patient's view.
- Past psychiatric history.
- Impact.
- **Coping skills:** Alcohol and substance misuse history.
- **Risk to self:** Background, presence of severe enduring mental illness, comorbidity, alcohol and substance misuse, deliberate self-harm, past or current history of abuse, presence or absence of relapse indicators and insight and disengagement.
- **Risk to patient's safety:** Vulnerability and exploitation.
- **Risk to others:** Aggression and agitation, forensic history.
- Management Plan

	Immediate	Short-term	Long-term
Bio			
Psycho			
Social			

- Appropriate use of Mental Health Act/Mental Capacity Act.

5. **Areas of importance to pass the station:**
   - Summary (33%).
   - Risk assessment (33%).
   - Risk management (33%).
6. **Equipment checklist if applicable**

   None

Linked Stations 3 and 4

Station 3: Link 1: Conversion disorder: Assess

Station 4: Link 2: Conversion disorder: Explain care plan and prognosis

Station 3: Link 1: Conversion disorder: Assess

Theme: Elicit History of Conversion Disorder from The Patient

1. **Instructions to candidates:**

   Patient's name: Miss Sarah Ford

   You are assessing a 20-year-old female patient in the medical ward who presented with inability to move the right arm and left leg. The ward doctors have informed you that she was investigated but there is no physical cause for her problem. Elicit psychiatric history, current symptoms and their relationship to the stressors.

   His father is waiting in the next station to talk to you.

2. **Instructions to the role player:**
   - You are Miss Sarah Ford. You started modelling when you were 14 years old and you have been working as a model in Paris. You always wanted to become a model but did not realise the pressures of working in this industry.
   - You are beautiful and good looking. You have not had a proper meal since the age of 14 in order to maintain your figure.
   - Initially, you enjoyed the profession but you could not cope with the pressure of work.
   - Your mother is nagging and wants you to continue working so that the family could have extra money flowing in for their luxuries.
   - Recently, you have been having arguments with your boyfriend who is also interested in your money. You want to marry him but he wants you to continue working so that you can enjoy holidays.
   - In general, there was no emotional support from the family which would allow you to leave work.
   - Yesterday night, you had strong arguments with your mother who was rather pushing you to sign a new contract with a big modelling agency. You wanted to continue with your studies and lead a life of a normal girl, enjoy going out with your friends, eat as much as you like without too many constraints arising out of your modelling career.
   - Today in the morning you realised that you could not move your right hand and left leg. You were brought to the hospital.
   - Ever since you have been in the hospital the whole family has come around. Your boyfriend has been bringing you flowers and chocolates. Your mother has calmed down. Yesterday she visited you and became very emotional. She even fed you with her own hands. She wants you to eat and drink properly so that you recover physically. Your mother now feels that she was very harsh on you and she wants you to continue with your studies so that you can change your career.

3. **Construct:**

   The station tests the candidate's ability to elicit the stressors precipitating the event. Candidate should elicit and differentiate conversion disorder from other disorders, such as, malingering, somatisation disorder, hypochondriasis and mood disorders. In this disorder, it is important to elicit 'la belle indifference', primary and secondary gains.

4. **Expanded construct:**
   - Explain your role and explain why you are seeing her.
   - Use good communication skills in establishing a rapport, showing empathy and use a non-judgmental approach.
   - Explore the reason for admission – Loss of power in right arm and left leg.
   - Onset, duration, progression.
   - Establish temporal relationship with stressors.
   - Find out the change in the stressors and the circumstances following the event.

- Explore patient's view, emotions (la belle indifference) and insight.
- Rule out comorbidity – Mood disorders, neurotic, stress-related and somatoform disorders. Alcohol and substance misuse.
- Try to find out about:
  - **Predisposing factors:** Premorbid personality, physical health and past experiences, attitude of family members towards the illness.
  - **Perpetuating factors:** Primary and secondary gains.
  - **Precipitating factors:** Psychosocial stressors.
- Impact.
- Coping skills.

5. **Areas of importance to pass the station:**
   - Communication (10%).
   - Elicit the diagnostic feature of dissociative disorder by ruling out other comorbidity (40%).
   - Elicit the aetiology stressors and its temporal relationship with the event (30%).
   - Elicit insight, impact and coping (20%).
6. **Equipment check:**
   Not applicable.

Station 4: Link 2: Conversion disorder: Explain care plan and prognosis

Theme: Management of conversion disorder

1. **Instructions to candidates:**

   You have assessed Miss Ford in the previous station. She has given consent to talk to her dad. Her father wants to talk to you. Explain the illness and its management plan including care plan and prognosis. Address his views, ideas and concerns.

2. **Instructions to the role player:**

   Go along with the candidate, if he is able to show empathy and he is able to make a good rapport with you. You are supposed to ask the following questions:
   - **Why is my daughter seeing a psychiatrist?**
   - **Is she going mad?**
   - **What has happened to her?**
   - **What is the cause?**
   - **Are you trying to say that everything is there in her head?**
   - **Is she making it up?**
   - **Is it my fault?**
   - **Why everyone does not develop the same problem?**
   - **Could there be any other explanation for her presentation?**
   - **What is the treatment like?**

- **Is she going to get better?**
- **What is the evidence in favour of the psychological therapy?**
- **How long is it going to take her to overcome the problem?**
- **What is the prognosis?**
- **What can I do for my daughter?**
- **How she can help herself?**

3. **Construct:**
Candidate demonstrate his ability to explain the management of conversion disorder including its prognosis.

4. **Expanded construct:**
   - Establishes rapport.
   - Elicits his ideas, explores his expectations and addresses his concerns.
   - Summarises and explains the diagnosis in jargon-free language by giving examples.
   - Explains that the symptoms are real, happening at unconscious level.
   - Mentions about exclusion of neurological cause.
   - Explains the aetiology. It is triggered by stressors.
   - Explains the psychopathology. Explain how the development of physical symptoms has reduced the distress.
   - Explores the gains associated with the condition.
   - Rules out comorbidity.
   - Explains short-term, medium-term and long-term management plan.
   - Discusses limited and short-term role of physical aid/physiotherapy, etc.
   - Discusses role of psychotherapy and resolution of symptoms.

5. **Areas of importance to pass the station:**
   - Communication (40%).
   - Empathy (20%).
   - Explanation (40%).

6. **Equipment checklist :**
Not applicable.

Linked Stations 5 and 6

Station 5: Link 1: Social phobia: History

Station 6: Link 2: Social phobia: Management

Station 5: Link 1: Social phobia: History

Theme: Elicit history of social phobia

1. **Instructions to candidates:**

Tony Atkinson, a 32-year-old man, has been referred to you by his GP for an assessment. He has been avoiding work recently, feeling low and has mentioned of resigning from his job.

Take a history from Mr Atkinson and arrive at a diagnosis. You may wish to take some notes as you are expected to discuss the management plan with his partner.

2. **Instructions to role player:**

- You are Tony Atkinson, 32-year-old, live with your partner and are employed as an accountant. Recently, you have been feeling increasingly anxious, are avoiding work and even contemplating taking another job.
- When asked you describe the following:
  - You like the present job and want to continue. You have been awarded the best employee of the year. Your boss has asked you to give a speech on an awards party. This has increased your anxiety and you fear the worst possible scenario.
  - You want to do the presentation, socialise, go to parties and 'have a relaxing evening'. But you are nervous about meeting and talking to people. In the party there will be 'lots of people' and "I cannot bear it".
  - You think that you will make a fool of yourself, people will stare at you, reject you outright, notice your nervousness and "feel like an outcast". You feel they will "judge me and criticise me".
  - You have always stayed away from social situation, meetings and parties for the past 5 years. You cannot bear to be the focus of attention as you are sure to embarrass and humiliate yourself.
  - When you are in such a situation your heart starts beating faster, palms are sweating. You have a dry mouth and you are unable to talk or have slurred speech. You are even more embarrassed as you start blushing and feel like vomiting.
  - You avoid these situations, spend most of the time at home watching TV and don't go anywhere with your partner which has strained your relationship.
  - You are aware this behaviour does not make any sense and is unreasonable.
  - Now, the thought of giving a speech, being amongst people makes you anxious and have brought back these symptoms.
  - You do not drink, smoke or use illicit substances. You do not have physical health problem, previous psychiatric history or any other phobia/anxiety.

3. **Construct:**

This station assesses candidate's knowledge of anxiety disorder and ability to elicit history from a man who has social phobia.

4. **Expanded construct:**
   - The candidate should be able to demonstrate skill in eliciting a history in a patient who has anxiety disorder.
   - The candidate should be able to elicit origin, duration, progress, severity and associated factors of social phobia.
   - The candidate should inquire into relevant differential diagnosis like organic cause, agoraphobia, specific phobia, depression, illicit substance use, and other relevant conditions.
   - They should establish the impact of the disorder on social life and functioning.
   - They should allay patient's anxiety, worries and fears.

5. **Areas of importance to pass the station:**
   - Communication (20%).
   - Eliciting accurate and sufficient information about social phobia, severity of episodes and impact on social life and functioning (50%).
   - Elicit history to rule out relevant differential diagnosis of social phobia (30%).

6. **Equipment checklist if applicable**
   Not applicable.

Station 6: Link 2: Social phobia: Management

Theme: Discussion of management of social phobia with partner

1. **Instructions to candidates:**
   You have seen Tony Atkinson. You have consent from him to discuss your assessment with his partner Sarah Brown.
   Talk to Sarah Brown to discuss your findings and further management plan.

2. **Instructions to the role player:**
   You are Sarah Brown, partner of Tony for the past 4 years. You are 'fed up' with Tony as he does not like going out or socialise. You love him and don't know what to do. Situation has deteriorated in the past month.
   When asked you describe the following:
   - Tony does not like talking to people when he is in a group. He can talk to someone one to one.
   - He did not attend your sister's wedding and you had to make an excuse for his absence.
   - You want to help him if there is a genuine problem. Otherwise, you will have to consider separation.

   You ask following questions:
   - **What is wrong with Tony? Why is he behaving like this?**
   - **Does he have a personality problem?**
   - **What is he scared of? I am always with him.**
   - **What is the cause of this problem? How common is it?**

- **What is the treatment?**
- **Will he get better? How quickly will he get better?**
- **Is the cure permanent?**
- **What do I have to do to make him better?**

3. **Construct:**

This station assesses candidate's knowledge of aetiology, evidence-based management and prognosis of social phobia.

4. **Expanded construct:**

The candidate should:

- Be able to demonstrate skills in discussing the aetiology, management and prognosis of social phobia.
- Consider possible differential diagnosis if relevant.
- Establish the impact of the disorder on social life and functioning from partner including relationship difficulties.
- Discuss evidence-based management of social phobia that include pharmacotherapy (e.g., antidepressant, beta blockers, tranquillisers) and psychotherapy (e.g., CBT, social skills training, graded exposure, stress management, relaxation, behaviour therapy) and other available treatment.
- Allay patient's as well as partner's anxiety, worries and fears.

5. **Areas of importance to pass the station:**

- Discussion of evidence-based management and offer appropriate treatment in this case (50%).
- Allay partner's anxiety, worries and fear and includes aetiology and prognosis of the social phobia (30%).
- Communication (20%).

6. **Equipment checklist if applicable:**

Not applicable.

Linked Stations 7 and 8

Station 7: Link 1: Anorexia nervosa: Aetiological factors

Station 8: Link 2: Anorexia nervosa: Explain care plan and prognosis

Station 7: Link 1: Anorexia nervosa: Aetiological factors

Theme: Anorexia nervosa: Assess aetiological factors

1. **Instructions to candidates:**

A 19-year-old college student Kate Parker has been referred to your outpatient clinic by her GP. Her mother is concerned that she is thin and losing too much weight.

Talk to Kate Parker to identify relevant aaetiological factors for her condition.

You may wish to take notes as you will be required to speak to her mother in the next station.

2. **Instructions to the role player:**

You are Kate Parker, 19-year-old college student and live with a roommate in university accommodation. Your mother took you to see the GP, who did some routine blood tests and referred you to see a psychiatrist. You do not wish to see a doctor, but are polite and answer questions.

- Over the last 6 months, you have restricted the amount you eat so that you lose weight to be six stone. When looking at yourself in the mirror, you do not like your body shape and feel your arms, stomach and bottom are fat. You weigh yourself regularly to check if you have lost weight.
- Daily intake for a week has been one slice of toast and a glass of fresh orange juice for breakfast and a leafy salad for lunch and a banana in the evening.
- You cut your food into tiny pieces and eat when you are alone in your room as you do not like eating in front of people.
- You do not mind being around food and spending time preparing meals for others.
- You spend three hours a day at the gym and exercise in your room in evening.
- You stopped menstruating 3 months ago, have cold hands and feet. You are more irritable about little things but do not have any significant disturbances in your mood. You are unable to pay attention and find it difficult to learn new information at university.
- You are not depressed and have no thoughts of self-harm. You do not use alcohol, drugs or smoking.
- Your father is alcoholic and mother suffers from anxiety. There are regular arguments and fights at home. You feel you have low self-confidence and you relate this to your early childhood experiences and to being only child.
- You are a high achiever academically and perfectionist. You have been through a relationship break up as he started dating an aspiring model. You have decided "to give him back by becoming a model".

3. **Construct:**

This station assesses whether the candidate is able to take a brief history of eating disorder, focusing on the aetiological factors associated with eating disorder, in particular anorexia nervosa.

4. **Expanded construct:**

- The candidate should take a brief history of eating disorder.
- Its origin, duration and progress.
- They should carry out a focused, fluent history into the aetiological factors of anorexia nervosa including relevant maintaining factors for anorexia nervosa, e.g., biological, genetic, and psychosocial like morbid fear of fatness/conflict/role change, personality like perfectionism/ negative self-evaluation and family dynamics.
- They should demonstrate empathy and sensitivity to patient's experience.

5. **Areas of importance to pass the station:**
   Eliciting aetiological factors, such as, psychological, biological, family dynamics and personality (60%).
   - Eliciting a brief history of eating disorder to establish anorexia nervosa (20%).
   - Communication (20%).
6. **Equipment checklist if applicable:**
   Not applicable.

Anorexia Nervosa: Aetiological factors
Genetic–Concordance rate MZ: DZ = 65% : 32%
Biological
– Possible hypothalamic dysfunction.
– Neuropsychological deficit like reduced vigilance, attention, visuospatial abilities and associative memory. These deficits improve with weight gain.
Family dynamics: Enmeshment, rigidity, overprotectiveness, lack of conflict resolution.
Personality: Perfectionism, negative self-evaluation.
Psychosocial: Fear of fatness, disturbed body image, parent's preoccupation with food, lack of sense of identity, issues with control.
Analytical: Regression to childhood, fixation at oral stage, escape from problems of adolescence.
Ref: Semple D, Smyth R. Oxford Handbook of Psychiatry, 3rd edn. Oxford University Press 2013; 398-399.

Station 8: Link 2: Anorexia nervosa: Explain care plan and prognosis

Theme: Anorexia nervosa: Management and prognosis

1. **Instructions to candidates:**

   You have recently assessed Kate in your outpatient clinic. Please speak to Kate's mother, Ms Jessica Parker, who is concerned about her daughter's condition. You have Kate's full consent to discuss her illness with her mother.

   Talk to Ms Parker and discuss the further management plan and prognosis. Address her anxieties, concerns and expectations.

2. **Instructions to the role player:**

   You are Kate's mother, Jessica Parker. You are a Head Teacher in primary school and are devoted to your work. Kate has an eating disorder, her problem has been bothering you for some time and this is affecting your work. You suffer from anxiety and live with your husband, Dave who is an alcoholic. Your daughter, Kate moved out of the house a year ago. You have noticed that she has lost a lot of weight and you are very concerned.

   You should ask the doctor:
   - **What is wrong with her?**
   - **Have I done anything wrong that she has developed eating disorder?**
   - **Why can't she understand that she is losing weight?**
   - **Is she punishing herself or us by doing this?**
   - **What can I do to help?**

- **How do you treat it?**
- **Does she need to be in hospital?**
- **Can I give her a tablet to make it better?**
- **What will happen to her in the future?**
- **Does she need to drop out of university?**
- **Would it help if I encouraged her to eat a lot of take-away which she may enjoy?**
- **Can she die from this?**
- **What if she gets worse and loses more weight?**

You become tearful and start to blame yourself, but accept reassurance from the doctor.

3. **Construct:**
This station assesses whether the candidate is able to establish a rapport with a distressed mother and deal with the situation sensitively. It tests the ability to explain the nature, aetiological factors, treatment and prognosis of anorexia nervosa. It tests the ability to make sure the person (patient's mother) understands the information provided.

4. **Expanded construct:**
   - The candidate should be able to explain nature, aetiological factors, treatment and management of anorexia nervosa in simple and jargon free language.
   - They should be able to alleviate mother's anxieties, concerns and expectation by providing relevant response.
   - They should ensure a full understanding of what has been discussed.
   - They should allow two-way communication rather than anyone dictating the interview.
   - They should demonstrate advanced listening skills, empathy and sensitive approach to the interview.
   - They should demonstrate an ability to listen, identify and respond to concerns.

5. **Areas of importance to pass the station:**
   - Discussing the nature, management and prognosis of anorexia nervosa (40%).
   - Discussing mother's fears, anxieties, concerns and expectations by appropriate responses (40%).
   - Communication (20%).

6. **Equipment checklist if applicable:**
Not applicable.

Prognosis of anorexia nervosa:

If untreated

High risk of mortality of about 10–15%

1/3 full recovery, 1/3 partial recovery, 1/3 chronic problems

Poor prognostic factors:

Male

Chronic course of illness

Presence of bulimic features

Late age of onset

Anxiety when eating with others

Excessive weight loss

Poor childhood adjustment and parental relationships

Ref: Semple D, Smyth R. Oxford Handbook of Psychiatry, 3rd edn., Oxford University Press 2013; 398–399.

Linked Stations 9 and 10

Station 9: Link 1: Frontal lobe syndrome: Collateral history from a carer

Station 10: Link 2. Frontal lobe syndrome: Explain care plan and prognosis to consultant, staff member, family member

Station 9: Link 1: Frontal lobe syndrome: Collateral history from a carer

Theme: Frontal lobe syndrome: Collateral history of head injury from a carer

1. **Instructions to candidates:**

   You have been asked to see Mr David Symonds a 45-year-old patient in the out-patient clinic. He is not interested in talking to you. While you were interviewing him, he left the outpatient clinic room abruptly and sits with his daughter in the reception area. He is accompanied by his wife Dorothy Symonds who is agreeable to provide an account of problems.

   Take a focused collateral history from Mrs Symonds and address her concerns.

   You may wish take notes as you are expected to discuss with the consultant in the next station.

2. **Instructions to the role player:**

   You are Dorothy Symonds, a 45-year-old married woman living with your husband, David Symonds. Two weeks ago, you contacted your GP who made a referral to the urgent psychiatric assessment clinic. During the interview, at times you feel overwhelmed and have tears in your eyes.

   You provide the following information:

   - "He is not David anymore."
   - Four months ago, your husband was robbed and assaulted on his head with a baseball bat by some young men when he was returning from work. He was taken to a hospital and was unconscious for 12 hours. Following a period of observation, he was discharged back home with follow-up and no major problems were identified.
   - You are concerned as your husband has been behaving strangely since then.
   - At first you noticed that he was forgetful, started losing his keys and missed his days to work. Then you have noticed that he has become increasingly disorganized at work and at home. He needed prompting to dress, shower and eat his food. His behaviour has changed and he becomes increasingly irritable, snappy and highly emotional frequently. For the past 2 months, he does not like talking to anyone and wants to spend time by himself.
   - He has been doing things that are embarrassing and you are ashamed of talking about. **Only give these answers if asked by the doctor to give some examples.**
     - Few days after accident, he started swearing at people and family for no reason.
     - He makes sexual remarks and gestures towards women including young girls.
     - Two months ago, he was in the office when he stripped himself naked and started masturbating in front of his female colleagues. Since then, he has been off sick and his boss has asked for a disciplinary action.

- Prior to the accident, he had been working as an accountant. He was caring, affectionate and never ever swore at anyone. He was a well-respected colleague in office and has had several awards for commitment and dedication to his work. You cannot believe that he is not this man anymore and you start crying.

3. Construct:

The station assesses the candidate's ability to gather a collateral history in a sensitive manner and establish frontal lobe syndrome due to acquired brain injury.

4. Expanded construct:

- The candidate should elicit history and clinical features suggestive of frontal lobe syndrome due to acquired brain injury.
- They should ask about behaviour and personality and ascertain the cause for the change, i.e., acquired brain injury.
- They should ask about cognitive symptoms of frontal lobe syndrome, e.g., short attention span, poor working and short-term memory, difficulty in planning and organisation.
- They should ask about emotional symptoms of frontal lobe syndrome, e.g., irritability, impulsivity, apathy, mood changes.
- They should ask about behavioural symptoms, e.g., utilisation, perseveration, inappropriate aggression and sexual behaviour, inappropriate humor (Witzelsucht).
- They should establish post-traumatic amnesia, pattern of recovery.
- They should establish premorbid personality and brief risk assessment.

5. Areas of importance to pass the station:

- Eliciting collateral history of signs and symptoms of frontal lobe syndrome and post-traumatic amnesia following an acquired brain injury. This should include the behavioural, cognitive and emotional symptoms and signs of frontal lobe syndrome (60%).
- Elicit premorbid personality and risk assessment (20%).
- Communication (20%).

6. Equipment checklist if applicable:

Not applicable.

Station 10: Link 2. Frontal lobe syndrome: Explain care plan and prognosis to consultant, staff member, family member

Theme: Frontal lobe syndrome: Explain care plan and prognosis to consultant, staff member, family member

1. Instructions to candidates:

You have gathered collateral history from Mrs Symonds.

Discuss your findings and further management plan with Dr Thompson, Consultant Psychiatrist.

2. **Instructions to the role player:**

You are Dr David Thompson, Consultant Psychiatrist. Your trainee doctor has gathered collateral history from Mr David Symonds wife and would like to discuss findings with you.

You ask the following questions once the doctor has summarised the relevant findings:

- **What is your likely differential diagnosis?**
- **What are the symptoms and signs of frontal lobe syndrome?**
- **Is there a significance of post-traumatic amnesia?**
- **What is the relationship between traumatic brain injury and psychiatric illness?**
- **How will you assess this patient further?**
- **How would you like to manage this patient?**
- **What is the long-term prognosis?**

3. **Construct:**

This station assesses the candidate's ability to discuss his/her assessment and further management plan with the consultant psychiatrist in a professional and comprehensive manner.

4. **Expanded construct:**

- They should discuss their assessment findings with the consultant in a professional, focused and comprehensive manner.
- They should discuss the symptoms and signs of frontal lobe disorder/dysexecutive syndrome due to acquired brain injury and comorbid mental health problem.
- They should discuss further management that may include neuroimaging, assessment of comorbidities, inpatient admission to manage risks and neuropsychological assessment including frontal lobe test.
- They should discuss medium to long-term prognosis.
- They should discuss the importance of family education, rehabilitation programme and possible future accommodation including respite care.

5. **Areas of importance to pass the station:**

- Discussion of collateral history, aetiology, investigations and management of frontal lobe syndrome and acquired brain syndrome (40%).
- Discussing the significance of post-traumatic amnesia and relevance to this case (20%).
- Discussing the prognosis of the acquired brain injury and its neuropsychiatric manifestations (20%).
- Communication (20%).

6. **Equipment checklist:**

Not applicable

Linked Stations 11 and 12

Station 11: Link 1: Hypochondriasis: Assessment

Station 12: Link 2: Hypochondriasis: Explanation

Station 11: Link 1: Hypochondriasis: Assessment

Theme: Hypochondriasis: Assess and take past medical history

1. **Instructions to candidates:**

   Mr Jake West is 34-year-old man who has attended the cardiology department requesting an investigation as he is convinced he has a cardiac disease. He had complained of palpitations in the past, though this is not persistent. He was not satisfied with the consultation and the physicians have requested your input in his management.

   - **Take a relevant history to understand this presentation.**
   - **You may wish to take notes to discuss your findings and the management with his wife in the next station.**

2. **Instructions to the role player:**

   You are Jake West, a 34-year-old full-time accountant. You have good relationship with your wife Amelia, with whom you have two children, Sylvia and Jessica. You are not sure why a psychiatrist has been called to see you.

   "You are wasting your time doctor, I am not crazy". However, you are prepared to talk.

   - You first noticed palpitations almost 14 months ago when you were at work during a meeting with your boss. You are under extreme stress at work and several of your colleagues are off sick.
   - Since then you occasionally experience palpitations and have visited your general practitioner several times. He has undertaken blood tests, ECG and other tests but there have been no significant findings.
   - You have seen three cardiologists so far who has done several investigations including 24 hours ECG. "They think I am normal and do not have any physical problem". You are disappointed and resentful that no one can identify what is wrong with your heart and refuse to accept any reassurance.
   - You are convinced that you have a problem with your heart. You have researched on the Internet and now believe that you have an arrhythmia that is going to kill you.
   - You have occasional palpitations, mild chest pain, and "dizziness due to reduced blood flow due to arrhythmia". You have bought small ECG monitoring instrument that you use every hour to check if you are ok. You have seen two private doctors who were 'incompetent' in helping you.
   - You came to emergency department today to have another ECG and echocardiogram. The cardiologist has 'dismissed your concerns' and sent a psychiatrist.
   - You spend most of the time at home alone in bed monitoring your heart rate and ECG. Your wife is angry and bitter about this behaviour.
   - When you were 12 years old, your doctor noticed a 'benign murmur'. As your father had died of a sudden cardiac arrest they investigated you thoroughly. Doctors were convinced that "I was ok." But, you started fearing that they have 'missed something' and became preoccupied for the past 3 years.

- There are no concerns about your mood and you do not have any psychotic symptoms (paranoid thoughts or unusual experiences). You have never seen a psychiatrist before. There is no family history of mental illness. There is no history of illicit drug or alcohol use.

3. **Construct:**

The station is assessing the candidate's ability to engage a patient who does not wish to see a psychiatrist and explore the appropriate history of hypochondriasis.

4. **Expanded construct:**
   - They should take a history of the presenting complaint focusing on the individual's experience of symptoms and associated beliefs.
   - Its onset, duration, progress, aggravating and relieving factors.
   - They should explore clinical features of hypochondriasis, such as:
     - Persistent belief of more than 6 months of at least two separate physical illnesses, one of which should be named.
     - Preoccupation with this belief causing distress and affecting activities of daily living.
     - Seek medical treatment and investigations.
     - Refusal to accept reassurance even if no identifiable physical cause is found.
   - They should inquire about possible differential diagnosis, such as, organic cause, depression, anxiety disorder, psychosis, drug/alcohol abuse.
   - They should inquire into past medical, psychiatric and relevant family history.
   - They should inquire about predisposing, precipitating and perpetuating factors if relevant.
   - They should be able to contain the patient's anxiety and address concerns and fears appropriately.

5. **Areas of importance to pass the station:**
   - Eliciting accurate and sufficient information about hypochondriasis/hypochondriacal disorder according to ICD-10 criteria (50%).
   - Eliciting maintaining factors, relevant family, past psychiatric and medical history (30%).
   - Communication (20%).

6. **Equipment checklist if applicable:**

Not applicable.

Station 12: Link 2: Hypochondriasis: Explanation

Theme: Hypochondriasis: Discuss findings and management

1. **Instructions to candidates:**

You have assessed Mr Jake West who is convinced that he has a cardiac disease in the previous station.

Discuss your findings and the management with his wife Mrs Amelia West.

2. **Instructions to the role player:**

You are a 28-year-old, Mrs Amelia West, and you live with your husband Jake West. You are concerned about your husband's health. He has been spending most of the time on his bed, looking at an ECG machine that he has purchased. He looks distressed and you are worried about his behaviour.

You listen to the doctor but are concerned about the possibility of him actually having an underlying physical illness.

You ask the following questions:

- **What is the problem?**
- **Is he making it up?**
- **How can you be sure that there is no illness?**
- **How can mind affect the body?**
- **What is the cause for this?**
- **How do you treat this?**
- **Is there a tablet he can take?**
- **How can I help?**
- **His father died of heart problem. I am worried.**

3. **Construct:**

This station assesses the candidate's ability to explain the findings of the clinical presentation and management of hypochondriasis in a fluent and jargon free manner.

4. **Expanded construct:**

- The candidate should discuss the nature and clinical features of hypochondriasis in a simple and jargon free manner.
- They should discuss aetiology, such as childhood illness, parental illness or excess medical attention–seeking in parents, predisposition to misattribute physical symptoms.
- They should discuss management of hypochondriasis, such as, developing therapeutic relationship, allowing patient to ventilate health-related anxieties, psychotherapy (behavioural therapy, CBT), pharmacotherapy, such as, antidepressant medication.
- They should check the understanding and clarify any misunderstandings.
- They should demonstrate empathy, sensitivity and provide appropriate reassurance.
- They need to elicit wife's fears, concerns and expectations and address them appropriately.

5. **Areas of importance to pass the station:**

- Demonstrating a knowledge of the clinical presentation and aetiology of hypochondriasis (40%).
- Demonstrating an understanding of management of hypochondriasis (40%).
- Discussing wife's fears, anxieties, concerns and expectations (20%).

6. **Equipment checklist if applicable:**

Not applicable.

Linked Stations 13 and 14

Station 13: Link 1: Erotomania: Assess the problem and the risk

Station 14: Link 2: Erotomania: Discuss the management with the potential victim

Station 13: Link 1: Erotomania: Assess the problem and the risk

Theme: Erotomania: Thought content, mental state and risk assessment

1. **Instructions to candidates:**

   Casey Smith is a 48-year-old, unemployed woman who has presented to reception at the mental health unit requesting to see Dr John Cline, foundation doctor in psychiatry placement. Casey had become increasingly irritable and aggressive. Security staff was called to assist the receptionist. You are on call doctor and you have been asked to assess her urgently.

   - **Talk to Ms Smith to discuss her problem and do a risk assessment.**
   - **You may wish to take any necessary notes to discuss the case with the doctor involved in the next station.**

2. **Instructions to the role player:**

   You are Casey Smith, 48-year-old, single unemployed woman currently living alone in a council house. You do not want to speak to anyone except 'John'. You are irritable, agitated and restless. Throughout the interview you interrupt and shout "Can I see John now?", "Where is John, I don't want to be kept waiting?", "Will you let me see John?", "I have to see John, no-one can stop me", "Why am I seeing you?"

   - You have long-standing problem of 'anxiety', alcohol abuse and occasional cocaine use.
   - You attended A and E last week feeling anxious and were seen by "lovely Dr John Cline". You call him John.
   - 'Dashing and handsome John' showed a deep interest in your personal life, childhood and interests. Further to your assessment, you have received a letter from John confirming that he is interested in you.
   - You show this letter to the doctor during the consultation; this is an assessment letter sent to your GP and you were copied into it.
   - You have found out John works in the mental health unit. You have attempted to get John's phone number and contact details but the staff have refused to give it you. You have been waiting outside the unit for the last 3 days, trying to catch a glimpse of John and finally saw him today. You want to speak to John and express your feelings of love.
   - You are convinced that John loves you and wants to marry you. "We are going to have a baby together".
   - If anybody interferes in your business you are "committed to take matters into your own hands". You do not discuss this further but say "I have got stuff that I can use".
   - Your ex-partner was a nurse but he left you for another woman. Your previous relationships have never lasted for more than a few months.

- You have been prescribed citalopram which you do not take. You have tried to kill yourself few times, but John told you not to hurt yourself and speak to him if needed.

3. **Construct:**

This station tests the candidate's ability to elicit thought content, brief mental state and risk assessment of a patient with erotomania in a challenging and volatile situation.

4. **Expanded construct:**

- The candidate should be able demonstrate skill in eliciting thought content and mental state.
- They should demonstrate an ability to carry out a detailed risk assessment to self and others, focusing on the risk to the doctor.
- They should demonstrate control of the interview in a safe manner.
- They should use an appropriate mix of closed and open questions.
- They should demonstrate ability to engage with an agitated patient and diffuse a potentially volatile situation.

5. **Areas of importance to pass the station:**

- Eliciting accurate information of the thought content, mental state and establish symptoms of erotomania (40%).
- Perform a thorough risk assessment identifying risk to others or self (30%).
- Communication and control of interview (30%).

6. **Equipment checklist if applicable:**
None applicable.

Station 14: Link 2: Erotomania: Discuss the management with the potential victim

Theme: Erotomania: Discuss the management with the potential victim

1. **Instructions to candidates:**

You have assessed Ms Casey Smith and arranged for a Mental Health Act assessment for an admission. However, Ms Smith left the mental health unit and has not been found for several hours. You are not aware of her whereabouts at this present time. You are asked to see Dr John Cline, foundation doctor in psychiatry placement, who is unaware of the current situation.

Talk to Dr John Cline and discuss the management.

2. **Instructions to the role player:**

You are John Cline, foundation year 2 doctor, who has assessed Ms Casey in A and E department one week ago on your own call duty. You are shocked to hear of the developments in the case and worried about your personal safety. You cannot recall saying anything that indicated you were interested in her apart from in a professional capacity. You are worried that this will lead to an enquiry into your conduct and affect your training. You are seeking further clarification and advice on the matter. You have several questions for the doctor and during the interview ask the following:

- **Will I go through an enquiry?**
- **This is my third week in Psychiatry. Have I done anything wrong?**
- **Do you know where the patient is at the moment?**
- **I am worried about my safety. What should I do now?**
- **I am frightened and what would you suggest to keep myself safe?**
- **I cannot miss any days. It will affect my training. Do you think I made a wrong choice coming into psychiatry?**
- **Does she know where I work or live?**
- **What does she know about me or my family?**
- **What is going to happen now?**

3. Construct:

This station assess whether the candidate has the knowledge about issues of confidentiality. This case involves breaking confidentiality due to risk to others and a practical discussion with a member of staff who is worried and fears for his safety.

4. Expanded construct:

- The candidate should demonstrate knowledge regarding confidentiality in case where there is risk to third party.
- They should provide information about the case that is relevant. They should discuss the clinical features, nature and management of the case suggestive of erotomania.
- They should provide information of further management plan, such as, involvement of police due to risks, mental health act assessment and admission to hospital.
- They should clearly state the risks to the doctor and avoid false reassurance. They should demonstrate sensitivity, empathy and ensure that the foundation doctor does not feel that he is responsible for the situation.
- They should discuss practical methods of risk management and safety for the involved doctor, e.g., involving line manager, security, Trust support, practical issues around personal safety and involvement of the police. This list is not exhaustive and the candidate should provide additional practical solutions and offer support to the foundation doctor.

5. Areas of importance to pass the station:

- Appropriate level of breaking confidentiality and discussion of the case (20%).
- Discussing the clinical features and management of erotomania (30%).
- Supporting and discussing practical risk management (20%).
- Communication, avoiding false reassurance, demonstrates empathy (30%).

6. Equipment checklist if applicable:

Not applicable.

Linked Stations 15 and 16

Station 15: Link 1: Morbid Jealousy: History and risk assessment
Station 16: Link 2: Morbid Jealousy: Discuss care plan

Station 15: Link 1: Morbid Jealousy: History and risk assessment

Theme: Morbid Jealousy: Take history and do risk assessment of a man who believes that his wife is having an affair

1. **Instructions to candidates:**

   You have been asked to see James Smith, 42-year-old man, who has been referred by his GP. He has been anxious and has not been coping at work due to poor concentration.

   Take a history from him to explore his current difficulties and do an appropriate risk assessment. You may wish to take notes, as you will be required to speak to his wife later.

2. **Instructions to the role player:**

   You are James Smith 42-year-old, married to Gloria Smith for 15 years and have two children aged 10 and 12 years. You and your wife are publicans. You look after the pub finances whereas your wife runs the front of the house. You are not sure why you have to see the psychiatrist as you don't think you are 'mental'. You begin by saying, "I don't need to see a 'shrink'. I can sort my own problems out". You are reluctant to give information, but if asked empathetically, you will disclose.

   - You have been anxious and upset in the last 6 months because of your wife's behaviour.
   - Over the last 6 months you have noticed that she has become particularly friendly with a man who visits the pub regularly.
   - You believe your wife is 'excessively friendly' with him than others. You know this because she "sees him in a special way". You have seen her waving to him in a seductive manner 'calling for sex'.
   - You are convinced that your wife might be having an affair with him for the past 6 months.
   - You are trying to get evidence to prove that she is having an affair with this man. You follow her when she goes out, hoping to catch them red-handed. You have been checking her cell phone, underwear and handbag to see if you will get any clues. You think they are clever and have managed to hide this from you.
   - You have confronted your wife but she has denied the allegation. This has led to arguments between the two of you. On two occasions you lost your temper and pushed and slapped her. She had a bruise on her forehead but you did not mean to hurt her.
   - Due to this preoccupation you are not able to concentrate in the pub business and as a result is running in losses.
   - You sleep in a separate room; don't share a bed with her for the past few weeks. You don't want your children to be influenced by 'her infidelity', but don't know how to keep this secret. May be when you have 'solid evidence', you will inform them.
   - You are convinced of your wife's infidelity and are not prepared to consider any other explanation.

- You are aware that she has had an affair with your neighbour 5 years ago, but she denied that as well.
- You have been drinking alcohol every day. You have been feeling low in mood, have poor sleep and appetite. You have been treated for depression with Fluoxetine for the past 5 years, but have stopped medication 1 year ago.
- You are angry with the man and want him out of your life. You have tried to follow him around with a hammer, but never managed to catch him alone. You feel if you can get your hands on him, you might teach him a lesson. But you don't want to end up in prison, as you had a terrible time in prison a year ago, when you hit someone at the pub following an argument.

3. **Construct:**

This station assesses whether the candidate is able to recognise the core features of morbid jealousy and establish the potential risks involved.

4. **Expanded construct:**

- The candidate should be able to take a detailed history and explore form of morbid jealousy, associated psychopathology and consider an organic disorder.
- They should establish the psychopathology of delusion against obsession and overvalued idea.
- They should explore and identify the symptoms of depression, anxiety, psychosis or other mental illness.
- They should explore the impact of his symptoms on his social and marital life.
- They should identify the risk of self-harm/suicide.
- They should identify risk to others including wife, children and third party. The risks to others should include domestic violence, threatened or perpetrated violence.
- They should explore past relationships, psychiatric, forensic and substance misuse history.

5. **Areas of importance to pass the station:**

- Eliciting accurate and sufficient information of psychopathology of morbid jealousy (40%).
- Eliciting risk to self and other including wife, third party and risk to children (40%).
- Communication (20%).

6. **Equipment checklist if applicable:**

None applicable

Station 16: Link 2: Morbid Jealousy: Discuss care plan

Theme: Morbid jealousy: Talk to the man's wife about your findings and discuss the care plan

1. **Instructions to candidates:**

You have just seen James Smith in the outpatient clinic. He has given permission for you to speak to his wife, who is anxiously waiting to hear what is wrong with him.

- **Speak to her and discuss your assessment and management plan. Address her concerns and expectations.**

2. Instructions to the role player:

You are Gloria Smith and you run the pub along with your husband James Smith.

- You have noticed that for the past 3 months James is more irritable and not quiet himself.
- Both of you have been having arguments. He has pushed, slapped and threatened you few times but you minimise these incidents saying "every married couple have ups and downs".
- There are times when your husband has passed comments like "I know what you are up to behind my back". But you don't take this seriously. You think your husband is stressed because the pub has been losing money, and therefore, that has affected your relationship.
- You want to help him, but are worried that James will be labelled with some 'mental problem' and that will ruin the pub business.
- If the doctor says he has some psychiatric problem, you disagree and say that he is just stressed and if you go on a holiday, things will be back to normal. You don't think he needs to be in a 'mental hospital'. You feel your husband loves you and he would not harm anyone, let alone you.
- You get angry if the doctor suggests that your husband should be in the hospital, as you don't have anyone to help you to run the business. You attempt to reassure the doctor that your husband was behaving similarly few years ago when he was suspicious that she might be having an affair with the neighbour. But he soon realised that was not the case and "it was back to normal". You think he is possessive because he loves you.
- You believe he will soon realise his mistakes and they will get on alright. You don't agree that you, your children or anyone else are at risk from him.
- If the doctor explains to you about the potential risks in a calm and sensitive manner, you show some willingness to work with the doctor. You may wish to agree for admission but only after you and your family return from holiday to France.

3. Construct:

This station assesses candidate's ability to alleviate the anxiety of a concerned relative and discuss the nature of morbid jealousy, associated risks and management plan in a sensitive manner.

4. Expanded construct:

- The candidate should be able to address wife's concerns, anxiety and expectations listening and providing appropriate information in clear, jargon free language.
- They should discuss the characteristics of delusion of morbid jealousy that the thoughts are patient's own, not resisted and ego syntonic.
- They should discuss the possible aetiology of morbid jealousy, e.g., depression, psychosis, stressful situations, alcohol misuse, sexual and marital difficulties, etc.
- They should be able to explain the risk to self and others clearly.

- They should discuss the management plan that includes treatment of mental disorder and management of risk. Treatment may involve pharmacotherapy (antipsychotic, antidepressant), psychotherapy (cognitive behaviour therapy, couple therapy, and dynamic psychotherapy), admission to hospital informally or under an appropriate Mental Health Act legislation. In some cases, child protection proceedings and/or geographical separation may need to be considered. Management plan should be guided by the history and clinical situation.
- They should discuss the prognosis of morbid jealousy.

5. **Areas of importance to pass the station:**
   - Explaining symptoms/signs and aetiology of morbid jealousy (20%).
   - Discussing the management plan and prognosis (20%).
   - Explaining the risk to self and risk to wife, children and third party (40%).
   - Communication (20%).
6. **Equipment checklist if applicable:**
   Not applicable

Linked Stations 17 and 18

Station 17: Link 1: Postpartum psychosis: History and risk assessment
Station 18: Link 2: Postpartum psychosis: Discuss care plan

Station 17: Link 1: Postpartum psychosis: History and risk assessment

Theme: Postpartum psychosis: Take history from a woman who is 8 weeks pregnant and has a 10-month-old child

1. **Instructions to candidates:**
   You are asked to see Mrs Jane Adams, a 24-year-old mother who has 11 months old child. She is also currently 6 weeks pregnant. She has been referred by her GP, who is worried that she may be depressed.
   - Take a comprehensive history from her and do a risk assessment.
   - You may wish to take notes as you will be expected to speak to her husband in the next station.
2. **Instructions to the role player:**
   You are 24-year-old Jane Adams and you live with your husband and 11 months old son Jack. You are now 6 weeks pregnant which was unplanned.
   - You work as a secretary in an office but currently you are on extended maternity leave.
   - You have been worried about the Jack for 6 months and hence, are feeling low and distressed.
   - It all began when the baby started losing his hair. You realised that he looked somewhat different. This got worse and you were contemplating what was wrong with him. Then it occurred to you

one day that you might be poisoning him with your breast milk. So you weaned him off when Jack was 3 months old and bottle fed him. However, you feel the damage has already been done and the 'thing' inside him is starting to grow. You feel if you starve him, perhaps this 'thing' will die. You have tried this on occasions but then he cries, so you eventually have to feed him. You believe that this 'thing' is an evil spirit.

- For the past 4 weeks, you hear voice of a devil who says that you are a cruel mother and should be burnt alive. At times the voice comes from inside your stomach and you are wondering if the unborn child is devil himself. As the pregnancy is progressing, the voice is becoming more intense and frequent.
- You have poor sleep and appetite and unable to do household chores.
- Your husband has been annoyed with your behaviour resulting in arguments. You don't feel like talking to anyone about your worries as they won't understand.
- You do not have any physical health problem. You have been depressed in the past which was treated by your GP with antidepressants.
- Your mother suffers from bipolar affective disorder. So you can't really expect her to help you.
- You want the doctor to help you by examining Jack and doing an ultrasound to make sure that the unborn child is not a devil.
- You do not have thoughts of self-harm/suicide as you want to help Jack. However, if it is confirmed that your unborn baby is a devil you will not hesitate to kill 'devil' by stabbing.

3. **Construct:**
This station assesses candidate's ability to elicit the symptoms of postpartum psychosis and do thorough risk assessment to self and baby including the unborn.

4. **Expanded construct:**
- The candidate should elicit the psychopathology of postpartum psychosis.
- They should explore the onset, duration and progression of the symptomatology.
- The candidate should carry out a thorough risk assessment to self (self-harm/suicide) and to others including 11-month-old son and unborn foetus.
- They should elicit comprehensive history to rule out any appropriate differential diagnosis.
- They should demonstrate empathy and sensitive inquiry into patient's problem.

5. **Areas of importance to pass the station:**
- Eliciting an accurate and systematic history of postpartum psychosis (40%).
- Carrying out a thorough risk assessment to self and others including an infant and unborn foetus (40%).
- Communication (20%).

6. **Equipment checklist:**
Not applicable

Station 18: Link 2: Postpartum psychosis: Discuss care plan

Theme: Postpartum psychosis: Explanation of management of psychosis and associated risks

1. **Instructions to candidates:**

   You have just seen Jane Adams in your outpatient clinic. Her husband, Nick Adams, is anxiously waiting to speak to you about her condition and what can be done about it.

   Discuss your findings and further management plan with Jane's husband.

2. **Instructions to the role player:**

   You are Jane's husband Nick Adams. You live with your wife and your 11 months old baby. You are worried about Jane for the past few months. You initially thought that she was stressed due to another pregnancy.

   Jane is not 'herself' and you are concerned about her and Jack.

   You are at work most of the day. You have financial difficulties at the moment as Jane is on extended maternity leave. You express your disappointment at Jane not contributing to household chores and not taking care of Jack. She expects you to earn money, do household chores and take care of Jack. You have tried to talk to her but she refuses to discuss her worries.

   She has been feeling tired and lethargic ever since the Jack was born but you thought it was normal after childbirth.

   For the past few weeks, she spends most of the time in her bedroom, rocking and muttering to herself. She seems to be preoccupied with thoughts. You have noticed that she talks to herself and hits her stomach when she is agitated.

   You ask the following questions:

   - **Why is Jane behaving like this?**
   - **Jack is not safe with her. Should I send him to my mother's house?**
   - **Is she angry at me for this second baby?**
   - **What are your views on abortion of this baby?**
   - **What should I do now?**
   - **I have done all I can. I cannot deal with this anymore. What do you suggest?**
   - **What is the reason for this illness/behaviour?**
   - **What is the treatment?**
   - **What is the chance of this illness coming back once treated?**

3. **Construct:**

   This station assesses the candidate's ability to discuss the presentation of postpartum psychosis sensitively and management plan including the associated risk.

4. **Expanded construct:**

   - The candidate should be able to establish a rapport with an anxious and distressed husband.
   - They should explain the diagnosis and aetiology of postpartum psychosis.

- They should be able to explain the prognosis. They should discuss that the risk of recurrence is high (30–60%) and demonstrate knowledge of risk factors of postpartum psychosis.
- Discuss the risk involved to the child, unborn foetus and to the patient.
- They should formulate a management plan with a biopsychosocial approach including admission (mother and baby unit) if necessary.

5. Areas of importance to pass the station:

- Discussion of diagnosis and aetiology of postpartum psychosis (20%).
- Discussion of risk to patient, child and unborn foetus (30%).
- Explaining appropriate management plan (30%).
- Discussing husband's fears and concerns appropriately (20%).

6. Equipment checklist if applicable:

Not applicable

Linked Stations 19 and 20

Station 19: Link 1: Body dysmorphic disorder: Assess
Station 20: Link 2: Body dysmorphic disorder: Discuss management plan

Station 19: Link 1: Body dysmorphic disorder: Assess

Theme: Body dysmorphic disorder: Assessment

1. Instructions to candidates:

GP refers Mr James, a 21-year-old unemployed man to your outpatient clinic. He has complained that his jaw is too small and that he does not look masculine enough. He has presented at the GP surgery on numerous occasions asking for a referral to a plastic surgeon.

Conduct a diagnostic assessment.

2. Instructions to the role player:

You are Mr James, a 21-year-old unemployed man. You are not in a relationship as you believe women do not find you attractive as you think your jaw is too small and that you need surgery. Various doctors have examined your jaw and say it is normal but whilst you are reassured for a while, you don't believe them. Sometimes your jaw clicks and you are fairly sure that this is a sign that it is too small.

You are very distressed about the look of your jawline and often stay indoors, but if you have to leave the house, you often wear a scarf around your neck covering the jawline. Your confidence has been severely affected, and you think jaw implants will mean you will be able to lead a normal active social life.

You have asked your GP on a number of occasions to refer you to a plastic surgeon for jaw implants, but he refuses. You recently purchased saline and syringes so that you could inject your jawline.

You have also researched a clinic in Germany which has accepted you for surgery in a couple of months' time. You've taken a loan to cover the fees.

You are unemployed and spend most of your day looking in the mirror. Over the last year your mood has dropped and you feel hopeless and worthless. You have been drinking heavily and smoking cannabis. Your sleep is fitful and you lack motivation and interest. You have no suicidal thoughts.

You are not happy about being referred to a psychiatrist as you feel your GP is not taking your problem seriously. You hope the psychiatrist will back your decision to have surgery and refer you to the plastic surgery department.

3. **Construct:**

The station tests the candidate's ability to elicit a history from a patient with Body dysmorphic disorder and to focus on the salient features.

4. **Expanded construct:**

The candidate should:

- Show an appropriate mix of open and closed questions.
- Demonstrate advanced communication skills and empathy.
- Acknowledge the patient's feelings about the referral and not argue with the patient.
- Examine the patient's mental state and demonstrate empathy with the patient's experience.
- Remain focussed throughout the interview, maintaining control whilst avoiding being drawn in to in-depth discussions about the size of the patient's jaw.
- Not collude with the patient and promise a referral to a plastic surgeon.
- Identify current risks.

5. **Areas of importance to pass the station:**
- Interview/communication skills (30%).
- Ability to elicit symptoms of body dysmorphic disorder (30%).
- Risk assessment (40%).

6. **Equipment checklist if applicable:**

Not applicable

Station 20: Link 2: Body dysmorphic disorder: Discuss management plan

Theme: Management of body dysmorphic disorder: Discuss with the relative

1. **Instructions to candidates:**

You recently assessed Mr James, a 21-year-old patient with body dysmorphic disorder. His mother, Mrs James has come to see you to discuss treatment. Her son cannot face leaving the house and so has sent his mother on his behalf.

Discuss the management of body dysmorphic disorder with the patient's mother.

2. **Instructions to the role player:**
- You are Mrs James, the mother of James. You are very concerned about him.
- Over the last 5 months, his mental state has worsened and he has become more and more pre-occupied with his physical appearance. He is now completely obsessional about the size of his jaw and that women will not find him attractive.

- You worry that he will go to any length to improve his appearance. He does not work and spends all day looking at himself in the mirror.
- You have tried repeatedly to reassure him that he looks normal but he just won't believe you. You are at your wits end.
- You are desperate that your son receives help and does not get a referral to a plastic surgeon.

3. **Construct:**
This station tests the candidate's ability to discuss the management of body dysmorphic disorder with a distressed relative.

4. **Expanded construct:**
   - The candidate should be able to establish a rapport with a distressed relative.
   - They should explain the diagnosis and aetiology of body dysmorphic disorder.
   - They should formulate a management plan with a bio-psychosocial approach including medications, such as, SSRIs, clomipramine or an antipsychotic where appropriate. There is a clear role for CBT.
   - They should be able to explain the prognosis, i.e., full remission may not be possible and body dysmorphic disorder runs a chronic course. Even if patient undergoes corrective surgery there is a risk that the overvalued thoughts shift to some other body part. Alternatively patient may be left dissatisfied with scarring or imperfection following surgery.

5. **Areas of importance to pass the station:**
   - Communication skills (30%).
   - Discuss the diagnosis of body dysmorphic disorder (30%).
   - Discuss the management and prognosis of body dysmorphic disorder (40%).

6. **Equipment checklist if applicable:**
Not applicable.

Single Stations 21–56

Station 21: Generalised anxiety disorder

Theme: Generalised anxiety disorder: History

1. **Instructions to candidates:**
You are talking to Rebecca Smith, 32-year-old woman, who is very anxious and referred to you by her GP for advice. She is worried that she will develop some form of illness. She is happy to talk to you.

   Take a history of her problems and address her fears, concerns and expectations.

2. **Instructions to role player:**
You are 32-year-old Rebecca Smith. You are extremely anxious and worried in the interview. You are fidgety, restless and require lot of reassurance from the doctor. You answer questions only if the doctor is empathetic and understanding.

When asked you describe the following:

- You have always been a worrier. Since you were 18 years old, you worry about everything: work, family, cooking, finance, etc. "You name it and I worry about it." "My mother was a big worrier, maybe I have picked this up from her." There is no reason for you to worry as your life is more or less perfect and this makes it even more distressing. There are no significant life stressors.
- Your friends call you 'high strung' and that you 'overreact to small problems'.
- You get anxious in any particular situation, time or place. You are aware that stress makes it worse.
- When anxious your heart beats 'faster than a train'. You start sweating, feel nauseous, dizzy and 'lose control'. You get irritable and a bit confused.
- You are unable to sleep as you worry about the next day and activities. You resort to few drinks at night to help you sleep but are fearful of self-medicating with alcohol.
- You do not have any physical health issues. You do not smoke, abuse alcohol or drugs.

You ask:

- **How can I stop worrying?**
- **Am I losing my head?**
- **How can you help me?**
- **What is the treatment?**

3. Construct:

This station assesses candidate's knowledge of generalised anxiety disorder and ability to manage interview with an anxious patient.

4. Expanded construct:

The candidate should:

- Be able to demonstrate skill in eliciting history of anxiety disorder from an anxious person.
- Elicit onset, duration, progress, aggravating and relieving factors of generalised anxiety disorder. Elicit associated problems and comorbid conditions, if present.
- Elicit possible differential diagnosis of anxiety disorder including the possibility of an organic cause.
- Establish the impact of the disorder on social life and functioning.
- Discuss briefly evidence-based management of generalised anxiety disorder that include pharmacotherapy and psychotherapy.
- They should allay patient's partner's anxiety, worries and fears.

5. Areas of importance to pass the station:

- Elicit history of generalised anxiety disorder and differential diagnosis (50%).
- Allay patient's anxiety, worries and fear by providing appropriate explanation to patient's questions (30%).
- Communication (20%).

6. Equipment checklist:

Not applicable.

Station 22: Non-organic vaginismus: History

Theme: Young woman with vaginismus and difficulty in entering long-term relationship

1. **Instructions to candidates:**

   Naomi Saunders is a 30-year-old woman referred by her GP to your services. She has difficulty to enter a long-term relationship. She was reluctant to discuss about this with the GP who felt that the problem could be of sexual nature.

   - **Assess the nature and extent of her problem.**
   - **You need not do a Mental State Examination or risk assessment.**

2. **Instructions to the role player:**

   You are 30-year-old Naomi Saunders. You are a barrister and own a firm. Two years ago, you fell in love with a software engineer. He proposed to marry you. You are also keen to marry and have children. However, you are worried about your difficulties on the sexual side of life.

   - At the age of 21 you were raped by a gang of four people. This was a very traumatising experience. The perpetrators were arrested and convicted. You had counselling and support. Your family also supported you well.
   - You recovered from trauma in 18 months' time. You went back to work, started enjoying things. You do not get flashbacks or night mares any more. You do not feel depressed.
   - However, you started noticing that you have difficulty wearing tampons.
   - You went to gynaecologist who could not find any abnormality except that they had difficulty using speculum.
   - About a year ago, you went on holidays to LA with your boyfriend. You both were in romantic mood. But as you both started making love you started feeling discomfort in the vaginal area. You thought that this could be due to anxiety. But next day same thing happened. Even though you wanted to continue, your boyfriend had difficulty penetrating into you. Hence, you both decided not to explore further.
   - When you watch videos with sexual content you get aroused. You stimulated yourself on many occasions and even though you had mild vaginal discomfort you had orgasm and climax.
   - Six months ago, you and your boyfriend tried to make love again. This time, he stimulated you and with this you had orgasm and climax and you thoroughly enjoyed it. However, when he tried to enter again you had the same difficulty. You thought at length about this and approached your GP for help.
   - You had your first sexual encounter at the age of 18 years. You were in a stable relationship from 18–20 years of age and had no difficulty in having sex.

3. **Construct:**

   Candidate explores the symptoms of vaginismus sensitively.

4. **Expanded construct:**

   - Candidate should be sensitive in eliciting the psychosexual history.

- Candidate should be able to elicit symptoms of vaginismus.
- Candidate should be able to rule out secondary causes of vaginismus.
- Candidate should be able to rule out other causes of sexual dysfunction.
- Candidate should be able to rule out axis I mental disorders like PTSD, depression and phobia.
- Good candidate may identify the type of vaginismus, i.e., generalised or specific; lifelong type or acquired type; due to psychological factors or combined factors.

5. **Areas of importance to pass the station:**
   - Advanced communication skills (30%).
   - Eliciting symptoms of vaginismus (50%).
   - Eliciting psychosexual history (10%).
   - Rule out axis I mental disorders and secondary causes (10%).

6. **Equipment checklist:**
   Not applicable

Station 23: Restless leg syndrome: History

Theme: Assessment of a patient presenting to the outpatient clinic with restless leg movement

1. **Instructions to candidates:**

   You are a CT3 trainee in psychiatry. You received a referral from the GP about 50-year-old Mrs Trudy Gibbens. She had difficulties in initiating sleep. She presented to the GP with cramp like sensation in the legs. The symptoms improved with a short course of temazepam but symptoms have relapsed after stopping temazepam. GP is worried about her getting addicted to temazepam; hence made this referral.

   - **Elicit history to arrive at a provisional diagnosis.**
   - **You need not do a mental state examination or risk assessment.**

2. **Instructions to the role player:**
   - You are Trudy Gibbens. You are 50-year-old and you live with your husband. You work as a typing assistant in a private company. You do not feel depressed or anxious.
   - You have difficulty initiating sleep for the past 5–6 years. You have strange sensations in your legs when you lie down for 5–10 minutes. These are either like insects crawling in your legs or cramp like sensation in the legs. You feel better when you move your legs. When the problem started, you could sleep after one hour of moving around in the bed. But now-a-days, it takes 3–4 hours for you to sleep. You massage your legs which gives temporary relief. When you have a drink in the party or in functions this sensation becomes better.
   - Your husband has noticed that on and off you kick him in sleep. Now-a-days, you can't sit still at work place. When you do typing, you keep moving your legs. People started commenting about this and this annoys you. If you try to stop your legs, you get pain in the legs. So you

started walking around to avoid criticism. Your husband also noticed that you snore during sleep. He has not witnessed apnoea or excessive day time sleepiness.

- You consulted your GP. He did blood tests and told that you are not anaemic. You do not suffer from diabetes or peripheral neuropathy. You are not on any regular medication. GP gave you sleeping pills which relieved your problems. But you are worried about getting addicted to the tablets and stopped it. But the symptoms have come back. Hence, the GP has referred you to the psychiatrist.
- You remember your mother telling you about her leg pains. You used to massage her legs and she felt better with this. You are not on any medication. You do not smoke, drink excessively or misuse drugs.

3. **Construct:**

Candidate demonstrates skills in assessing a patient with sleep difficulties and restless legs.

4. **Expanded construct:**

- Candidate should demonstrate advanced listening skills.
- Candidate should elicit history of normal sleep pattern.
- Candidate should be able to identify the type of sleep disturbance.
- Candidate should be able to elicit the history of restless leg syndrome.
- Candidate should be able to rule out secondary causes of restless legs.

Diagnostic criteria for restless leg syndrome (Acronym URGE):

(i) U: Urge to move limbs caused by cramp like or unpleasant sensations in the limbs.

(ii) R: Rest worsens the symptoms.

(iii) G: Getting up or movement gives temporary relief from the symptoms.

(iv) E: Evening worsening of symptoms.

(Ref: www.rls.org)

5. **Areas of importance to pass the station:**

- Communication skills (20%).
- Through history of present illness (60%).
- Considering differential diagnosis, i.e., rule out medical causes, drugs and other causes of sleep difficulties (20%).

6. **Equipment checklist:**

Not applicable

Station 24: Lithium in pregnancy

Theme: Talking to 25-year-old female patient suffering from bipolar affective disorder and stable on lithium, and planning for pregnancy

1. **Instructions to candidates:**

   GP has referred Sally Johns, a 25-year-old woman, to you. She suffers from bipolar affective disorder and is managed well on lithium carbonate 800 mg nocte. She is in a stable relationship and wants to start a family now.

   Talk to her and address her concerns.

2. **Instructions to the role player:**

   You are Sally Johns, a 25-year-old patient. You suffer from bipolar affective disorder and are managed well on lithium carbonate 800 mg at night. You are in a stable relationship and want to plan for pregnancy. You do not have any children. You are worried that you might relapse if you stop lithium as it happened few years ago.

   Ask the following questions to the candidate:

   - **How long do I need to take lithium?**
   - **I want to become pregnant, is it safe to continue lithium in pregnancy?**
   - **What are the effects of lithium on the foetus? What are the chances of baby developing birth defects?**
   - **How would you monitor this?**
   - **Do I need to take more lithium in pregnancy?**
   - **I have been stable for 3 years now, can I stop lithium?**
   - **What is the medication option when I become pregnant?**
   - **What precautions I need to take if I stop lithium?**
   - **Can I breast feed the baby while on lithium?**
   - **Any useful source of information.**

3. **Construct:**

   Candidate should discuss the issues around the use of lithium in pregnancy.

4. **Expanded construct:**

   - Candidate should be able to address patient's concern sensitively.
   - Candidate should be fluent in giving information regarding lithium in pregnancy.
   - Candidate should be giving information regarding teratogenic effects of lithium as well as precautions that can be taken.
   - Candidate should be discussing risk of relapse and other options available in case lithium were to be stopped.
   - Candidate should be discussing lithium/anti-psychotics usage and breastfeeding.

5. **Areas of importance to pass the station:**
   - Sensitively addressing patient's concerns (20%).
   - Discussing about lithium, alternatives in pregnancy (70%).
   - Discussing about breastfeeding and psychotropic medication (10%).

6. **Equipment checklist:**
   Not applicable.

Station 25: History from a patient with PTSD

Theme: Post-Traumatic Stress Disorder (PTSD): History taking

1. **Instructions to candidates:**

   Patient's name: Mr Hooper

   A GP has asked you to see Mr Hooper, a 35-year-old man, van driver who is struggling at work after a road traffic accident 4 months ago. Please conduct a diagnostic assessment focusing on the salient features of PTSD and its differential diagnoses.

2. **Instructions to the role player:**
   - You are Mr Hooper, a 35 years old man, who works as a van driver. Four months ago whilst driving home from Peterborough, a lorry veered across the road in front of you, hitting you head on. You thought you were going to die. Fortunately you only sustained cuts and bruises and a minor head injury, and have now completely recovered physically. You seem to suffer with more headaches than before the accident and wonder if you have done any lasting damage to your brain.
   - You are now off sick from work as you are struggling with vivid flashbacks of the accident. You tried to return to work but you were hypervigilant for lorries on the road. You have only been back to the site of the accident once. As you experienced such intense anxiety and now avoid it. You have daily flashbacks of the accident. You feel anxious and on edge most of the time and tend to be startled easily.
   - Your sleep is now disturbed, whereas before you used to sleep easily, you now find it hard to fall asleep. You also have nightmares about the accident three times a week on average. You find this strange because when you try and think about the accident you find it hard to recall all the details.
   - You are not low in mood but at times you feel very irritable, especially now you're off work. Your appetite is normal, you are not suicidal and you have good energy levels.
   - Prior to the accident you did not suffer from anxiety and would have described yourself as a perfectionist. You are able to get out of the house to visit friends but only if you walk. Being driven by friends or family now makes you anxious. You do not take drugs and only drink alcohol occasionally. You have never had any mental health problems in the past.

3. **Construct:**

   The station tests the candidate's ability to elicit a history from a patient with suspected PTSD and to distinguish it from other differential diagnoses.

4. **Expanded construct:**

   The candidate should:

   - Demonstrate advanced listening skills, ask questions which are structured, focused and fluent.
   - Examine the patient's mental state and demonstrate empathy with the patient's experience and elicit the key features of PTSD.
   - Identify ongoing compensation claims.
   - Differentiate PTSD from depression, anxiety disorders and substance misuse. Also elicit whether patient could be suffering from a comorbid psychiatric disorder.
   - Do a focused risk assessment and assess the impact of symptoms on driving.

5. **Areas of importance to pass the station:**
   - Interview/communication skills (30%).
   - Ability to elicit symptoms of PTSD and screen for differential diagnoses (50%).
   - Risk assessment (20%).

6. **Equipment checklist:**

   Not applicable.

Station 26: History and Mental State Examination of a manic patient

Theme: History and mental state of a manic patient

1. **Instructions to candidates:**

   Patient's name: Mrs Highbrow

   You have been asked to see Mrs Highbrow, a 50-year-old woman who works as a cleaner in a supermarket. Her GP referred her because she has suspected mania.

   Explore this patient's symptoms and mental state.

2. **Instructions to the role player:**
   - You are Mrs Highbrow, a 50-year-old cleaner. You went to the GP because your friend asked you to do so. You feel totally well, but your colleagues feel you are ill.
   - For the last few weeks you have been putting in extra hours at work, unpaid, because you wanted to get the supermarket totally clean. You get irritable with the customers for making your supermarket dirty. You were disciplined for this and you are now on your final warning at work.
   - For the last 2 weeks you have been feeling very well, energetic, irritable, a bit flirtatious, self-important, sociable, etc. You won't wear the staff uniform as it seems drab, you prefer bright clothes. You have been buying lots of clothes recently.
   - Your colleagues say you talk too much. They've complained that your behaviour is over friendly and occasionally, socially inappropriate and flirtatious with customers. They say you behave as if you are a very important person, which you think you are.
   - You are the best cleaner in the world and you're going to win an award for the cleanest supermarket. The prize is a lot of money, which is why you can justify spending lots of money on clothes.

- You don't hear voices and you won't take medication. You drink alcohol to get you off to sleep. You sleep for 2 hours before you wake up and feel raring to go again. You're not interested in food as you're too busy cleaning. Your new hobbies include researching the best cleaning products available on the internet.
- Your sister has problems with her mood but you don't know the details. You don't take drugs.
- You have been flirting with the customers and have recently asked some of the men who shop there for sex. You feel very attractive and you are keen to find the man of your dreams. You have noticed that you have become more efficient at cleaning and time seems to have speeded up.
- You have felt low in the past and had highs but never this high.
- You are not and have never been suicidal. You are not a violent person, but when customers mess up your supermarket you have shouted at them and at times felt like hitting them.

3. **Construct:**

The station tests the candidate's ability to elicit a history from a patient with suspected mania and to focus on the salient features.

4. **Expanded construct:**

The candidate should:

- Demonstrate advanced listening skills, ask questions which are structured, remain focussed throughout the interview, maintaining control whilst conducting self in a calm and polite manner.
- Be non-judgmental and do not argue with the patient.
- Examine the patient's mental state and demonstrate empathy with the patient's experience.
- Elicit the salient features of mania, stressors, substance misuse, past history, family history and a focussed medical history.
- Identify current risks.

5. **Areas of importance to pass the station:**
   - Interview/communication skills (30%).
   - Ability to elicit appropriate history and symptoms of mania (30%).
   - Risk assessment (40%).
6. **Equipment checklist:**
   Not applicable

Station 27: Assessment of dissocial/antisocial personality disorder

Theme: Assess a patient with dissocial/antisocial personality disorder with a view to referring to personality disorder service

1. **Instructions to candidates:**

Patient's name: Paul Goodman

A GP has referred a 21-year-old man named Paul Goodman. He has a long history of police involvement, mainly breaching the peace. The GP is concerned that he suffers with personality disorder and wonders whether he would benefit from a referral to a personality disorder service. Please conduct a diagnostic assessment and assess his suitability for referral to a personality disorder service.

2. Instructions to the role player:

- You are Paul Goodman, a 21-year-old man who is currently unemployed. You do not want to be at this assessment. You live with your mum and often use her car but she has threatened to take this away unless you get some help. You are only here to please her and to get her off your back. You see nothing wrong and wish your mum would stop badgering you. It frustrates you that she can't accept that it is your decision not to work and claim benefits. You blame her for how your life has turned out. You don't think that being lazy is a reason to be referred to a psychiatrist.
- You like going out late at night with your friends, drinking alcohol in excess and think it is fun to wake the neighbourhood in the early hours of the morning. You have been issued with a number of anti-social behaviour orders (ASBOs) for breach of the peace, fines and a community order, but nothing will stop you from having a good time with your friends. You don't care about your neighbours' feelings. They have challenged you over the noise you make at night, but this irritates you and often your friends have to hold you back from punching the neighbours.
- You are currently single as your girlfriend just left you for cheating on her. You don't care because you know you can always get another girlfriend any time you want. You have two children by different mothers but you don't have anything to do with them because you don't want to be saddled with the responsibility of kids.
- Your opinion of psychiatrists is that they meddle in things that are none of their business. You don't want any medication and certainly don't want to talk to any more do-gooders. The only pills you're willing to take are those bought off the street.

3. Construct:

This station tests the candidate's ability to take a history focusing on the salient features of dissocial personality disorder and whether referral to a personality disorder service is appropriate.

4. Expanded construct:

The candidate should:

- Demonstrate advanced communication skills, deflect anger and be non-confrontational.
- Take appropriate history including features of dissocial personality disorder, alcohol and substance misuse as well as comorbidity.
- Do a focussed risk assessment.
- May use motivational interviewing style to assess insight and motivation to change.

5. Areas of importance to pass the station:

- Interview/communication skills (30%).
- Ability to elicit the features of dissocial personality disorder (30%).
- Recognize the appropriateness of a referral to a personality disorder service (10%).
- Risk assessment (30%).

6. Equipment checklist:

Not applicable

Station 28: Assessment of a mute patient

Theme: Collateral history about a mute patient from a prison officer

1. **Instructions to candidates:**

   Prison Officer's name: Mr Neil Mills

   You have been asked to take a collateral history from prison officer after one of their inmates, a 39-year-old man named James became mute. The patient has already been seen by the prison doctor and a full examination has taken place revealing no neurological, biochemical or endocrine cause for this patient's presentation.

   Take a collateral history from the prison officer in order to evaluate the current mental state.

2. **Instructions to the role player:**
   - You are Mr Mills, the prison officer at Wormwood scrubs. A few weeks ago, James was remanded to prison awaiting sentencing for a series of violent armed burglaries. Initially he was full of bravado, was arrogant and had a high disregard for authority. He bragged to officers that he knew his sentence would be short.
   - One week ago, after his trial, he was told by the judge that he would serve 15 years without parole. He was overheard talking to another inmate that he intended to get out of prison one way or another, even if it meant a spell in hospital.
   - Shortly afterwards he became mute, but was fully conscious and alert. This happened suddenly, there was no history of assault prior to him becoming mute. Since becoming mute his appetite has reduced, but his self-care is good, as is his sleep.
   - Around officers he appears low in mood and tries to cry at times, although no tears come. On a couple of occasions, he has been observed smiling and winking at other inmates, but quickly reverts to appearing low. He sits for long periods staring blankly, but when one of the other inmates threatened to punch him he ducked out of the way.
   - He has been seen by the prison doctor who examined him and could find no cause for his mutism. You know that blood tests were taken but you are not sure which tests were done. The prison doctor confirmed with the GP that James has no previous psychiatric history and is usually fit and well.

3. **Construct:**

   This station tests the candidate's ability to obtain a history from a prison officer about a mute patient, asking questions in a structured manner which gives insight into the patient's mental state.

4. **Expanded construct:**

   The candidate should:
   - **Use a systematic approach to questioning, structured, focused and fluent.**
   - **Demonstrate advanced listening skills.**
   - **Understand that psychiatric assessment is not the prison officers' area of expertise so ask questions which are simple, understandable and jargon-free.**
   - **Check that a full physical as well as neurological assessment has been carried out and organic causes have been ruled out.**

- **Attempt to ascertain any behaviour indicative of a psychiatric illness in the inmate.**
- **Have a high level of suspicion that this inmate is malingering when psychiatric symptoms are absent.**
- **Elicit history of alcohol, substance misuse and prescribed medications.**

5. **Areas of importance to pass the station:**
   - Interview/communication skills (30%).
   - Ability to quickly screen organic causes of unresponsiveness had been ruled out (20%).
   - Ability to screen for psychiatric symptoms using the collateral history as a witness (30%).
   - Correctly identify malingering (20%).
6. **Equipment checklist:**
   Not applicable

Station 29: Depressed man with a history of recent myocardial infarction

Theme: Assessment of post-myocardial infarction (MI) depression

1. **Instructions to candidates:**

   Patient's name: Mr Benson

   A GP has referred Mr Benson, a 50-year-old builder who has experienced low mood since his recent myocardial infarction. The GP is concerned that his mental state is deteriorating and that he may be neglecting his medical needs.
   - **Carry out psychiatric assessment and assess his attitude towards and self-management of his ischaemic heart disease.**
   - **Do not do a physical examination.**
   - **Do not assess cognitive functions.**
2. **Instructions to the role player:**
   - You are Mr Benson, a 50-year-old married builder. You have always been a physically active man as your job is physically demanding. Before the heart attack, you used to work long days and then you would unwind in the pub with your colleagues. You smoked 40 cigarettes per day and drank an average of three pints each night.
   - Six months ago you noticed chest pains when lifting heavy building materials, but these went away after rest. At first you thought it was muscular pain. You immediately stopped smoking and drinking on advice from your GP and you were referred to a cardiologist.
   - A few weeks later you suffered with an MI while walking the dog with your wife. You were taken to A and E and given an injection to thin the blood and were admitted to the coronary care unit. You had a three-vessel angioplasty 4 months ago and are now on tablets, but you can't remember the name of them. The cardiology consultant came to see you and told you to permanently stop smoking, drink only a moderate amount of alcohol, take moderate exercise and take your heart medications as prescribed.

- Seven weeks after the heart attack, whilst still off work, your wife and friends noticed that your mood was getting bad, particularly in the mornings. Sometimes you don't get out of bed all day. You have been told you can return to work but don't feel you have the energy. You no longer enjoy the things you used to, e.g., socializing with your friends in the pub. Also you don't feel like being around lots of people. Your libido has dropped and you feel hopelessness and helplessness. You can't see a future but are not suicidal. You are tearful, your sleep is poor and you wake up several hours earlier than usual. You've lost weight and your appetite and concentration are poor.
- At the moment you are taking your tablets as prescribed and not drinking or smoking, but you are close to going against the doctor's orders as following their advice isn't making you feel any better either.

3. **Construct:**

The station tests the candidate's ability to elicit a history from a depressed patient who has a recent history of MI, focusing on the depressive symptoms and the patient's attitude to self-management of the confirmed ischaemic heart disease.

4. **Expanded construct:**

The candidate should:

- Demonstrate advanced listening skills.
- Be reassuring, avoid lecturing the patient.
- Use language which is simple and understandable.
- Examine the patient's mental state and demonstrate empathy with the patient's experience.
- Identify that this patient's depression may be affecting his judgment regarding his attitude towards his physical needs.
- Identify current risks.

5. **Areas of importance to pass the station:**

- Interview/communication skills (20%).
- Ability to elicit symptoms of depression (30%).
- Ability to recognise this patient's judgment is impaired and may be impacting on his physical needs and explaining this to the patient (30%).
- Risk assessment (20%).

6. **Equipment checklist:**

Not applicable

Station 30: Somatization disorder: Assess

Theme: Assessment of somatization disorder

1. **Instructions to the candidates:**

You are a Specialist Registrar in psychiatry. You are going to assess Mrs Jas Kaur, a 48-

year-old woman of Asian origin in the outpatient clinic. She has presented to her GP with history of headaches, dizziness, and chest pain. The GP could not find any physical causes for her symptoms and has referred her to you.

- **Elicit history of presenting illness.**
- **Do not do a risk assessment.**
- **Address her concerns and expectations.**

2. **Instructions to the role player:**

You are Mrs Jas Kaur, 48-year-old woman of Asian origin. You live with your husband Kamal Singh and two daughters. You work as a cook in a nearby school.

- Mr Singh has not been working for the past 5 years. He used to work as a taxi driver. Unfortunately he met with an accident 5 years ago and became disabled. Now, you are the sole bread-winner for your family.
- You have two daughters aged 26 and 20 years. As you are from a traditional Indian family, you wanted to make sure that they are married within your own culture.
- You approached your GP as you have been suffering from headaches for the past 3 years. They are dull and all over the head. At times it seems like heaviness or a tight band around the head. You still get these headaches on and off.
- You feel dizzy at times. You try to ignore these symptoms and continue to work.
- One year ago, your daughter disclosed to you that she is in love with Danny Spencer. You had your first episode of chest pain on that day. You started getting tightness in the chest and you started panicking. Six months ago, they broke up and your daughter took a serious overdose. You did not tell anything to your husband, as you were worried that he may not be able to cope with the news. Gradually, you started getting tightness in the chest almost every day.
- You went to the GP who did ECG and blood tests. He could not find any physical cause for your difficulties. He prescribed you some tablets that you took for a week as they made you drowsy.
- You are annoyed, as you don't feel that you have a mental illness, but reluctantly agreed to see the psychiatrist when the GP suggested.
- You suffer from sleep disturbance, irritability and loss of appetite for the past 6 months. You feel sick on and off for no reason. You have been suffering from back pain, neck pain, pain in the hands and legs for years.
- You have burning sensations while passing water. You also have irregular periods for the past 2 years.
- In your 20's, you used to lose your speech whenever you had arguments at home. You disclose this to the doctor only if the doctor asks you specifically.

3. **Construct:**

The station assesses the candidate's ability to explore symptoms of somatization disorder, possible aetiological factors and communication with a distressed person.

4. **Expanded construct:**

- Candidate should be able to open the topic sensitively and demonstrate advanced communication skills.

- They should be able to demonstrate knowledge of criteria of somatization disorder according to ICD-10.
- They should be able to elicit the symptoms of somatization disorder.
- They should be able to rule out depression, medical causes and secondary causes of multiple somatic symptoms.
- They should be able to address the patient's concerns without colluding with the patient, i.e., agreeing for more investigations, physician referral, etc.

5. **Areas of importance to pass the station:**
   - Advanced communication skills (20%).
   - Eliciting symptoms of somatization disorder (60%).
   - Ruling out depression, medical causes and other relevant differential diagnosis (10%).
   - Addressing patient concerns and expectations (10%).
6. **Equipment checklist:**
   Not applicable

Station 31: Organic personality disorder: Collateral information

Theme: Collateral history of organic personality disorder

1. **Instructions to the candidates:**
   You are a 3rd year Core Trainee in psychiatry. You are advised to take a collateral history from Mrs Carpenter. She is worried about the changes in her husband's personality following a serious accident at his work.
   - **Take a history to arrive at a diagnosis.**
   - **Address her fears, anxieties and concerns.**
2. **Instructions to the role player:**
   You are wife of 34-year-old Mr Carpenter. You have been married for the past 12 years and have two sons.
   - When asked, you mention that your husband used to be a loving and caring person. He was altruistic in nature. He was a fireman by occupation. He worked hard to support his family.
   - About 2 years ago, he had a fall from the first floor of a house where he was trying to save three children from fire. He sustained a head injury following the fall. He was unconscious for an hour and had a convulsion. He was admitted to his local hospital. Fortunately, the scans and other tests were normal and he was discharged home following observation for 48 hours.
   - However, for the last 18 months, you have noticed the following change in his personality, which are unusual for him.
   - He is unable to maintain focus and attention at his work. He is getting increasingly forgetful. The other day you asked him to get bread and milk. He went to the shop and returned home empty handed. He totally forgot the purpose of going to the shop.
   - About 6 months ago, you went with him and children to Robinson Swimming pool. He asked you for sex while at the swimming pool. You were shocked, as he appeared serious about it.

- He has started making inappropriate comments in front of the children. You were watching a movie the other day and he made a sexual comment in front of the children, which was embarrassing.
- Nowadays, you noticed that he has lost his patience. If he needed something he should have it immediately. Otherwise, he would be angry and start swearing.
- Recently, his friends started commenting that soon he would be giving up the job and turn religious full time. You found him spending hours and hours reading Bible. Last week, he was found reading Bible in work place and not focusing on work. However, you could not understand many things he discussed and claimed to be in Bible.
- He would talk about the same topic repeatedly and you can't make anything out of it. This also puzzles children.
- He does not misuse alcohol or drugs. He does not have a medical problem. He did not suffer from mental illness in the past.
- You are worried about him as well as your marriage.

3. **Construct:**

The station assesses the candidate's ability to elicit features of personality disorder change following a traumatic brain injury, in particular frontal lobe disorder.

4. **Expanded construct:**
   - The candidate should approach the topic sensitively.
   - The candidate should be able to elicit premorbid personality.
   - The candidate should elicit the details of head injury.
   - The candidate should elicit personality changes following head injury.
   - The candidate should rule out major psychiatric illnesses and medical problems.
   - The candidate should rule out alcohol or substance misuse.

5. **Areas of importance to pass the station:**
   - Candidate should demonstrate advanced listening skills (20%).
   - Sensitively explores change in personality post head injury including premorbid personality (60%).
   - Rules out comorbid mental illness, physical health problems, alcohol and drug misuse (20%).

6. **Equipment checklist:**

Not applicable

Station 32: Post-concussion syndrome: Collateral history

Theme: Collateral history from mother of a patient with post-concussion syndrome following minor head injury

1. **Instructions to the candidates:**

You are going to speak to 56-year-old school teacher Mrs Nancy Thatcher. Her 21-year-old daughter

Mary has dropped out of university recently. Mrs Thatcher is worried about the changes in her daughter's personality following a minor head injury.

- **Elicit history of present illness.**
- **Address her concerns.**

2. **Instructions to the role player:**
   - Mary was a very ambitious girl. She was a high achiever in GCSEs as well as 'A' levels following which she joined medical school 2 years ago. She was doing well in her studies.
   - She went on an expedition with her friends at the beginning of last year and met with an accident. Fortunately no one was seriously injured.
   - Mary had an injury on her forehead and was unconscious for approximately 30 minutes. She recovered well in the hospital. Doctors did some scans and tests. Everything was normal and she was discharged home.
   - Over a period of 2 to 3 months, she started complaining of headache and dizziness. She lost her self-confidence. She was anxious and nervous about minor things. For example, about 3 months ago she panicked on seeing the electricity bill.
   - She told that suddenly she felt as if everything was new. She could not concentrate on her studies as well. She dropped out of her university course.
   - She gets irritated easily. She is usually withdrawn and tearful.
   - Last Christmas, she had a glass of wine and became very aggressive and agitated.
   - No past history of mental or physical illness.
   - No history of alcohol or substance misuse.

3. **Construct:**
   The station assesses the candidate's ability to elicit features of personality and behavioural change following a traumatic brain injury from a relative/mother who is anxious, worried and concerned.

4. **Expanded construct:**
   - Candidate should be sensitive and demonstrate advanced listening skills.
   - Candidate should explore premorbid functioning of the patient.
   - Candidate should take a detailed history about the nature and severity of head injury.
   - Candidate should take detailed history of the changes in the patient following head injury.
   - Candidate should rule out medical problems, mental illness as well as alcohol and substance misuse.

5. **Areas of importance to pass the station:**
   - Demonstrating advanced listening skills (20%).
   - Eliciting the history of behavioural change following head injury (60%).
   - Rule out other causes of behavioural change (10%).
   - Addressing mother's concerns without giving false reassurance (10%).

6. **Equipment checklist:**
   Not applicable.

Station 33: Patient with chronic pain: History taking

Theme: Psychological issues associated with chronic pain

1. **Instructions to candidates:**

   You are asked to assess 32-year-old Mr James Gregory who has been referred by pain clinic. He has been complaining of chronic back pain for the past 5 years following a road traffic accident. There is no identifiable organic cause for persistence of pain. The consultant in pain clinic wonders if this is related to psychological issues.

   Take a history to establish underlying psychological issues contributing to his pain.

2. **Instructions to the role player:**

   You are 32-year-old, James Gregory, who has chronic pain for the past 5 years following a road traffic accident.

   - You don't understand why you have been referred to a psychiatrist and you sometimes wonder whether the doctors in pain clinic feel that you are 'making it up'. You want to make it clear to the psychiatrist that the pain is real and that you are not imagining things.

   When asked you describe following:

   - You had a road traffic accident 5 years ago. Your wife Karen and two children aged 10 and 12 were in the car. Fortunately, no one was injured though you started having back pain few hours later.
   - At the time of accident you were working in a high paid job as a sales manager. Following the accident you went off sick for some time.
   - Incidentally, before the accident your wife found out that you were having an affair with a work colleague. You and Karen had a discussion. She was 'understanding' and agreed that 'we need to work on relationship'. The matter was put to a close following discussion.
   - During this period, your mother was unwell and you were 'trying' to take care of her. However, your sister who lived 100 miles away had to come regularly to help mother due to your inability to support her due to pain. Your sister accused you of 'you are not doing enough' which you think was 'unfair'. "I needed help and sympathy rather than accusation. I was not making it up".
   - Six months later, when you returned to work you found it stressful and committed several errors. You were made redundant 2 years ago.
   - Your wife has taken a full time job since your redundancy. You think you 'have to' contribute to home finances. Hence, you took a night shift job of a porter in a university, which was the only available position a year ago.
   - Karen leaves for work early and returns late due to travel. You return home in the morning when she is leaving. You take children to school, do some household chores and catch on some sleep for few hours. You think it is 'unfair' that you have to do household chores, take care of children following a night shift when you suffer from excruciating pain.
   - If you 'overdo' some work, you end up having 'more pain' and you end up 'crippled' in bed for a couple of days. Because of this, you fear 'overdoing' things. This situation is putting a lot of pressure in the relationship with your wife as she ends up doing the bulk of household chores.

- You drink socially. No drugs or smoking. No other physical health problems.
- You have been visiting pain clinic for the past 4 years. You have taken various painkillers that seem to work in the beginning but later on 'stop working'. You wish there was a painkiller that could magically cure your pain so that you could contribute to your family.

You ask the doctor:

- **What is the cause of this pain?**
- **Can you write to my doctor saying that I am not crazy and not making this pain up?**

3. **Construct:**
The station tests the candidate's ability to take a relevant history to establish underlying psychological issues being a perpetuating factor for chronic pain.

4. **Expanded construct:**
   - The candidate should elicit the history to establish underlying psychological issues.
   - They should establish the association between the psychological issues and pain.

5. **Areas of importance to pass the station:**
   - Eliciting psychological process involved in maintaining chronic pain (60%).
   - Address patient's concerns and expectations (20%).
   - Communication (20%).

6. **Equipment checklist:**
Not applicable.

Station 34: Bulimia nervosa: History taking

Theme: Take history about diagnosis and prognostic factors of bulimia nervosa

1. **Instructions to candidates:**
You are asked to see 34-year-old school teacher Jane Simpson by her GP who is concerned about her low mood, recent change in eating habits and thinks she may have anorexia.
Assess the patient with a view to establishing the diagnosis and the prognostic factors.

2. **Instructions to the role player:**
You are a 34-year-old, single, school teacher Jane Simpson and have recently seen your GP due to low mood. You had two relationships break-ups at age 27 and 29 years.
When asked you describe following:
   - You have been binge eating every couple of days and it has been worse in the last 4 weeks.
   - Following a binge, you make yourself sick by sticking your fingers into your mouth and at times use laxative. You have not lost any weight.
   - You have also been self-harming by cutting since the age of 15 years but worse since last 4 weeks. This is worse when stressed.

- You have been feeling low with lack of interest and lack of energy. You lack motivation to finish your work. Your sleep is disturbed. You are tearful at times. You do not smoke or drink.
- Following an OFSTED inspection recently, you were told you improve your performance, as some of the targets were not met for which you were accountable. You tried to complete the required paper work, but found yourself to be increasingly stressed and are on sick leave since 3 weeks.
- You were admitted at the age of 17 under Mental Health Act, as your weight was dangerously low. You were weight conscious since the age of 14 when you went to ballet classes. You were slightly chubbier than the other girls.
- You were bullied at school for being 'fat and chubby'. This resulted in extreme dieting, exercise regime resulting in severe weight loss. This was worse while preparing for A level examination.
- You have been admitted to hospital three times, when you were 16, 27 and 29 years of age. First two admissions were due to significant loss of weight and were diagnosed with anorexia nervosa. Last admission was following a relationship breakup and you started binge eating and were diagnosed to have bulimia. Each admission has been precipitated due to exposure to a stressful situation. In between the episodes, you have remained well.
- You have been treated with family therapy and antidepressant medication. You are currently taking Fluoxetine 40 mg.
- Your family is of 'high achievers: Father is a GP, mother is a solicitor, elder sister is an executive and younger brother is a GP.
- Your mother has a history of depression. Your maternal aunt has anorexia.

3. Construct:

This station tests the candidate's ability to take a relevant history in a patient with eating disorder and to establish relevant prognostic factors.

4. Expanded construct:

- The candidate should be able to elicit brief history and clinical features suggestive of bulimia nervosa.
- Demonstrates knowledge of presentation of bulimia nervosa and differentiate from anorexia/ binge eating disorder.
- They should establish the severity of symptoms, past history of eating disorders, previous psychiatric history including treatment, comorbidity (e.g., depression, alcohol misuse).
- They should elicit past and present risk.

Bulimia nervosa prognostic factors:

- Low self-esteem.
- Duration of symptoms.
- High levels of weight and shape concerns.
- Impulsivity.
- Social adjustment.
- Substance misuse.
- Personal difficulty.

5. **Areas of importance to pass the station:**
   - Ability to elicit and explore the criteria (60%).
   - Subsidiary elements are: Interviewing/communication skills (20%).
   - Appropriate risk assessment (20%).

6. **Equipment checklist:**
   Not applicable

Station 35: Temporal lobe epilepsy: Assessment

Theme: Assessment of temporal lobe epilepsy

1. **Instructions to candidates:**

   You have been asked to assess Martin Jones who has been started on amitriptyline recently for depression. The patient has developed funny turns following the initiation of medication. GP needs your advice on further management.

   Talk to Mr Martin Jones and take a history of his problems.

2. **Instructions to the role player:**
   You are 40-year-old, Martin Jones and live with your wife and children.
   - For the past 9 months, you have been stressed at work due to increasing demands. Over last 8 weeks you have been feeling low in mood, unable to enjoy things and have low energy. You were diagnosed with depression by your GP who started you on Amitriptyline, the dose of which was increased last week.
   - Since then you have noticed 'funny turns'. You get strange smells at home and you tried to find out whether there is any putrid food in the fridge. However, there is none. You have experienced strange things like objects around you would be large in size and faces are distorted.
   - Your wife has noticed that you are found staring at the walls and smacking your lip, "it is as if you are in a trance". This is distressing, as you do not remember much of the episode.
   - Recently, you found yourself in a shopping complex and "I don't know how and why I went there". The last thing you remember was trying to start the car.
   - These days, before the funny attacks, you could feel the stomach churning and a 'feel' that 'something' was going to happen. You get a feeling of déjà vu.
   - You have experienced four 'funny turns' so far and think "I am going crazy" or "someone is trying to play games with my mind".
   - You used to suffer from frequent infections as a child and you suffered from febrile convulsions as a child.
   - You do not have epilepsy. You do not have any significant medical problems.

3. **Construct:**
   The station tests the candidate's ability to take a history to diagnose temporal lobe epilepsy.

4. **Expanded construct:**
   - The candidate should be able to demonstrate the skill in eliciting the history and clinical features suggestive of temporal lobe epilepsy.
   - Its origin, duration and progress including relationship with antidepressant medication.
   - They should ask a range of questions to establish aura, characteristic signs and symptoms of temporal lobe epilepsy like aura, post-seizure confusion, déjà vu, jamais vu, macropsia, etc.
   - They should ask relevant questions to elicit behavioural and other relevant psychiatric signs associated with temporal lobe epilepsy.
   - They should enquire about past history of epilepsy, febrile seizures and family history of psychiatric problems.

5. **Areas of importance to pass the station:**
   - Eliciting accurate and sufficient information about temporal lobe epilepsy including associated neurobehavioural symptoms and signs (50%).
   - Eliciting relevant past medical, psychiatric history and establishing a link between antidepressant and temporal lobe epilepsy (30%).
   - Communication (20%).

6. **Equipment checklist:**
   Not applicable

Station 36: Panic disorder: History taking

Theme: History of panic disorder

1. **Instructions to candidates**
   Mrs Perry Smith, 43-year-old, has been referred to your clinic by her GP. She has been complaining of anxiety and has attended GP surgery every week for the past 2 months. She has been investigated for physical health problems and no cause has been identified.

   Take a history from Mrs Smith and address her fears, concerns and expectations.

2. **Instructions to the role player:**
   You are Perry Smith, 43-year-old teacher, living with your husband and two children. You are anxious, fidgety as you just had an anxiety attack before entering the clinic. You need reassurance from doctor before you can relax. You have come to the clinic as you think it will give you some answers regarding treatment.

   When asked you describe the following:
   - Four months ago, when you were standing in a queue to get a train ticket you suddenly started feeling uneasy. Initially, you thought it was due to tiredness. But within few minutes, your heart started racing, you had sweaty palms and bouts of shortness of breath. You felt funny in your stomach and felt that everything around you was unreal. You felt you were 'going crazy' with a fear of 'losing control'. You felt dizzy and had to sit down. This lasted for 10–15 minutes.

- You felt you were going to die due to a heart attack or stroke.
- You cannot identify any reason for this episode.
- Since then you have been experiencing at least one episode every week.
- In this month, you had four attacks in a week and you are terrified that something is seriously wrong, but don't know what.
- These episodes are not related to any specific situation or event. You may be standing in a queue, cooking, watching TV or shopping.
- You are avoiding driving and going out as often as you fear the attack will start anytime. You are on sick leave since 3 weeks.
- You do not have any other phobias, anxiety or worries. You do not have particular stress, physical health or mental health problem.
- You do not fear social situations, crowded places, shopping areas or public places.

You ask the doctor the following questions:

- **What is wrong with me?**
- **I do not have any worries or stress. Why do I get anxious?**
- **Is it going to get worse?**
- **Could this be a warning sign of stroke? I have family history of stroke.**
- **What is the treatment?**

3. **Construct:**

This station assesses candidate's knowledge of anxiety disorder and ability to elicit history from a woman who had a panic attack minutes before clinic appointment and requiring reassurance.

4. **Expanded construct:**

- The candidate should be able to demonstrate skill in eliciting a history a patient who has anxiety disorder.
- The candidate should be able to elicit origin, duration, progress, severity and associated factors of panic attacks.
- The candidate should inquire into relevant differential diagnosis like organic cause, social phobia, agoraphobia, specific phobia, depression, illicit substance use, and other relevant conditions.
- They should establish the number of panic attacks per week to grade the severity of panic disorder.

  Moderate: At least four panic attacks in 4-week period.

  Severe: At least four panic attacks per week over a 4-week period.
- They should establish the impact of the disorder on social life and functioning.
- They should allay patient's anxiety, worries and fears. They should discuss the aetiology, management and prognosis of panic disorder.

5. **Areas of importance to pass the station:**

- Eliciting accurate and sufficient information about panic disorder, severity of episodes and impact on social life and functioning (40%).

- Elicit history to rule out relevant differential diagnosis of panic disorder (20%).
- Allay patient's anxieties, fears and concerns (20%).
- Communication (20%).

6. **Equipment checklist:**
   Not applicable

Station 37: Depression with psychotic symptoms

Theme: History taking: Severe depressive episode with psychotic symptoms

1. **Instructions to candidates:**
   Mrs Jane Parker, 38-year-old was brought to accident and emergency department by her sister. She has being talking of devil and sin for the past few days. Her husband has found it increasingly difficult to manage her at home. She refuses to talk to the mental health nurse and junior doctor, and hence, as a specialty registrar your input has been requested.
   Talk to her with a view of taking a history and appropriate risk assessment.
2. **Instructions to the role player:**
   You are 38-year-old Mrs Jane Parker. You are scared, irritable and guarded. You sit with head down, shoulders shrugged and do not maintain eye contact. You keep on repeating 'sin sinner, sin sinner'. You talk only if the doctor is sensitive and empathetic.
   When asked you describe the following:
   - You repeat "sin sinner, sin sinner". When asked what it means you reply that you have committed a sin and you are a sinner.
   - You believe that your husband died prematurely due to cancer, as you did not take enough care of him, which is a 'sin'. You had been the main carer for a year, but the cancer of pancreas was aggressive and spread rapidly. If think that he could have lived longer if you were more caring and supportive. You did not even tell him how much you loved him before he died. You are unable to explain what else you could have done for him.
   - You blame yourself for his death, have significant guilt, and feel worthless.
   - You have low mood, are not able to enjoy things and poor energy levels.
   - You hear devils voice saying that "Jane you are a sinner, you are responsible for Ben's death", "you should die and your body should rot for the sin". The voice is always there, clear and derogatory.
   - You see a dark shadow of the devil with horns staring at you with bloodshot eyes.
   - You don't want to kill yourself as you think your body will rot and decompose on its own due to your sin. Hence, you have stopped eating, drinking and taking care of yourself. You can already smell rotten flesh. You are not scared of death, but are terrified to think that you will not be with your husband in heaven due to your sin.
   - You keep on asking "can I go home now, I cannot talk to you, and please let me go I am a sinner". You make attempts to leave on a couple of occasions.
   - You do not answer any other questions.

3. **Construct:**

This station assesses candidate's knowledge of depressive episode and to elicit a history of a severe depressive episode with psychotic symptoms, including consideration of differential diagnosis.

4. **Expanded construct:**

- The candidate should be able to demonstrate skill in eliciting a history a patient who is irritable, guarded and distressed.
- The candidate should be able to elicit origin, duration, progress, severity and associated factors of the depressive episode with psychotic symptoms.
- The candidate should explore the delusion, hallucinations and other psychotic symptoms and signs.
- They should assess the risk of suicide/self-harm, self-neglect, vulnerability and other relevant risk areas.
- The candidate should explore symptomatology of other relevant differential diagnosis.

5. **Areas of importance to pass the station:**

- Eliciting accurate and sufficient information about depressive episode including severity, differential diagnosis (40%).
- Assess risk of suicide/self-harm (30%).
- Communication (30%).

6. **Equipment checklist:**

Not applicable

Station 38: Recurrent depressive disorder: History taking

Theme: History taking and discussion with patient suffering from recurrent depressive disorder

1. **Instructions to candidates:**

Mrs Deborah Jones, 62 years of age, has been referred to your outpatient clinic her general practitioner (GP). She has been complaining of feeling numb, having headache and body aches for which no cause is found. Her GP thinks that it is most probably psychosomatic in origin.

- **Talk to her with a view to taking her clinical history.**
- **Address her fears, anxieties, concerns and expectations.**

2. **Instructions to the role player:**

You are 62-year-old Mrs Deborah Jones. You live alone and your three children live locally. You are a retired teacher and presently governor of a school. You take some time to answer the questions as your thinking is slower than usual. You are keen to know what is wrong with you and agreeable to any treatment offered. Your main complaints are headache and body ache, though answer other questions asked appropriately.

When asked you describe the following:

- You have been having constant headache and body ache for the past 3 weeks. You have been taking painkillers that help marginally. You do not have any other physical health problems of significance.
- You have been feeling low in mood and extremely tired for the past 2 months.
- You find it difficult to manage your day-to-day activities. You sit on the sofa for most of the day and think 'have lost motivation and enthusiasm'. You are not able to perform your duties as a governor and have not been involved with school activities for 3 weeks.
- You have been using take away, seem to have lost appetite and possibly lost some weight.
- You are unable to sleep due to body ache and headache.
- You do not feel hopeless or worthless. You do not have thoughts of suicide or self-harm. You do not have any psychotic symptoms.
- Your husband died 4 months ago due to heart attack. You were married for 34 years and miss him, but have come to terms with his death. You have grieved appropriately. However, you have to manage all the bills, collect rent from tenants, etc. that he used to do and at times find it overwhelming and stressful.
- In the past you had similar symptoms and signs. You have had two separate episodes – first when you were 53 years and another at 58 years of age. On both occasions, you were dealing with stressful situations and were not able to cope with them. The second episode was severe and you had felt suicidal though never acted on them. Each episode lasted for about 4 months. You do not have any manic or hypomanic episode.
- You were treated with antidepressants like Sertraline for 3 months (first episode) and then Mirtazapine for 3–4 months (second episode) with good effect by your GP.
- You have been completely well in between the episodes.
- Presently you are taking Mirtazapine for the past 6 weeks but do not have any benefit.

You should ask the following questions:

- **Why am I getting depressed again?**
- **What is the diagnosis?**
- **How can I stop this?**
- **I am completely well in between the episodes, so I stop medication. How long will I have to take medication this time?**

3. **Construct:**

This station assesses candidate's knowledge of recurrent depressive disorder and ability to elicit a history suggestive of recurrent depressive disorder, moderate type with somatic symptoms.

4. **Expanded construct:**

- The candidate should be able to demonstrate skill in eliciting a history a patient who is pre-occupied with somatic symptoms.
- The candidate should be able to elicit origin, duration, progress, severity and associated factors of the recurrent depressive disorder.

- The candidate should explore the likely precipitating factors for present and past depressive episodes.
- The candidate should inquire into past history, treatment, family history and remission in between the depressive episodes.
- They should assess the risk of suicide/self-harm, self-neglect, vulnerability and other relevant risk areas.
- They should elicit if there are any manic/hypomanic episodes in the past. If there is mild mood elevation and over activity that may fulfill criteria of hypomania immediately after a depressive episode, still the diagnosis of recurrent depressive disorder can be used. The rational is that this episode may be precipitated by treatment of depression rather than being a true hypomanic episode of bipolar disorder.

5. **Areas of importance to pass the station:**
   - Eliciting accurate and sufficient information about depressive episode including severity, somatic complaints and differential diagnosis (30%).
   - Past history of depressive episodes, remission in between the episodes and management (30%).
   - Assess risk of suicide/self-harm (20%).
   - Communication (20%).
6. **Equipment checklist:**
   Not applicable

Station 39: Electroconvulsive therapy (ECT): Consent

Theme: Consent for electroconvulsive therapy (ECT)

1. **Instructions to candidates:**
   Mr Robert Lee is a 58-year-old gentleman admitted to in-patient ward for the past 6 weeks. He has been tried on various antidepressants, which have not helped him. He was seen in the ward rounds and your consultant has suggested ECT. He remains low in mood and thinks everybody will be better off if he is dead.
   Give information about ECT with a view to helping him making a decision to receive ECT. You are not expected to take a history.
2. **Instructions to the role player:**
   You are 58-year-old, admitted Robert Lee who was admitted to the hospital about 6 weeks ago. You have been feeling very depressed and do not want to live any more. Anti-depressants have not helped and you are sick of feeling miserable and worthless.
   You speak in low tone and ask following questions:
   - **What is ECT?**
   - **How is ECT given?**
   - **What happens during ECT?**

- **Why is it better than medication?**
- **Could I die from it?**
- **You have read that it causes brain damage and severe memory problems.**
- **What are the side effects of ECT?**
- **What if I really don't want ECT?**

3. **Construct:**
The station tests the candidate's ability to explain about ECT and respond appropriately to the concerns of a patient who is severely depressed.

4. **Expanded construct:**
- Explain about ECT

They should:
- Show the ability to give information and demonstrate empathy with the patient.
- Answer range of questions that demonstrate knowledge about ECT and be able to explain this to the patient in terms that he will understand.

5. **Areas of importance to pass the station:**
- Ability to answer the concerns of the patient (40%).
- Ability to explain the procedure of ECT (40%).
- Subsidiary elements are: Interviewing/communication skills (20%).

6. **Equipment checklist:**
Not applicable

Station 40: Lithium augmentation: Discuss

Theme: Explain about lithium augmentation and obtain consent from the patient

1. **Instructions to candidates:**
Mr Tom Bellhouse is a 55-year-old man with three previous episodes of depression. He is currently taking sertraline and your consultant has suggested lithium augmentation. Your task is:
- **To explain what is lithium and its augmentation and obtain consent.**
- **Address his beliefs, concerns and expectations.**

2. **Instructions to the role player:**
You are 55-year-old Tom Bellhouse who had three episodes of depression in the past 10 years.
- You are currently taking a third antidepressant, sertraline 200 mg per day and still do not feel any better.
- A decision has been made to add another drug, lithium to your prescription.
- You are an occasional drinker.
- The doctor is going to discuss as to why this decision has been considered and answer your questions. If doctor asks you about your kidneys, tell him that you are prone to kidney infection.

You should ask the following questions:

- **How does lithium work?**
- **What tests do I need before starting lithium?**
- **Why must I take a blood test?**
- **Is lithium dangerous?**
- **What are the side effects?**
- **How can I be careful?**
- **How effective is lithium?**
- **Could I drink alcohol if I am taking lithium?**
- **Will it affect my sex life?**
- **If I have another bout of depression does that mean lithium is not working?**

Finally, you agree to the addition of lithium if your concerns are answered adequately.

3. **Construct:**
The station tests candidate's ability to give information about lithium including its efficacy, side effects and necessary precautions. They should avoid medical jargon and be able to explain this to the patient in the language he understands.

4. **Expanded construct:**
   - To discuss about lithium therapy.
   - To explain the benefits and common side effects of lithium.

   They should:
   - Check the understanding of patient and answer his concern.
   - Check the past medical history especially thyroid and renal disease.

   Interview/Communication skills
   They should include:
   - o Show an appropriate mix of open and close questioning.
   - o Demonstrate advanced listening skills.
   - o Ask questions that are structured, focused and fluent.
   - o Diplomacy and empathy with the patient.
   - o Use language, i.e., simple and understandable and avoid jargon.

5. **Areas of importance to pass the station:**
   - Interview/communication skills (20%).
   - Ability to explain lithium therapy and its side effects (60%).
   - Demonstrate ability to address patient's fears (20%).

6. **Equipment checklist:**
Not applicable

Station 41: Antipsychotic depot injections: Consent

Theme: Explain about antipsychotic depot injections and obtain consent

1. **Instructions to candidates:**

   Mr Paul Read is 28-year-old man, who has paranoid schizophrenia and is known to the community mental health team. This is his third admission in inpatient unit as a result of non-adherence to medications. When unwell, he stops going out of the house due to the belief that FBI is after him. He has stopped eating, as he believes his spine and belly are stolen as part of a plot against him. He constantly hears voices telling him he is not safe. He is settled in the unit after being recommenced on quetiapine. Your consultant has suggested depot antipsychotic injection for him in the ward round.

   Discuss with Mr Read the need for antipsychotic depot injections.
   Explain the rationale for initiation of antipsychotic depot injections.
   Answer any specific questions and concerns to obtain consent.

2. **Instructions to the role player:**

   - You are 28-year-old man, Mr Paul Read. You were diagnosed with paranoid schizophrenia 2 years ago and are under care of the community mental health team.
   - You don't like taking tablets and also at times forget to take them. This makes you unwell and gets you admitted to hospital. This is your third admission.
   - When unwell you stop going out of the house as voices tells you that you are not safe. You believe FBI is following you and their agents have stolen your spine and belly. As result of this you have stopped eating.
   - In the hospital, the doctors have started you back on antipsychotic tablets called Quetiapine. A decision is made to consider starting you on an antipsychotic depot injection. This is slow release injection given into buttock or upper arm at a frequency of 4 weeks. Once you are on this injection you don't need to take tablets.
   - The doctor is going to see you and explain about antipsychotic depot injection to obtain your consent.

     You agree to take injection if all concerns and questions are answered.

     You should ask the following questions:

     - **What is antipsychotic depot injection?**
     - **How does it work?**
     - **How are the injections given?**
     - **What are the side effects?**
     - **What are the advantages of taking the depot?**
     - **How will you start the injection and what will happen to tablets?**
     - **Will I have to take injection for the rest of my life?**
     - **What if I forget my appointment for injection?**
     - **Can I stop taking it if I change my mind?**

     In the end you agree to take medication if all your concerns are answered.

3. **Construct:**

This station assesses candidate's knowledge of long acting antipsychotic injection with a view to assisting patient in making the decision.

4. **Expanded construct:**

- Give information about antipsychotic depot injection.
- Check understanding of the patient and address all concerns.

They should:

- Give appropriate information and discuss all side effects.
- Check the patient's ability to understand, retain and make the decision in light of the information given.
- Take medical history (enquire about heart problems and diabetes), relevant to commencing on antipsychotic depot injection.
- Check previous non-pharmacological treatments (such as, psychotherapy, family therapy) considered or offered.

Interview/communication skills:

They should include:

- Demonstrate advanced listening skills.
- Listening and responding appropriately to patient's concerns.
- Discuss appropriate choices of treatments available.

5. **Areas of importance to pass the station:**

- Ability to address the patient's fears about treatment. A good candidate will take a medical history (40%).
- Able to assess the capacity of patient in decision-making (20%).
- Avoid use of technical terms and medical jargons (20%).
- Use of appropriate mix of open and closed questions (20%).

6. **Equipment checklist:**

Not applicable.

Station 42: Antipsychotics: Side-effects

Theme: Explanation of extrapyramidal and other side effects of antipsychotics

1. **Instructions to candidates:**

Thirtytwo-year-old Andrea Cummins has a diagnosis of schizophrenia. She was commenced on antipsychotic depot injection and is currently stable with regards to her mental health. She has started experiencing rigidity and tremors. Her husband Alex is quite concerned and came today to see you in the outpatient clinic. Andrea has agreed to your discussing her medical details with her husband.

Explain about your diagnosis and its management.

Explain about side effects of antipsychotics.

Address ideas, concerns and expectations.

2. **Instructions to the role player:**
   - You are the husband of 32-year-old patient Andrea who is diagnosed with schizophrenia.
   - Recently, she was started on an antipsychotic injection which has been prescribed once every two weeks. You have noticed that her movements have slowed down and she has tremors in her hands. She is also tired most of the day.
   - You are going to see the doctor today in the clinic to discuss your concerns about this injection.
   - You are very annoyed and blame yourself for her condition as you agreed to the doctor's advice and persuaded her to accept the depot injection.
   - You are meeting her doctor today for an explanation about her side effects and medication.

   Opening statement: She is like a robot. It's my fault entirely.

   You should then ask the following questions:
   - **What is wrong with her?**
   - **What can we do about it?**
   - **What are other side effects of antipsychotics?**
   - **How long should she need to take this injection for?**
   - **We were planning to start a family; how does medication affect this?**
   - **How can I support her?**

3. **Construct:**

   This station tests the candidate's ability to provide explanation about short-term and long-term side effects of antipsychotics.

4. **Expanded construct:**
   - To develop rapport with the concerned relative.
   - To explain wide range of side effects of antipsychotics.

   They should:
   - Explain to the relative with the information tin the language he understands.
   - Address the concerns with empathetic responses.
   - Explain the common and uncommon side effects, i.e., EPSEs, hyperprolactinaemia, anticholinergic side effects, metabolic syndrome and lowered seizure threshold.
   - A good candidate will also discuss the risk factors.

   Interview/Communication skills:

   They should include:
   - Demonstration of advance listening skills.
   - Diplomacy and empathy with the relative.
   - Use language, i.e., simple and avoid jargon.

5. **Areas of importance to pass the station:**
   - Ability to discuss about side effects with concerned relative (40%).
   - Interview and communication skills (40%).
   - Able to discuss the risk factors (20%).
6. **Equipment checklist:**
   Not applicable

Station 43: Lithium and other mood stabilizers: Side-effects

Theme: Explain side effects of lithium and other mood stabilizer medication

1. **Instructions to candidates:**

   You are meeting with Alison Clark, 24-year-old lady, who is an inpatient on your ward. She was admitted with elated mood, overspending, increased energy, not sleeping and promiscuous behaviour. She had two previous episodes of depression. She is treated with benzodiazepines and haloperidol during her current admission. The plan is to commence her on a mood stabilizer. Your role is to see her and explain the side effects of lithium and other mood stabilizers.

   Explain about the diagnosis and its management with mood stabilizers.

   Address patient's beliefs, concerns and expectations.

2. **Instructions to the role player:**
   - You are Alison Clark, 24-year-old patient, who is currently in hospital.
   - You were admitted to hospital as you was very hyperactive, talking continuously, spending too much money on your credit card. You were not sleeping and because of increased sexual energy you were involved in promiscuous behaviour.
   - Previously you had two episodes of depression.
   - In hospital, you are treated with haloperidol and anti-anxiety tablets.
   - The plan is to start you on a mood stabilizer to manage mood swings.
   - You have no physical health problem and do not use drugs.
   - You are meeting the doctor who should explain the diagnosis and go through the side effects of mood stabilizer.

   You should ask the following questions:
   - **What is wrong with me?**
   - **How you are going to treat this?**
   - **What is a mood stabilizer?**
   - **How does it work?**
   - **What are different types of mood stabilizers?**
   - **What are their side effects?**
   - **Do I need to have blood tests before or during when I am on them?**
   - **How long I need to continue this treatment?**
   - **Will I be able to have children?**
   - **How I can decide which is best for me?**

- **Will I be allowed to drive?**
- **Will I be allowed to drink?**
- **What other type of treatments are available?**

3. Construct:

This station tests the ability of the candidate to explain about short-term and long-term side effects of mood stabilizers.

4. Expanded construct:

- To develop rapport with the patient.
- To explain side effects of lithium, anticonvulsants and antipsychotic mood stabilizers.

They should:

- Explain to the patient with the information the way she understands.
- Address the concerns with empathetic responses.
- Explain the pre-workup of lithium and regular monitoring, pre-workup of anticonvulsants and atypical antipsychotics, side effects especially in pregnancy.

Interview/Communication skills:

They should include:

- Demonstration of advance listening skills.
- Diplomacy and empathy with the patient.
- Use language, i.e., simple and avoid jargon.

5. Areas of importance to pass the station:

The core task at this station is to provide information about management of bipolar affective disorder.

- Ability to discuss about side effects of mood stabilizers (40%).
- Interview and communication skills (40%).
- Able to keep in consideration patient's young age and gender in deciding mood stabilizer (20%).

6. Equipment checklist:

Not applicable.

Station 44: Clozapine: Side-effects

Theme: Explain side-effects of clozapine

1. Instructions to candidates:

You are meeting with Tom Clark, 38-year-old man, suffering from schizophrenia. He was admitted for initiation of clozapine as he continued to be troubled by voices telling him to kill himself. He believes that IRA is broadcasting his thoughts through airwaves. He has not responded to treatment in the past.

Explain about the rationale of initiation of clozapine and its side effects.

Address patient's beliefs, concerns and expectations.

2. **Instructions to the role player:**
   - You are Tom Clark, 38-year-old patient, who is currently in hospital.
   - You are suffering from treatment-resistant schizophrenia.
   - You are admitted to the hospital as you continue to hear voices telling you to kill yourself. You believe IRA is broadcasting your past through air waves. You have not responded to any treatment in the past.
   - The plan is to start you on new medication called clozapine that may help to get rid of voices.
   - The main serious side effect is that it can affect your bone marrow, causing to a shortage of white cells. This makes you susceptible to infection. If this happens, the medication is stopped at once so that the bone marrow can recover.
   - If you take clozapine you will need weekly blood tests for the first 18 weeks and 2 weekly blood tests after that for 34 weeks. It can also cause weight gain, excessive saliva and cause epileptic fits more likely.

   The doctor is going to explain the diagnosis and go through the side effects of clozapine.

   You should ask the following questions:
   - **Do I need tests before starting clozapine?**
   - **Is clozapine dangerous?**
   - **What are the side effects?**
   - **What are serious side effects?**
   - **What are the things I need to be careful of?**
   - **What if I forget taking it?**
   - **How soon will I notice its effect?**
   - **How long do I need to take?**
   - **What other type of treatments are available?**
   - **Will it affect my sex life?**

3. **Construct:**

   This station tests the knowledge and ability of the candidate to explain side-effects of clozapine in a clear manner without use of medical jargons.

4. **Expanded construct:**
   - To develop rapport with the patient.
   - To explain immediate, short-term and long-term side effects of clozapine.
   - Check understanding of patient.

   They should:
   - Explain to the patient with the information the way he understands.
   - Address the concerns with empathetic responses.

- Explain the pre-workup of clozapine and regular monitoring.
- Good candidate will take medical history and history about caffeine and smoking.

Interview/Communication skills:

They should include:

- Demonstration of advance listening skills.
- Diplomacy and empathy with the patient.
- Use language, i.e., simple and avoid jargon.

5. **Areas of importance to pass the station:**
   - Ability to discuss about side effects of clozapine (40%).
   - Interview and communication skills (40%).
   - Able to take patient's medical history along with smoking and caffeine habits (20%).
6. **Equipment checklist:**
   Not applicable.

Station: 45: Antidepressants: Side-effects

Theme: Explain side-effects of antidepressants

1. **Instructions to candidates:**
   You are seeing Mr Jenkins 40-year-old married man who is referred by his GP to your outpatient clinic. He has been suffering from low mood for last 4 months and been signed off from work 2 weeks ago.
   Take history with a view of commencing on an antidepressant.
   Explain about antidepressants and its side effects.
   Address patient's beliefs, concerns and expectations.
2. **Instructions to the role player:**
   - You are Mr Jenkins, 40 years of age, married and lorry driver by profession.
   - You are referred to outpatient clinic by your GP.
   - You had been suffering from low mood for last 4 months with no apparent reason. You find hard to concentrate and not motivated to go to work or gym. You are up early in the morning and unable to go back to sleep.
   - The doctor has signed you off from work 2 weeks ago.
   - You have no thoughts to end your life, as you cannot "do this to your beloved wife".
   - You have no medical problem and you don't drink alcohol.
   - The doctor is going to see you to assess how you are feeling, explain the diagnosis and offer you to consider antidepressant. He will also explain how they work and their side effects.
     If the doctor suggests an antidepressant that can cause sedation, remind him that you are lorry driver.

- **You will also like to try an antidepressant that will not affect your sexual life.**

You should ask the following questions:

- **How do antidepressants work?**
- **Are they addictive?**
- **What different types of antidepressants are available?**
- **What are their side effects?**
- **How effective they are and how long do I have to continue?**
- **Which antidepressant you have in mind?**
- **Will I be able to drive?**
- **Will it affect my sex life?**

3. **Construct:**

This station tests the ability of the candidate to explain about antidepressants and its side effects.

4. **Expanded construct:**

- To develop rapport with the patient.
- To able to address patient's fears regarding treatment.

They should:

- Explain to the patient with the information the way he understands.
- Address the concerns with empathetic responses.
- Candidate is expected to take the history before suggesting antidepressant therapy.
- Good candidate is expected to take medical history.

Interview/Communication skills:

They should include:

- Demonstration of advance listening skills.
- Diplomacy and empathy with the patient.
- Use language, i.e., simple and avoid jargon.

5. **Areas of importance to pass the station:**

- Ability to discuss about antidepressant treatment with the patient (40%).
- Interview and communication skills (40%).
- Able to take patient's circumstances into consideration when suggesting treatment (20%).

6. **Equipment checklist:**

Not applicable

Station 46: Schizophrenia: Management

Theme: Explain about management of schizophrenia to the relative

1. **Instructions to candidates:**

You are meeting with mother of 26-year-old patient Dean Scott who is currently an inpatient on your ward for 6 weeks. He was admitted following complaints of auditory hallucinations, persecutory delusions and verbally aggressive behaviour towards his neighbour. He is diagnosed with schizophrenia and treated with olanzapine. Her mother wants to meet you and discuss his treatment. Mr Scott has provided his permission to talk to his mother.

Explain about the diagnosis and its management.

Address beliefs, concerns and expectations.

2. **Instructions to the role player:**
   - You are mother of 26-year-old patient Dean Scott who is in hospital for the past 6 weeks.
   - He was admitted as a result of hearing voices. He was paranoid towards his neighbour and verbally aggressive towards him.
   - He studies in university but for last 1 year he was falling behind his assignments. He does not use drugs or drink excessively.
   - He is diagnosed with schizophrenia.

   The doctor is going to come and explain the diagnosis and discuss the management plan.

You should ask the following questions:

- **What is wrong with Dean?**
- **How common is schizophrenia?**
- **What treatment he is on?**
- **How does it work?**
- **How long will he have to take medication?**
- **Can he become violent towards family or others?**
- **Is he a risk to himself?**
- **What other type of treatments are available?**
- **What support is available after discharge?**
- **Will he be able to work again?**
- **Can he have children?**
- **Will he be allowed to drive?**
- **What support family can provide?**
- **What support is available for carer like me?**

3. **Construct:**

   The core task at this station is to check the ability of the candidate to explain about immediate/short-term and long-term management of schizophrenia.

4. **Expanded construct:**
   - To develop rapport with concerned relative.
   - To explain management plan using biopsychosocial model.

   They should:
   - Explain to the relative with the information the way she understands.
   - Address the concerns with empathetic responses.
   - Explain the medical management, mainly medication.

- Explain psychological management, such as, psychoeducation of patient and family, CBT, family therapy.
- Social management, such as, occupational therapist, CPN, Social worker.
- Predischarge care program approach meetings and care plan.
- Involvement of other services.
- Give information about coping with stigma, help and support for the family.

Interview/Communication skills:

They should include:

- Demonstration of advance listening skills.
- Diplomacy and empathy with the relative.
- Use language, i.e., simple and avoid jargon.

5. **Areas of importance to pass the station:**
   - Ability to discuss about management plan with concerned relative (40%).
   - Interview and communication skills (40%).
   - Inform parent about other services and their role (20%).
6. **Equipment checklist:**
   Not applicable

Station 47: Social phobia: Management

Theme: Explain about management of social phobia to the relative

1. **Instructions to candidates:**
   You have assessed 24-year-old Anthony Slade in your outpatient clinic following a referral from his GP. He works in an IT company. His boss has asked him to do a presentation to Board of Directors and other employees while he is on leave. He is feeling very anxious since he had heard this. His partner Lynn is waiting outside to see you to discuss the diagnosis and treatment. The patient has agreed that you can discuss his case with his wife.
   Explain about the diagnosis and its management.
   Address her ideas, concerns and expectations.
2. **Instructions to the role player:**
   - You are Lynn, partner of 24-year-old Anthony Slade.
   - You have been together for the past 5 years.
   - Anthony is a shy person and prefers his own company. If you both go to the restaurant, Anthony will like to sit in the corner table. He generally avoids rush hours.
   - Now since he has heard about his presentation, he is very anxious and thinking of not turning up on the day. He fears that he has to talk in front of lot of people and they will be watching him.
   - Previously whenever he is in gatherings, he would blush and his heart starts pounding. He starts trembling and unable to speak.
   - At the age of 11, he was ridiculed in school assembly giving a speech.

- He has no medical problems and drinks alcohol occasionally.
- He does not use street drugs.

You suggested to him to go to his GP who then referred him to this clinic. You want to know what is wrong with Anthony and how you can help him.

You should ask the following questions:

- **What is wrong with him?**
- **Why he behaves this way?**
- **Does he have to take tablets?**
- **What other type of treatments are available?**
- **Who will give psychotherapy and for how long?**
- **How I can support him?**

3. Construct:

This station tests the ability of the candidate to explain about immediate, short-term and long-term management of social phobia to a relative in a sensitive and empathic manner.

4. Expanded construct:

- To develop rapport with concerned relative.
- To explain management plan using biopsychosocial model.

They should:

- Explain to the relative with the information the way she understands.
- Address the concerns with empathetic responses.
- Explain the medical management, such as, SSRIs, buspirone, beta-blockers.
- Explain psychological management, such as, CBT using graded exposure and relaxation.
- Social management, such as, self-help, social skill training.
- A good candidate will ask about aetiological factor from relative.

Interview/Communication skills:

They should include:

- Demonstration of advance listening skills.
- Diplomacy and empathy with the relative.
- Use language, i.e., simple and avoid jargon.

5. Areas of importance to pass the station:

- Ability to discuss about management plan with concerned relative (40%).
- Interview and communication skills (40%).
- Able to address psychological factors (20%).

6. Equipment checklist:

Not applicable.

Station 48: Discharge planning

Theme: Discuss discharge planning with patient's mother

1. **Instructions to candidates:**

You are meeting with mother of 36-year-old patient Ricky Scott with chronic schizophrenia who is currently an inpatient on your ward as a result of non-adherence to clozapine. On his previous admission, he was discharged to his brother Martin's address. He was unable to cope because of his brother's excessive drinking habit and stopped taking his medication. The agreed plan for him is to go to rehabilitation unit following discharge.

Your role is to discuss the discharge planning with his mother. You have Mr Scott's permission to discuss his management with his mother.

Discuss discharge planning.

2. **Instructions to the role player:**

- You are mother of 36-year-old patient Ricky Stott who is in hospital. He suffers from chronic schizophrenia. On his previous admission, he was discharged to your younger son Martin.
- You are aware that Martin drinks heavily. Ricky was unable to cope with Martin's behaviour and stopped his medication. This results Ricky to be back in hospital within 2 months of discharge. Now the doctors have decided that Ricky should go to a rehabilitation unit until he is ready for discharge in the community.
- The doctor is going to come to see you to discuss discharge planning.
- You are annoyed. You tell the doctor you don't think he is mentally ill. You think he is just being lazy and talk rubbish.
- You heard about clozapine from a friend and know there are horrendous side effects.
- You don't want your son to get dependent on drugs, especially when no one knows how they work. You want to take him home.

You should ask the following questions:

- **Why you are treating him with dangerous drug?**
- **I know psychiatrists always blame parents.**
- **What is rehabilitation?**
- **How long he need to take medication?**
- **Will he ever get better?**
- **Can he be violent towards family and others?**
- **What are his chances of getting unwell again?**
- **Will he be able to have children?**
- **Will he be able to drive?**
- **Will he be able to work?**
- **What is care programme approach?**
- **Who will be involved into his discharge planning?**

- **What is the role of psychiatrist in aftercare?**
- **What other type of treatments are available to him?**
- **Who will help him with his accommodation and benefits?**
- **What support is available for carer like me?**
- **How I can support him?**

3. **Construct:**

This station tests the ability of the candidate to discuss about discharge planning, demonstrate knowledge of care programme approach and psychosocial rehabilitation.

4. **Expanded construct:**

- To develop rapport with concerned relative.
- To explain discharge planning using care programme approach.

They should:

- Explain to the relative with the information the way she understands.
- Address the concerns with empathetic responses.
- Explain discharge planning meeting, who will be involved and role of that person.
- Explain role of other services, such as, rehabilitation/crisis team.
- Explain role of voluntary agencies, i.e., MIND, Schizophrenia Fellowship, Rethink etc.
- Explain high expressed emotions.

Interview/Communication skills:

They should include:

- Demonstration of advance listening skills.
- Diplomacy and empathy with the relative.
- Use language, i.e., simple and avoid jargon.

5. **Areas of importance to pass the station:**

- Ability to discuss about discharge planning using care programme approach with concerned relative (40%).
- Interview and communication skills (40%).
- Explain high expressed emotions, role of voluntary organizations (20%).

6. **Equipment checklist:**

Not applicable

Station 49: Breaking bad news

Theme: Breaking bad news to the relative

1. **Instructions to candidates:**

You are meeting with Mr Stuart son of 70-year-old patient Elizabeth Grace who is currently an inpatient on your ward. She was found wandering on the street by police and subsequently admitted to your ward. During investigations, it was identified on CT scan that she has a large tumor mass covering the left temporoparietal area. Her son is very concerned about her mother to be discharged back home and wants to discuss about her diagnosis and management.

Explain about the diagnosis and its management.

Address any concerns and expectations of relative.

2. **Instructions to the role player:**
   - You are Mr Stuart, son of 70-year-old patient Elizabeth Grace who is in hospital. She was admitted in hospital following being picked up by police who found her wandering on the street.
   - She was fine until 4 months ago when she started getting confused.
   - Your father died 6 years ago and she was living alone. You made her agreed to move with your family.
   - Her confusion got rapidly worse in few months.
   - You normally keep the door locked. Unfortunately the door was left open and she walked out and was found on a busy road. You know she had a CT scan.
   - The doctor haş arranged to see you. You suspect it is not good news. The doctor is going to tell you that scan has shown cancer in her brain.

   You will feel upset and will ask following questions for further clarification.

   Questions:
   - **Where has the cancer come from?**
   - **Can we do further tests to find the origin of cancer?**
   - **Are any further tests going to be uncomfortable for her?**
   - **Is the cancer making her confused?**
   - **Can anything be done to make her less confused?**
   - **How long has she left to live?**
   - **Will she be in pain?**
   - **Will she remain in hospital or move to a nursing home?**

3. **Construct:**

   This station tests the ability of the candidate to break bad news in a sensitive and empathetic manner.

4. **Expanded construct:**
   - To break bad news in compassionate manner.
   - Giving realistic opinion.

   They should:
   - Explain to the relative with the information the way he understands.
   - Address the concerns with empathetic responses.
   - The candidates should follow six steps of SPIKES:

1. Setting up the interview, such as, mental rehearsal of how one will handle emotional reactions and difficult questions.
2. *Perception:* Check understanding of situation.
3. *Obtaining invitation:* Check how much patient/relative would like to know.
4. *Giving knowledge:* Warning that bad news is coming lessens the shock.
5. Addressing patient's emotions with empathic responses.
6. *Strategy and summary:* Treatment/care plan.

- Candidates should give realistic opinion and should not take over the role of oncologist.

Interview/Communication skills:

They should include:

- Demonstration of advance listening skills.
- Diplomacy and empathy with the relative.
- Use language, i.e., simple and avoid jargon.

5. **Areas of importance to pass the station:**
   - Ability to break bad news in compassionate manner to concerned relative (40%).
   - Interview and communication skills (40%).
   - Explain role of oncologist (20%).
6. **Equipment checklist:**
   Not applicable

Station 50: Management: Agoraphobia

Theme: Explain about management of agoraphobia to the relative

1. **Instructions to candidates:**
   You have seen Elizabeth Smith, a 45-year-old housewife, in the outpatient clinic, following a referral by her GP. She suffered from a panic attack 4 months ago in super market. Since then she has stopped going out of the house on her own and is now virtually house bound. Four months ago her daughter moved out of the house. You have diagnosed her with agoraphobia. Her husband is waiting outside to see you to discuss her diagnosis and treatment. The patient has agreed to your discussing her medical details with her husband.
   Explain about the diagnosis and its management.
   Address ideas, concerns and expectations.
2. **Instructions to the role player:**
   - You are Mr Michael Smith, husband of 45-year-old patient Elizabeth.
   - She went for shopping 4 months ago to local super market where she almost fainted. She was rushed to the local Accident and Emergency department, where she was investigated but no medical reason was found for her 'fainting'. Since then she is house bound and does not leave the house on her own. You work long hours and find difficult to cope with additional responsibilities.

- Recently, you have found bottles of wine missing from cabinet.
- You consulted with your family doctor who referred her to this clinic.
- You want to know what is wrong with Elizabeth and how she can get better.
- You are somewhat puzzled and a bit annoyed that she is referred to a psychiatrist instead of a referral to a specialist physician.

The doctor is going to explain her diagnosis and go through the management plan.

You should ask the following questions:

- **What is wrong with her?**
- **How can she get better?**
- **Does she have to take tablets?**
- **What other type of treatments are available?**
- **Who will carry out the treatment?**
- **What support the family can provide?**

3. **Construct:**

The core task at this station is to test the ability of the candidate to explain the nature of agoraphobia and its immediate/short-term as well as long-term management.

4. **Expanded construct:**

- To develop rapport with concerned relative.
- To explain management plan using biopsychosocial model.

They should:

- Have knowledge of ICD-10 criteria for agoraphobia.
- Explain to the relative in simple, easy to understand manner without use of medical jargons.
- Address the concerns with empathetic responses.
- Explain the medical management, i.e., SSRIs, buspirone, beta-blockers.
- Explain psychological management, i.e., CBT using desensitization.
- Social management, i.e., self-help, family support.

Interview/Communication skills:

They should include:

- Demonstration of advanced listening skills.
- Diplomacy and empathy with the relative.
- Use language, i.e., simple and avoid jargon.

5. **Areas of importance to pass the station:**

- Explaining nature and aetiology of agoraphobia (30%).
- Discussion of management plan with a concerned relative (50%).
- Interview and communication skills (20%).

6. **Equipment checklist:**

Not applicable

Station 51: Bipolar affective disorder: Management

Theme: Explain about management of bipolar affective disorder to the relative

1. **Instructions to candidates:**

   You are meeting with the mother of 24-year-old patient, Elaine, who is currently an inpatient on your ward. She was admitted with elated mood, overspending, not sleeping and playing loud music throughout the night for the past 1 week. One and a half years ago, she was treated for depression.

   Explain about the diagnosis and its management.

   Address any other concerns mentioned.

2. **Instructions to the role player:**
   - You are Mrs Smith, mother of 24-year-old patient Elaine, who is currently in hospital.
   - Your daughter was admitted to the hospital, as she was very hyperactive, talking excessively, spending too much money on her credit card. She was not sleeping and disturbing the neighbours by playing loud music all night.
   - Fifteen months ago she was treated with anti-depressant for her depression.
   - She does not use illicit drugs or drink alcohol.
   - Her grandfather suffered from manic depression. She has no significant medical history.

     She is now diagnosed with bipolar affective disorder (Manic Depression).

     The doctor is going to come and explain the diagnosis and go through the management.

   You should ask the following questions:
   - **What is wrong with her?**
   - **What treatment is she on?**
   - **How long does she need to continue with this treatment?**
   - **Will she be able to get married and have children?**
   - **What other type of treatments are available?**
   - **What support is available after discharge?**
   - **What are her chances of getting unwell again?**
   - **Will she be able to work?**
   - **What support is available for carer like me?**
   - **Will she be allowed to drive?**
   - **How can the family help her?**
   - **Will the younger sister develop 'Bipolar'?**

3. **Construct:**

   The station tests the ability of the candidate to explain about immediate/short-term and long-term management of bipolar affective disorder.

4. **Expanded construct:**
   - To develop rapport with concerned relative.

- To explain management plan using biopsychosocial model.

They should:

- Explain to the relative with information in the language she understands.
- Address the concerns with empathetic responses.
- Know ICD-10 criteria for mood disorders.
- Explain the medical management, i.e., mood stabilizer, atypical antipsychotics, side-effects especially in pregnancy.
- Explain psychological management, i.e., Psychoeducation of patient and family, CBT.
- Social management, i.e., role of CPN, Social worker.
- Pre-discharge care programme approach (CPA) meetings and care plan.
- Involvement of other services in crisis, i.e., Crisis resolution and home treatment team.
- Give information about coping with stigma, help and support for the family.

Interview/Communication skills:

They should include:

- Demonstration of advanced listening skills.
- Diplomacy and empathy with the relative.
- Use language, i.e., simple and avoid jargon.

5. **Areas of importance to pass the station:**
   - Ability to discuss about management plan with concerned relative (40%).
   - Interview and communication skills (40%).
   - Inform parent about other services and their role (20%).

6. **Equipment checklist:**
   Not applicable

Station 52: Dementia: Management

Theme: Explain about management of dementia to the relative

1. **Instructions to candidates:**

   You are meeting with son of 68-year-old patient Sandy Smith who is currently an inpatient on your ward for 4 weeks. Police who found her wandering on a busy road brought her. She has been diagnosed with Alzheimer's dementia.

   Her son is very concerned about her mother and wants to discuss about her diagnosis and management.

   Explain about the diagnosis and its management.

   Address ideas, concerns and expectations.

2. **Instructions to the role player**
   - You are Jason Smith, son of 68-year-old patient Sandy Smith who is in hospital for last 4 weeks.

- She was admitted in hospital after the police found her.
- Your mother was well until 3 years ago when she started having problems with memory.
- You changed the gas cooker to electric and visit her every day.
- She manages her blood pressure tablets in a dosette box.
- She lives alone and you are concerned about her discharge back home.
- The doctor is going to come and explain the diagnosis and its management.

When the doctor tells you, your mum suffers from dementia you appear shocked and express "I can't believe".

You should ask the following questions:

- **What is wrong with my mum?**
- **Did she have any tests?**
- **What treatment she is on?**
- **What other type of treatments are available?**
- **I have read in newspaper about tablets that cure dementia.**
- **If she is discharged home what support is available?**
- **What support is available for carer like me?**
- **Will I get dementia?**
- **Will she be allowed to drive?**
- **Will she be able to look after her finances?**
- **How can the family provide support?**
- **How long will she live?**

3. Construct:

The core task at this station is to check the ability of the candidate to explain about immediate/short-term and after discharge management of dementia.

4. Expanded construct:

- To develop rapport with concerned relative.
- To explain management plan using biopsychosocial model.

They should:

- Explain to the relative with the information the way he understands.
- Address the concerns with empathetic responses.
- Explain dementia screening and neuropsychological assessment, occupational therapist assessment and assessment of social needs as part of management plan.
- Explain the medical management, such as, use of acetyl cholinesterase inhibitors, treatment of behavioural and psychological symptoms of dementia.
- Candidate is expected to know ICD-10 criteria for different dementias and be able to explain difference between normal aging and dementia.
- Explain non-pharmacological management, such as, reminiscence, reality orientation, validation

therapy and cognitive stimulation therapy. Alternative therapies for behaviour symptoms, such as, art, music, aromatherapy and multisensory approaches.

- Social management such as home care visits, meals-on-wheels, day center, respite care, long-term placement.
- Information about voluntary agencies, such as, Alzheimer's Society, Age Concern and Advocacy Services.
- Involvement of other services.
- Give information about financial and legal matters.

Interview/Communication skills:

They should include:

- Demonstration of advance listening skills.
- Diplomacy and empathy with the relative.
- Use simple and avoid jargon.

5. **Areas of importance to pass the station:**
   - Ability to discuss about assessment and management plan with concerned relative (30%).
   - Diagnosis explained fluently and succinctly (10%).
   - Interview and communication skills (40%).
   - Inform carer about voluntary agencies and support groups and their role (20%).
6. **Equipment checklist:**
   Not applicable.

Station 53: Obsessive Compulsive Disorder: Management

Theme: To explain management of Obsessive Compulsive Disorder (OCD) to the patient's relative

1. **Instructions to candidates:**
   Mr Wilson is husband of your patient Lorraine, who is 32-year-old and diagnosed with OCD. Her obsessional thoughts are mainly about contamination and she spends hours cleaning the house. Her husband finds it difficult to cope with her cleaning behaviours. He is attending your outpatient clinic today and intends to discuss his concerns.
   Explain about the diagnosis of Obsessive Compulsive Disorder.
   Explain about the management.
   Address Mr Wilson's concerns, beliefs and expectations.
2. **Instructions to the role player:**
   - Your wife Lorraine who is 32-year-old has been diagnosed with Obsessive Compulsive Disorder.
   - She gets repeated intrusive thoughts about spreading of germs. As a result, she spends hours dusting and cleaning the house.

- She also repeatedly washes her hands to ensure that they are clean and free from germs.
- You have 8 years old twins who are not allowed to play in back garden for fear of contamination.
- You are attending the outpatient clinic to see the doctor, who is going to explain the diagnosis and its management.

You should ask the following questions:

- **What's wrong with her?**
- **How common is OCD?**
- **How bad can OCD get?**
- **What causes OCD?**
- **What keep OCD going?**
- **How can it be treated?**
- **What other treatments are available?**
- **How I can help her?**

3. Construct:

The station checks candidate's ability to explain about OCD, its symptoms, causes and treatments both pharmacological and non-pharmacological.

4. Expanded construct:

- To develop rapport with distressed relative.
- To explain about diagnosis, symptoms, causes and different treatment options of OCD.

They should:

- Explain to the relative with information in the language he understands.
- Address the distress to the family with empathetic responses.
- Be able to see how the children are affected.
- Explain the medical management, i.e., SSRIs, clomipramine.
- Explain psychological management, i.e., Exposure and response prevention therapy (ERP).

Interview/Communication skills:

They should include:

- Demonstration of advanced listening skills.
- Diplomacy and empathy with the patient.
- Use language that is simple and avoid jargon.

5. Area of importance to pass the station:

- Ability to discuss about OCD with distressed relative (40%).
- Ability to identify stress to family (20%).
- Interview and communication skills (40%).

6. Equipment checklist:

Not applicable

Station 54: Angry and agitated patient: Management

Theme: To demonstrate an understanding and capacity to manage an acutely agitated patient suffering from paranoid schizophrenia

1. **Instructions to candidates:**

You have been asked to assess Mr Peter Parker, 22-year-old man, who has been brought to section 136 suite by police and Approved Mental Health Professional. The senior doctors have been delayed with another assessment. The police report that Mr Parker was found at a local shopping mall, talking to himself and when confronted by staff, he brandished a knife. No one was hurt, but police were called. He was observed to be talking gibberish, in the police car.

- **Talk to him to understand what is going on.**
- **Explain to him, what will happen as to further management.**
- **Address his views, expectations and concerns.**
- **Do not perform a risk assessment.**

2. **Instructions to the role player:**

- You are Peter Parker a 22-year-old man brought to a local section 136 suite by the police. You were found at a local shopping mall talking to yourself and when approached by staff, you brandished a knife. The police were called and you were brought to the section 136 suite. You are co-operative generally with the doctor.
- You know that you are an undercover agent for the secret service, MI5. You dropped out of university, physics course 2 years ago and since you have been on a secret mission as an agent for the MI5.
- You were on a special surveillance mission at the local shopping mall. You were disturbed by people and needed to scare them away before your cover was blown. You did not want to hurt anyone.
- You are very angry that the police and doctors don't understand that you are on a special mission and that they are holding you back from your job. Initially you are pleasant. As time progresses you receive messages from the secret service. You are distressed by the fact both the police and doctors don't understand despite your clear explanation.
- You generally hear voices telling you a commentary of your life as it progresses and occasionally you are told that certain people are enemies of the country and as a result you are suspicious towards them.
- You have never accessed mental health services. You are not on any medication.
- You are an only child. Your parents are separated and you have occasionally lived with your mother but often you spend time at an abandoned allotment shed, which you take as your office.
- You occasionally used cannabis at parties at university but you have not used any drugs or alcohol for 2 years.
- You don't feel you need any help and you need to get on with your job.

3. **Construct:**

The station tests the candidate's ability to build rapport with, explore and understand psychopathology in an acutely psychotic and agitated patient.

4. **Expanded construct:**
   - The candidate should be able to establish rapport with a patient suffering from acute psychosis.
   - Candidates should be able to demonstrate advanced communication skills with an acutely agitated and angry patient.
   - The candidate should be focussed, fluent and empathetic.
   - The candidate should be able to take a history and carry out the mental state examination.
   - The candidate should seek to understand what is happening and elicit symptoms of paranoid schizophrenia.

5. **Areas of importance to pass the station:**
   - Ability to elicit and explore symptoms of paranoid schizophrenia (40%).
   - Ability to manage an acutely agitated and angry patient (40%).
   - Interviewing/communication skills (20%).

6. **Equipment checklist:**
   Not applicable

Station 55: Neuroleptic Malignant Syndrome: Explanation

Theme: Explain Neuroleptic Malignant Syndrome to an angry relative

1. **Instructions to candidates:**
   You are a junior doctor looking after Erik Banna, who has a history of paranoid schizophrenia. A recent relapse of a psychotic episode was treated with haloperidol. However, Erik developed neuroleptic malignant syndrome that was promptly treated and has now fully recovered. You are due to see his father who has requested an appointment with you. The staff informed you that he appears to be angry and upset.
   - **Talk to the father and explain about Neuroleptic Malignant Syndrome (NMS).**
   - **Discuss the future management of Erik's schizophrenic illness.**
   - **Address his views, expectations and concerns.**

2. **Instructions to the role player:**
   - You are Mr Joe Banna, Erik's father. Erik suffers from paranoid schizophrenia.
   - Erik had a recent relapse after stopping his medication. He was admitted to hospital to support compliance with treatment.
   - Erik does not like coming into hospital and required compulsory detention.
   - Staff on the ward has informed you that Erik suffered NMS, which you are told is a condition that could be potentially fatal.
   - You are angry and want to see the doctors regarding this. You tell the doctors that you will make a formal complaint.
   - Erik was given haloperidol. You do not like medication and think, he may have been overdosed on the haloperidol.

- "You doctors brought him into hospital and jabbed him with medication. You're lucky, he's still alive."

You ask the following questions:

- **What is NMS?**
- **Is it life threatening?**
- **Why did you not tell me, that NMS is a side effect of the medication?**
- **I want to make a complaint.**
- **How did you treat the NMS and what will happen now?**

3. **Construct:**
The station tests the candidate's ability to explain clearly about Neuroleptic Malignant Syndrome to an angry relative and address the beliefs, concerns and expectations.

4. **Expanded construct:**
   - The candidate should be able to explain the symptoms and definition of neuroleptic malignant syndrome.
   - The candidate should be able to give a coherent explanation of the treatment and prognosis of NMS.
   - The candidate should be able to explain the need for re-challenge with antipsychotic medication in the future.
   - The candidate should be able to explain that treatment required admission to an acute hospital.
   - The candidate should be able to use language, i.e., simple and understandable and avoid jargon.

5. **Areas of importance to pass the station:**
   - Ability to respond appropriately to the questions posed (20%).
   - Ability to explain NMS in a sensitive manner (60%).
   - Communication skills (20%).

6. **Equipment checklist:**
Not applicable

Station 56: Psychodynamic psychotherapy: Explanation

Theme: To demonstrate understanding and capacity to explain psychodynamic psychotherapy

1. **Instructions to candidates:**
You are one of the psychiatric doctors working within the psychological services. The care co-ordinator of one of your patients wants to see you. You are providing psychodynamic psychotherapy to this patient. Scott Logan is due to be seen for a year and has attended once a week for the last month. You are aware of a history of sexual abuse, which has been the focus of the psychotherapy. Scott has recurrent suicidal ideation and self-harm thoughts especially in the context of breakdown in relationships.

The care co-ordinator is keen for you to take over care of the patient and discharge him from his/her caseload.

- **Talk to the care co-ordinator of Scott Logan about his/her concerns and explain psychodynamic psychotherapy principles to him/her.**

2. **Instructions to the role player:**

- You are a community psychiatric nurse whose main responsibilities have been in crisis and acute work. This has meant you have not really had the opportunity to work with patients on a longer term. Your knowledge of psychological therapy is limited.
- Scott Logan is one of your most challenging patients, who often contacts you claiming to have taken an overdose or after superficially cutting himself. He likes seeing you and does not want to be discharged from your care. You feel a lot of what he does is attention seeking and that he does not have "a real mental illness". You would prefer to discharge him from your workload. You are not sure why the psychological services cannot take over the patient. You wonder to yourself that maybe the psychological services are taking it easy.
- You are keen to discharge Scott Logan, despite a recent impulsive overdose, which he now regrets. You are due to have a meeting with the psychiatrist undergoing the psychodynamic psychotherapy with the patient.

You ask the following questions:

- **Will the psychological services take over the care of the patient?**
- **Why won't the psychological services see the patient after each overdose, in between therapy sessions?**
- **How does psychodynamic psychotherapy work?**
- **My role is pointless and I want to discharge him from my caseload.**

3. **Construct:**

The station tests the candidate's ability to explain psychodynamic psychotherapy to an anxious colleague clearly and address the beliefs, concerns and expectations.

4. **Expanded construct:**

- The candidate should be able to explain psychodynamic psychotherapy principles and methods.
- The candidate should be able to demonstrate knowledge of boundaries of length and timing of sessions.
- The candidate should be supportive and be able to explain the importance of keeping the care co-ordinator involved.
- Candidates should be able to demonstrate knowledge of the importance of containment and 'acting out'.
- The candidate should demonstrate advanced listening skills.
- The candidate should use language that is simple and understandable and avoid jargon.
- The candidate should be polite and respectful in communicating with a colleague.

5. **Areas of importance to pass the station:**
   - Ability to explain psychodynamic psychotherapy (60%).
   - Ability to respond appropriately to the questions posed (20%).
   - Communication skills (20%).

6. **Equipment checklist:**
   Not applicable

Linked Stations: 57 and 58

Station 57: Link 1: Explain: Schizophrenia and chronic cannabis use

Station 58: Link 2: Management: Schizophrenia and chronic cannabis use

Station 57: Link 1: Explain: Schizophrenia and chronic cannabis use

Theme: Explain the link between Schizophrenia and chronic cannabis use to father of a patient on your ward

1. **Instructions to candidates:**
   You are a junior doctor helping to look after Clark Lane, who has a history of paranoid schizophrenia. You are due to see his father who wants to see you, regarding his observation that Clark has been smoking cannabis for a long time. Mr Lane (Senior) believes that Clark's illness is due to his cannabis misuse.
   - **Talk to the father and explain about the link between his cannabis use and schizophrenia.**
   - **Address his views, expectations and concerns.**

2. **Instructions to the role player:**
   - You are Mr John Lane, Clark's father. Clark suffers from paranoid schizophrenia. He has been recently admitted to hospital after behaving in an odd and aggressive fashion.
   - You are angry with Clark and blame him for his illness. You are sure; his cannabis use has caused his schizophrenia. In the past, you have smelled cannabis and have challenged Clark about his smoking, but he has always denied it.
   - You are not sure how long he has been smoking cannabis for but you also have a number of relatives in your family who suffer from schizophrenia. You believe that if Clark stops his cannabis everything will be okay and he will not require any medication.

   You ask the following questions:
   - **What causes schizophrenia?**
   - **Can cannabis cause schizophrenia?**
   - **How does cannabis act?**
   - **Can cannabis cause depression?**
   - **Can schizophrenia cause cannabis addiction?**
   - **What will the doctors do now?**
   - **What can you do to help?**

3. Construct:

The station tests the candidate's ability to explain the link between prolonged cannabis use and paranoid schizophrenia to an angry relative clearly and addressing to the relatives beliefs, concerns and expectations.

4. Expanded construct:

- The candidate should be able to explain the causes of schizophrenia and the links with cannabis use.
- The candidate should be able to give a coherent explanation of the treatment and prognosis of schizophrenia, where cannabis misuse is also involved.
- The candidate should be able to explain the risk of relapse should cannabis use persist in a patient with underlying propensity for psychosis.
- The candidate should be able to explain the need for comprehensive management of schizophrenia on a long-term basis with medication and appropriate monitoring.
- The candidate should demonstrate advanced listening skills.
- The candidate should use language, i.e., simple and understandable and avoid jargon.
- The candidate should avoid a didactic pseudo-academic lecture.

5. Areas of importance to pass the station:

- Ability to explain the link between paranoid schizophrenia and prolonged cannabis misuse (60%).
- Communication skills (20%).
- Ability to respond appropriately to the questions posed (20%).

6. Equipment checklist:

Not applicable

Station 58: Link 2: Management: Schizophrenia and chronic cannabis use

Theme: Discuss the management of a patient recently diagnosed with schizophrenia with the ward consultant

1. Instructions to candidates:

You are a junior doctor helping to look after Clark Lane, who has recently been diagnosed with paranoid schizophrenia. You are due to discuss his case with the ward consultant.

- **Talk to the consultant.**
- **Discuss the management of first episode psychosis/early intervention in psychosis.**

2. Instructions to the role player:

- You are Dr Xavier, the ward consultant for Clark Lane. He suffers from paranoid schizophrenia. He has been recently admitted to hospital after behaving in an odd and aggressive fashion.
- Clark is a 24-year-old man with a long history of cannabis misuse. He smokes 20 pounds worth of cannabis daily for the last 2 years. He had a recent psychotic episode where he was hearing voices and reported being controlled by a 'presence'. He has disordered thoughts.
- He is suspicious of the doctors and believes that they are agents of the government.

You ask the following questions:

- **What would the doctor like to do to manage Clark's schizophrenia?**
- **What medication would they like to start?**
- **What alternatives to tablets are available?**
- **What would you advise regarding the risk of continued use of cannabis?**
- **What is DUP (Duration of untreated psychosis)?**
- **What scales can be used to assess the symptoms of schizophrenia?**
- **What is the prognosis?**

3. **Construct:**

The station tests the candidate's ability to explain the initial management of schizophrenia to a consultant.

4. **Expanded construct:**

- The candidate should be able to explain the acute management of schizophrenia using Biopsychosocial approach.
- The candidate should be able to explain the principles of early intervention in psychosis.
- The candidate should be able to explain the need to trial an atypical antipsychotic and trial period with options for treatment resistance.
- The candidate should be able to explain the need for monitoring on a regular basis and considerations for non-compliance.
- The candidate should be able to explain prognosis of schizophrenia.
- The candidate should be confident and fluent in his discussions.

5. **Areas of importance to pass the station:**

- Ability to explain the acute management of paranoid schizophrenia (60%).
- Communication skills (20%).
- Ability to respond appropriately to the questions posed (20%).

6. **Equipment checklist:**

Not applicable

Single Stations 59–61

Station 59: Somatisation disorder: Management

Theme: Explain somatisation disorder and its management to the husband of a patient on your ward

1. **Instructions to candidates:**

You are a junior doctor looking after Mrs Jubilee Storm, who was admitted with a sudden onset of weakness and stiffness in her right arm and left leg. These symptoms are still persisting. Neurological investigations including MRI scan of the head and spinal cord have all come back as normal. The neurologist has ruled out any physical cause of her symptoms. The staff has noticed that Mrs Storm is able to move her limbs whilst she is asleep. She has had a number of stresses in her life recently and has been diagnosed with somatisation disorder.

Steven Storm, husband of Jubilee Storm is waiting to see you to get a better understanding of his wife's condition and what can be done to help.

- **Talk to the husband and explain about somatisation disorder.**
- **Discuss the management of somatisation disorder.**
- **Address his views, expectations and concerns.**

2. Instructions to the role player:

- You are Mr Storm, Jubilee's husband who had been admitted to hospital but all the physical investigations have come back as normal.
- Jubilee is 34 and works as a manager at a local Sports Center. She has recently been promoted and she has struggled with the new management responsibilities. She is conscious that there are also likely to be redundancies.
- Jubilee's mother had a stroke recently and Jubilee acts as her main carer. Jubilee normally visits daily and helps with the shopping and cleaning. Her sister feels that care services would be more helpful and so does not get involved.
- You had also suggested to Jubilee that you should consider starting your own family, but Jubilee had felt things are very difficult with her work. There was a big row recently on the matter.
- You are also a manager at the local council and work long hours.

You have a number of questions for the doctor who has reviewed Jubilee:

- **What is somatisation disorder?**
- **Is it life threatening?**
- **How did it happen?**
- **What needs to be done to get her better?**
- **How can I help?**
- **Will she make a full recovery?**

3. Construct:

The station tests the candidate's ability to explain somatisation disorder to a relative clearly and addressing the relative's beliefs, concerns and expectations.

4. Expanded construct:

History, risk assessment and clinical features:

- The candidate should be able to explain the symptoms and definition of somatisation disorder.
- The candidate should be able to provide a coherent explanation of the treatment and prognosis of somatisation disorder.
- The candidate should demonstrate advanced listening skills.
- The candidate should be able to use language, i.e., simple and understandable and avoid jargon.
- The candidate should be able to avoid a didactic pseudoacademic lecture.

5. **Areas of importance to pass the station:**
   - Ability to explain somatisation disorder (40%).
   - Communication skills (40%).
   - Ability to respond appropriately to the questions posed (20%).

6. **Equipment checklist:**
   Not applicable.

Station 60: First episode psychosis

Theme: Discuss the aetiology of a patient recently diagnosed with first episode psychosis with the patient's mother and address her views, concerns and expectations

1. **Instructions to candidates:**

   You are a junior doctor looking after John Snow, who has recently been diagnosed with first episode psychosis. You are due to discuss the aetiology of first episode psychosis with the patient's mother.

   - **Talk to the mother.**
   - **Discuss the aetiology of first episode psychosis.**
   - **Address her views, expectations and concerns.**

2. **Instructions to the role player:**
   - You are Mrs Snow, John's mother. John has suffered a first episode of psychosis. He has been recently admitted to hospital after claiming he had received a message from the star Alpha Century, that he has been selected to bring back to life, Jesus.
   - John is a 24-year-old man who was working at the local nightclub as a bouncer. On one occasion he had let too many people in and as a result Russia will now invade Afghanistan. He feels he is responsible. He feels that news has now spread to Moscow and special agents have been sent to UK to track him down. He is under surveillance. He has seen spy vans and there are bugs on the telephones at home.
   - He has informed you of this. But you did not believe this. So he informed the police to arrest him for his crimes.
   - He feels that neighbours are talking about him. When he watches television he feels that the people are referring to him and it has all got too much for him to handle. He is not sleeping or eating well and lost interest in his self-care. He is not bathing or combing his hair.
   - He reported hearing two men talking about him and what he was doing. Sometimes they tell him that they are "out to get him".
   - He is suspicious of the doctors and feels that they are agents of the government.
   - He had a difficult birth and was born in January. He spent a few days in the special care baby unit but made a fast recovery and achieved normal milestones. He was a happy child but was often bullied at school for being 'odd'.

- You separated from John's father when John was seven. John dropped out of school after his GCSE's as he found studying too stressful. He does not have many friends.
- He occasionally has used cannabis but no other illicit drugs. He does not drink alcohol.

You are not sure about the diagnosis.

You ask the following questions:

- **What is the cause of John's psychosis?**
- **Did you have anything to do with it?**
- **Am I to blame?**
- **Did it start all of a sudden?**
- **Could you have done anything to prevent it?**
- **Does it only affect young people?**
- **Is there a chemical imbalance or anything twisted in his brain?**
- **Will he be cured?**

3. **Construct:**

The station tests the candidate's ability to explain the aetiology of psychosis.

4. **Expanded construct:**

- The candidate should be able to explain the aetiology of psychosis.
- The candidate should be able to explain multi-factorial causation of psychosis.
- The candidate should demonstrate advanced listening skills.
- The candidate should be able to ask questions that are structured, focused and fluent.
- The candidate should be able to use language, i.e., simple and understandable and avoid jargon.
- The candidate should be able to avoid a didactic pseudo-academic lecture.

5. **Areas of importance to pass the station:**

- Ability to explain the aetiology of psychosis (60%).
- Communication skills (20%).
- Ability to respond appropriately to the questions posed (20%).

6. **Equipment checklist:**

Not applicable

Station 61: Rapid tranquilisation

Theme: Explain rapid tranquilisation and its management to an angry and agitated father of a patient on your ward

1. **Instructions to candidates:**

You are specialist registrar looking after Anthony Stark, who has a history of bipolar affective disorder. A recent episode of severe agitation and aggression required rapid tranquilisation. You are due to see his father.

- **Talk to Anthony's father and explain about rapid tranquilisation.**
- **Address his views, expectations and concerns.**

2. **Instructions to the role player:**
   - You are Mr Stark, Anthony's father. Anthony suffers from bipolar affective disorder.
   - Anthony had a recent relapse after stopping his medication. He was admitted to hospital under compulsory detention to support compliance with treatment.
   - The staff on the ward has informed you that Anthony has not stopped talking since admission. He is running around the ward and even jumped up and down from the dining table. The staff tried to settle him down, but he became irritable and aggressive and started smashing the window to the exit.
   - The doctors were called and despite attempts to settle Anthony, he required an intramuscular injection of an antipsychotic medication to settle him down. He was heavily sedated and required to sleep for a few hours.

   You ask the following questions:
   - **Why did he need an injection?**
   - **Could he not have been nursed better?**
   - **Will he be ok, he is sleeping a lot?**
   - **Will he always be like this?**
   - **Are there any other side effects?**

3. **Construct:**
   The station tests the candidate's ability to explain rapid tranquilisation to an angry relative empathetically and clearly as well as address the relative's beliefs, concerns and expectations.

4. **Expanded construct:**
   History, risk assessment and clinical features:
   - The candidate should be able to explain the need for rapid tranquilisation.
   - The candidate should be able to give a coherent explanation of the treatment of acute agitation.
   - The candidate should be able to explain psychological and supportive methods used prior to medication.
   - The candidate should be able to explain appropriate safety procedures and monitoring of physical health.
   - The candidate should be able to explain urgency and risk assessment to self and others.
   - The candidate should be able to demonstrate advanced listening skills.
   - The candidate should be able to use language that is simple and understandable and avoid jargon.
   - The candidate should be able to avoid a didactic pseudo-academic lecture.

5. **Areas of importance to pass the station:**
   - Ability to explain rapid tranquilisation (60%).
   - Communication skills (20%).
   - Ability to respond appropriately to the questions posed (20%).

6. **Equipment checklist:**
   Not applicable

Linked Stations: 62 and 63

Station 62: Link 1: Schizotypal disorder: History taking

Station 63: Link 2: Schizotypal disorder: Differential diagnosis

Station 62: Link 1: Schizotypal disorder: History taking

Theme: Schizotypal disorder: History taking to arrive at a diagnosis and differential diagnosis

1. **Instructions to candidates:**

   You are asked to see Peter Riley who calls himself 'El-Thor' following a referral by social services as he refuses to move from his residence which was in a poorly maintained state. He is odd and seems quiet withdrawn. Social services are concerned about his mental health and have requested you for an assessment.

   Take a relevant history from Peter with a view of reaching a diagnosis/differential diagnosis. You may wish to take notes as you will be presenting your findings and management plan to the consultant in the next station.

2. **Instructions to the role player:**

   - You are 38-year-old Peter Riley. You prefer to be called 'El-Thor' and correct the doctor every time they call you Peter.
   - You have very little emotional expression on the face and appear cold and aloof. You say that you expected this appointment as you have seen it in the crystal ball.
   - When you were a child you had said a flying saucer and 'maybe' the aliens abducted you and sent you back with powers of 'sixth sense'. Since then you are 'my own company'.
   - You behave in an odd and peculiar manner, moving your hands in the air as if you were trying to read something and close your eyes intermittently. When asked you say that you have sixth sense and an ability of clairvoyance. You are trying to read the aura of the room.
   - You have a large mark on your forehead which you make every day to signify membership to an elite 'clairvoyance' group of chosen few who also believe in aliens and 'may be abducted by aliens at some point in the life'.
   - You do not have any friends, prefer to stay by yourself and spend most of the time in the room.
   - You do not trust people; at times feel they are laughing or talking about you. You have some degree of paranoia and suspiciousness.
   - At times you get out of body experience and you think you are not real.
   - You make comments in between the interview like 'You are like star, moon; have to make sure the world moves, round the sky, up and down'. When asked, you say it is a 'telepathic ritual' you have to do every half hour as a part of clairvoyance group.
   - You do not have any psychotic, depressive or other features of mental illness. No previous psychiatric treatment or admission. No drugs, alcohol or physical health concerns.
   - You are not bothered of what the social services think or do. You just prefer to be left alone.

3. **Construct:**

   This station assess whether candidate have knowledge and are able to take a history to elicit schizotypal personality disorder and consider other differential diagnosis.

4. **Expanded construct:**
   - The candidate should be able to demonstrate skill in eliciting a history from a patient who is odd, peculiar and behaving in a bizarre manner.
   - Its onset, duration, progress and associated factors.
   - Knowledge of ICD-10 and DSM-V criteria of schizotypal disorder. According to ICD-10, patients should have at least three or four typical features like being cold and aloof, odd behaviour, beliefs and thinking, paranoia and suspiciousness, ruminations without resistance, unusual perceptual experiences like depersonalisation, derealisation or illusions.
   - They should ask questions about differential diagnosis like depression, schizophrenia, physical illness, schizoaffective disorder and other relevant conditions.

5. **Areas of importance to pass the station:**
   - Eliciting accurate and sufficient information about schizotypal disorder and differential diagnosis (60%).
   - Eliciting relevant associated risk (20%).
   - Communication (20%).

6. **Equipment checklist:**

   Not applicable

Station 63: Link 2: Schizotypal disorder: Differential diagnosis

Theme: Schizotypal disorder and differential Diagnosis: Discussion with consultant psychiatrist

1. **Instructions to candidates:**

   You have seen Peter Riley in your outpatient clinic. As a part of case-based discussion, talk to the consultant psychiatrist about your assessment and management plan.

2. **Instructions to the role player:**
   - You are Dr David Smith, Consultant Psychiatrist (clinical supervisor) of the specialty registrar who has assessed Mr Riley and wants to discuss the case with you.
   - You are keen to know about the diagnosis, differential diagnosis and management plan.

   You ask the following questions:
   - **Tell me about the case.**
   - **What do you think is the diagnosis and differential diagnosis?**
   - **What criteria for diagnosis have you looked at and are there any differences (ICD-10 and DSM-V)?**

- **Have you considered any other diagnosis?**

  What are your views on the likely aetiology and prognosis of this condition?
- **Are there any risks involved? Ask this question only if not covered.**

  How will you proceed now?
- **What is your management plan?**
- **What about social services and their concerns?**

3. Construct:

This station assess whether candidate have knowledge about schizotypal disorder, differences in ICD-10 and DSM-V criteria, relevant differential diagnosis and management plan.

4. Expanded construct:

- The candidate should be able to communicate in a professional manner providing a comprehensive formulation and using appropriate jargon.
- Demonstrate knowledge of ICD -10 and DSM-V criteria and differences of schizotypal disorder. In ICD-10, it is classified along with schizophrenia and in DSM-V it is under personality disorder cluster (Cluster A).
- Demonstrate consideration or relevant differential diagnosis like depression, schizophrenia, physical illness, schizoaffective disorder and other relevant conditions.
- Knowledge of aetiology, management, prognosis, risks associated with schizotypal disorder and relationship with schizophrenia.
- Demonstrate importance of collateral history and involvement of other agencies where appropriate.

5. Areas of importance to pass the station/Examiner briefing notes:

- Discussion of diagnosis and differential diagnosis (40%).
- Differences in ICD-10 and DSM IV-criteria of Schizotypal disorder (20%) .
- Aetiology, prognosis, risks, management plan (20%).
- Communication in a professional manner (20%).

6. Equipment checklist:

Not applicable.

Single Stations: 64–80

Station 64: Persistent Delusional Disorder: Capgras' syndrome

Theme: Persistent delusional disorder/Capgras' syndrome: History taking

1. Instructions to candidates:

You are asked to see 62-year-old woman Simone Barry who has been referred by her GP following concerns regarding her mental health. For the last 1 year, she has been behaving in an odd fashion.

She locks herself in the bedroom every night and her husband has to sleep in the lounge.

Take a history and do a relevant risk assessment. Address her fears, anxieties and expectations.

2. **Instructions to the role player:**
    - You are Simone Barry, 62 years old and live with your husband Jacob (68 years).
    - You present as worried and fearful during the interview and need lot of reassurance that you are safe.
    - You have been married for 30 years and have three grown up children who live nearby. You have a good relationship with family.
    - You ask doctor repeatedly "take him away, take him away".

    You mentioned of the following when asked:
    - For the past 18 months, things have 'not being right' "something strange is happening to you".
    - You have realised that an imposter has replaced your husband Jacob. Initially you thought it was a daft idea. However, in the last 6 months you are convinced that this is true as you have noticed a change in his face, eyes are wider, nose is smaller and there is scar under this chin which was not there before. He talks like your husband but sometimes you can make out the difference in the voice.
    - You think he may be 'the one' who had abused you when you were a child.
    - You are fearful and do not want him anywhere near you. You are scared to be in the same house with him, lock the bedroom in the night sleeping by yourself and wake up at the slightest noise to make sure you are safe.
    - You have thought about keeping a knife with you for your safety, but did not go ahead as "he may get the hint and then attack me". You are too scared of him to go near him or hurt him.
    - All the other family members are the same. They believe he is your husband and "are easily fooled by him".
    - You are vigilant, fearful for your safety and are thinking of running away but not sure where and when. You do not intend to kill or harm yourself.
    - You do not have any other symptoms of depression or psychosis.
    - You suffer from diabetes and stroke. Presently, you are well and taking your physical medications as prescribed.

3. **Construct:**

    This station assess whether candidate have knowledge about delusion of misidentification mainly Capgras' disorder and other persistent delusional disorders.

4. **Expanded construct:**
    - The candidate should be able to elicit detailed and systematic history of delusion of misidentification.
    - Demonstrate knowledge by exploring differential diagnosis like schizophrenia and other psychotic disorders including organic cause.
    - Elicit onset, duration, progress and associated factors.
    - Able to elicit delusion and related set of delusions that do not meet criteria for schizophrenia, presence for more than 3 months, no major psychotic features.

- Knowledge of aetiology, management, prognosis, risks associated persistent delusional disorder.
- Elicit risks associated with this condition.

5. **Areas of importance to pass the station:**
   - Eliciting accurate and sufficient information about persistent delusional disorder/Capgras' syndrome and differential diagnosis (40%).
   - Assess risk of suicide/self-harm/harm to others (20%).
   - Address patient's concerns and expectations (20%).
   - Communication (20%).
6. **Equipment checklist:**
   Not applicable

Station 65: Persistent Delusional Disorder (Delusional Parasitosis): History taking

Theme: Persistent delusional disorder (Delusional Parasitosis): History Taking

1. **Instructions to candidates:**

   Mrs Lisa Berry, 42 years of age, has been referred to your psychiatric outpatient clinic from the dermatology clinic where she presented few years ago with complaints of pruritus all over her body. Following thorough investigations and various treatment regimes, no cause has been identified and the dermatologist thinks this is psychosomatic in nature. Mrs Berry has reluctantly agreed to see you in the clinic.

   Take a history with a view of reaching a differential diagnosis. Address her fears, anxieties, concerns and expectations.

2. **Instructions to the role player:**

   You are Lisa Berry, 42 years of age, living with your partner of 2 years in a council flat. You resigned from your job as a teacher 3 years ago, had to move into a council property due to financial difficulties and are on benefits, which you dislike due to the problem you are suffering. You are distracted, seem uncomfortable and scratch intermittently. You describe the following problem when asked:

   - Six years ago, while on holiday in Tanzania, you were admitted to the hospital following an insect bite that led to a 'reaction'.
   - Six months following your return to UK, you started experiencing itching at the site of insect bite. You noticed that this itching was spreading to other parts of your body. You spend nearly 8–10 hours scratching various parts of body, but to no relief.
   - You are convinced that following insect bite, eggs were deposited into your skin and there are several 'nasty bugs' floating in your body. You at times can feel them crawling under your skin. It seems as if "I have a skin under my skin where they live".
   - These bugs have infected your body fluids, which cause various symptoms like increased bleeding, headaches, intermittent fever and body aches. You have consulted your GP, gynaecologist, eye doctor and many other specialists but no one can 'help me'.

- You sleep on the chair at night, as you fear that these 'bugs' will enter into your brain if you lie down and damage it.
- You feel depressed and suicidal as no one can help you and you have lost your job and house.
- You do not have any other symptoms of psychosis or other mental illness.

You want to know if the doctor can help you to remove these bugs, may be by radiation, strong chemical inside your body or even 'electric therapy'.

3. **Construct:**

   This station assess whether candidate have knowledge and are able to take a history to elicit persistent delusional disorder (delusional parasitosis) and consider other differential diagnosis.

4. **Expanded construct:**
   - The candidate should be able to demonstrate skill in eliciting a detailed and systematic history of persistent delusional disorder from a patient who is worried, distressed and distracted due to her symptoms.
   - Demonstrate knowledge of persistent delusional disorder and criteria according to ICD-10 classification system. Able to elicit delusion and related set of delusions that do not meet criteria for schizophrenia, presence for more than 3 months, no major psychotic features.
   - Elicit origin, duration, progression and associated factors of the condition.
   - They should ask questions about differential diagnosis like depression, schizophrenia, and side effects of medications, physical illness and other relevant conditions.
   - They should assess the risk of suicide and self-harm.
   - They need to elicit the patient's concerns and expectations and address them accordingly.

5. **Areas of importance to pass the station:**
   - Eliciting accurate and sufficient information about persistent delusional disorder/Delusional Parasitosis and differential diagnosis (40%).
   - Assess risk of suicide/self-harm/harm to others (20%).
   - Address patient's fears, anxieties, concerns and expectations (20%).
   - Communication (20%).

6. **Equipment checklist:**

   Not applicable.

Station 66: Post-Schizophrenic depression

Theme: Post-Schizophrenic depression: History and discussion

1. **Instructions to candidates:**

   You are about to see Joseph Dent in the outpatient clinic. His care co-ordinator has expressed concerns that even though he is taking olanzapine 20 mg for schizophrenia, he spends most of his time in the room and refuses to engage in any other activities. He has recovered from most of his psychotic symptoms.

   Talk to him and take a brief history for his presentation and address his concerns and expectations.

2. **Instructions to the role player:**

You are 28-year-old Joseph Dent and suffer from schizophrenia for the past 5 years. You were discharged from the inpatient unit 8 weeks ago, following a brief admission. When unwell, you believe that you are a member of a secret society, the purpose of which is to prevent World War III and hear voice of devil, which is derogatory. You are taking olanzapine 20 mg regularly. When asked you describe following:

- Since discharge, the voice of devil has reduced in intensity and frequency and you do not believe that you are a member of secret society. There are no other psychotic symptoms.
- You have good insight into your illness, accept treatment and take olanzapine 20 mg regularly. You do not have any side effects except mild weight gain. You do not have any other physical health problems, stressors or worries.
- For the past 4 weeks you feel low in mood, don't enjoy activities and feel tired most of the time.
- You are unable to think clearly and have poor motivation, attention and concentration.
- You are unable to express your emotions, feel worthless and blame yourself for who you are feeling.
- You have been getting thoughts of suicide for the past 2 weeks. You do not have an intention to act on these thoughts.

You want to know what is wrong with you and what else can be done to get better.

3. **Construct:**

This station assess whether candidate are able to take a history to elicit post-schizophrenic depression and consider other differential diagnosis.

4. **Expanded construct:**

- The candidate should be able to demonstrate skill in eliciting a history a patient who has marked apathy and pick up relevant information about post-schizophrenic depression.
- Its origin, duration, progress and associated factors.
- They should ask questions about differential diagnosis like depression, negative symptoms of schizophrenia, side effects of medications, physical illness, schizophrenia with negative symptoms, schizoaffective disorder and other relevant conditions.
- They should assess the risk of suicide and self-harm.
- They need to elicit the patient's concerns and expectations and address them accordingly. For example, explaining what post-schizophrenic depression, aetiology, treatment, possible other differential diagnosis and further management.
- Demonstrate the knowledge in history taking that depression arising following schizophrenic illness where the psychotic symptoms are minimal is likely to be post-schizophrenic depression. Patients in this case are at a higher risk of suicide.
- If depression is associated with prominent schizophrenia symptoms, diagnosis should remain as schizophrenia. If depression is present in the absence of any schizophrenic symptoms, it should be diagnosed as a depressive episode.

5. **Areas of importance to pass the station:**

- Eliciting accurate and sufficient information about post-schizophrenic depression, differential diagnosis (40%).

- Assess risk of suicide/self-harm (20%).
- Address patient's concerns and expectations (20%).
- Communication (20%).

6. **Equipment checklist:**
   Not applicable.

Station 67: Residual schizophrenia

Theme: Residual Schizophrenia: Collateral History

1. **Instructions to candidates:**
   You are about to meet Jessica Parker, mother of David Parker, who has schizophrenia for the last 4 years. She is concerned about David and wants to talk to you about him.
   - **Take a relevant collateral history from Jessica Parker and**
   - **Address her fears, anxieties concerns and expectations about her son.**
2. **Instructions to the role player:**
   You are Jessica Parker, mother of 32-year-old David who has schizophrenia for the past 4 years. David has been admitted on two occasions with deterioration of mental health, last being 2 years ago. He lives with you and you are clearly concerned about his future and quality of life. You have following concerns when asked:
   - David has schizophrenia "a life changing condition" for the past 4 years.
   - He was doing a job as a teaching assistant before he became unwell.
   - When unwell, he hears voices, sees things, is paranoid and says that 'she' (Jessica) is a devil who wants to kill him. He will talk nonsensical, i.e., not make any sense and refuse to take his medication.
   - He has been well for the past year and a half and does not have these symptoms.
   - You are worried as he does not show emotions and has no facial expressions.
   - You think he has become very lazy and careless with a laissez faire attitude.
   - Speaks very little in monosyllables, does not maintain eye contact and does not engage in activities.
   - Needs lot of promoting to do his chores and take care of him. He does not eat unless offered, wears the same clothes every day and does not shave for days. He is neglecting his care and health.
   - He is on risperidone injection which he takes every 2 weeks, does not have any physical health problems or worries.

   You ask following questions after the history is taken:
   - **What is wrong with my son?**
   - **Will he ever work or have a family?**
   - **How can I motivate him?**
   - **Am I responsible for not pushing him harder?**

- **What is the treatment?**
- **What is the reason for this?**

3. **Construct:**

This station assess whether candidate have knowledge and are able to take a collateral history to elicit residual schizophrenia and consider other differential diagnosis.

4. **Expanded construct:**
   - The candidate should be able to demonstrate skill in eliciting a collateral history from mother of a patient who has marked negative symptoms of schizophrenia.
   - Its origin, duration of at least for a year, progress and associated factors.
   - Demonstrate the knowledge by eliciting that residual schizophrenia has at least four negative symptoms that are present for at least 12 months, general criteria of schizophrenia should have been met at some point in past but not presently.
   - They should ask questions about differential diagnosis like depression, side effects of medications, physical illness, schizoaffective disorder and other relevant conditions.
   - They should assess the risk of suicide and self-harm.
   - They need to elicit mother's fears, anxieties, concerns and expectations and address them accordingly.
   - Demonstrate knowledge of aetiology, prognosis and management of residual schizophrenia.

5. **Areas of importance to pass the station:**
   - Eliciting accurate and sufficient information about residual schizophrenia and differential diagnosis (50%).
   - Address mother's fears, anxieties, concerns and expectations (30%).
   - Communication (20%).

6. **Equipment checklist:**

Not applicable.

Station 68: Acute polymorphic psychotic disorder with symptoms of schizophrenia

Theme: Acute polymorphic psychotic disorder with symptoms of schizophrenia: Collateral history from patient's son

1. **Instructions to candidates:**

You are about to see Mr Benjamin France, son of Bernadette France (58 years) who apparently is unwell again for the third time and an inpatient in the psychiatric hospital. She was admitted following a bizarre behaviour, being motionless, irritable and impaired cognition.

Take a collateral history with a view of reaching a diagnosis/differential diagnosis. Address his fears, anxieties, concerns and expectations.

2. **Instructions to the role player:**

You are Benjamin France, son of 58-year-old Bernadette France. She has been admitted to a psychiatric hospital for the third time in past 10 years. Previous two admissions were about 4 and

6 years ago in France, initial country of residence. As the doctor has limited information of past history, you have been asked to see the doctor. You have following information to share when asked:

- Previous two admissions were 4 years and 6 years ago lasting for 1 week and then 3 weeks respectively.
- Prior to both admissions:
  - You saw your mother becoming rapidly unwell in a couple of days. She became confused and looked puzzled.
  - Initially, she was mute and motionless. Few hours later, she became restless, irritable and started talking in a language that made little sense.
  - She was wandering on the streets, moving furniture in the house, repeatedly filling and emptying water from a bottle and other bizarre behaviour.
  - She did not sleep or eat well. Once she woke up in the middle of the night and said that she has to go to work, as she is already late. She was very anxious and shaking.
  - Next day, she said that she is dying and was fearful. She reported seeing her dead uncle saying he has come to 'take her' and became obsessed with dying and death.
  - On both occasions she was admitted, thoroughly investigated and treated with anti-psychotic medication. She recovered within days and maintained full recovery without any problems in between the episodes.
  - She used to say that everyone was plotting against her and trying to kill her.
  - Doctors said that she had psychotic episode may be schizophrenia 'but not sure'.
- This admission:
  - Similar presentation but seemed happy and ecstatic for no reason initially before she stopped talking and moving. Rest of the presentation was same.
  - Knowing her condition, you think treating her with anti-psychotic for few days will make her completely normal.
- Your mother has no history of alcohol, drug use or smoking. She had one previous operation where a part of thyroid was removed due to raised thyroid hormones. She is presently taking thyroid hormones for low thyroid. No other significant family history.
- She has been completely normal in between the episodes.

You ask the doctor:

- **Does my mother suffer from schizophrenia?**
- **What else can it be if not schizophrenia?**
- **Can you treat this illness aggressively so that it does not come back?**

3. **Construct:**

This station assess the knowledge of the candidate and are ability to take a collateral history to elicit longitudinal history and symptomatology of acute polymorphic disorder with schizophrenia (Cycloid psychosis with symptoms of schizophrenia) and relevant differential diagnosis of acute and transient psychotic disorder.

4. **Expanded construct:**
   - The candidate should be able to demonstrate skill in eliciting a detailed and systematic collateral history of acute and transient psychotic disorder (according to ICD-10 criteria) mainly acute polymorphic disorder with and without symptoms of schizophrenia.
   - Elicit origin, duration, progression and associated factors of the condition that suggests cycloid psychosis with symptoms of schizophrenia.
   - They should ask questions regarding relevant differential diagnosis of psychotic disorder mainly acute transient psychotic disorders.
   - They need to elicit son's concerns and expectations and address them accordingly.
5. **Areas of importance to pass the station:**
   - Eliciting accurate and sufficient collateral information about acute and transient psychotic disorders – Acute polymorphic disorder with symptoms of schizophrenia and differential diagnosis (50%).
   - Address patient's fears, anxieties, concerns and expectations (30%).
   - Communication (20%).
6. **Equipment checklist:**
   Not applicable

Station 69: Schizoaffective disorder: Mixed type

Theme: Schizoaffective disorder, Mixed type: History from son

1. **Instructions to candidates:**

   You are about to see Mr Graham Bell, son of Jess Bell (42 years) who has been admitted to a psychiatric inpatient unit as she was shouting, disturbing neighbours and tried to jump out of her 5th floor apartment. She was admitted following a Section 136 MHA assessment (English Mental Health Act). You have not reviewed her yet in the ward, but are asked to gather collateral history form her son Mr Bell to guide further management plan.

   Take a collateral history from Mr Bell with a view of reaching a diagnosis/differential diagnosis to guide further management plan. Address his fears, anxieties, concerns and expectations.

2. **Instructions to the role player:**

   You are Graham Bell, son of 42-year-old Jess Bell. She lives alone in 5th floor apartment. She had two previous episodes of her illness in the past 8 years. You are in university and studying a course in business administration. You are on term break and have been staying with your mother for 4 weeks. You noticed that she has been behaving strangely for the past 3 weeks. You provide the following information when asked:

   - Three weeks ago, your mother told you that she could read your mind, fly like a bird and heal the world. You thought she was joking and 'out of her mind' figuratively.
   - In a couple of days she started talking very fast, was difficult to interrupt, had lots of new ideas, cleaned the whole flat three times in a day, did not sleep or eat and was talking 'gibberish'. She started throwing garbage out of the window and shouting at strangers.

- She thinks that people are interfering with her thoughts. She accuses me of stealing her ideas and thoughts and thinks that her ideas are on the TV and radio. She talks to herself and at times it appears that she is talking to someone who is not there. She believes that I and other people will kill her as she has special abilities of flying and reading mind.
- There have been periods, lasting for 3–4 days, when she becomes sad and depressed. She stops talking, does not eat and sits on the sofa with a vacant stare. It appears as if she lost all motivation, enthusiasm and energy. She has on a couple of occasions expressed thoughts of suicide.
- Last 2 days she has again been 'high' and 'full of energy'. She tried to jump out of the window to show you how she can fly. You stopped her, called an ambulance and police who took her to hospital.
- Your grandmother had depression. No other family history. No drugs, alcohol or physical health concerns.

You ask the doctor:

- **What is wrong with my mother?**
- **What is the reason for her problem?**
- **Will she get better and remain well for a long time?**
- **She tried to jump out of the window. Is the ward safe?**

3. **Construct:**

This station assesses whether candidate has knowledge of schizoaffective disorder and its different types. This station assesses the ability to elicit a detailed and systematic collateral history from a worried son about schizoaffective disorder and its differential diagnosis.

4. **Expanded construct:**

- The candidate should be able to demonstrate skill in eliciting a detailed and systematic collateral history of schizoaffective disorder.
- Elicit origin, duration, progression and associated factors of the condition that suggests schizoaffective disorder, mixed type.
- They should ask questions regarding relevant differential diagnosis of psychotic disorder and affective disorder.
- They need to elicit son's concerns and expectations and address them accordingly.

5. **Areas of importance to pass the station:**

- Eliciting accurate and sufficient collateral information of schizoaffective disorder and differential diagnosis (40%).
- Assessment of relevant risk factors (20%).
- Address patient's fears, anxieties, concerns and expectations (20%).
- Communication (20%).

6. **Equipment checklist:**

Not applicable

Station 70: Cyclothymia: History

Theme: Cyclothymia: History taking and discussion

1. **Instructions to candidates:**

   You are asked to see Sarah Parker, 26-year-old student, who is convinced that she has got bipolar affective disorder. She is referred to your clinic following her request to her general practitioner.

   Talk to her with a view of taking a history and address her fears, anxieties, concerns and expectations.

2. **Instructions to the role player:**

   You are Sarah, 26-years of age doing a university degree in architecture. You are worried that you have bipolar disorder and that you will "end up like your mother". Do not talk about your mother unless asked about your family and if there is any mental illness in family.

   When asked you describe the following:

   - Since the age of 16 years, you have noticed mood changes and fluctuations.
   - Most of the time you feel down, have low energy and motivation. You have low motivation and poor self-esteem. You are unable to make decisions easily without things going round and round in your head. Some days you just want to spend time by yourself and stare at the wall. However, you can make an effort to go out with friends, do your work and studies and take care of yourself.
   - In the past 4 years, you have noticed periods where your mood is 'high' and you feel 'happier in me'. You feel like you have got "new gush of enthusiasm and motivation". You are able to achieve most things in this state. These 'high' last for 3–4 days and then you feel low again.
   - At times you find it difficult to concentrate and do your assignments. However, you 'push' yourself and get things done. "But it is an effort".
   - You cannot identify any particular stressor, worry or reason for this fluctuation in mood.
   - You do not remember any period since you were 16 years, where you felt normal. It has been either low or high mood.
   - Your mood changes are "not as bad as my mother's". Your mother has been diagnosed to have Bipolar disorder for the past 12 years is taking mood stabiliser Lithium. When your mother is 'down' she stops taking care of her, does not meet or talk to anyone, is very low, does not enjoy anything and has suicidal thoughts. She has tried to kill herself twice since she has been unwell. When your mother is 'high' she talks very fast, has lots of ideas in her head, thinks she knows everything and can read peoples future, buys stuff that is not needed and does risky things. She has been admitted to hospital four times so far.
   - You are aware that your episodes of high and low are different and may be milder than your mother's mood changes.
   - You are frightened and worried that you have got Bipolar disorder and want to start treatment early so that you do not end up like 'my mother'.

   You ask the following:

   - **I have bipolar affective disorder, don't I?**

- **Can you start me on lithium? If not, something else to keep me sane.**
- **I don't like feel like this all the time. I don't even know why this is happening. Can you help me?**
- **What is going on if this is not bipolar affective disorder?**
- **Will I get bipolar disorder in future?**
- **How can I prevent bipolar disorder in future?**

3. **Construct:**
   This station assesses candidate's knowledge of persistent mood (affective) disorder and ability to elicit history from a worried woman and discuss the diagnosis of cyclothymia and other possible differential diagnoses.

4. **Expanded construct:**
   - The candidate should be able to demonstrate skill in eliciting a history a patient who is pre-occupied and worried that she has bipolar disorder.
   - The candidate should be able to elicit origin, duration, progress, severity and associated factors of the mood fluctuations.
   - The candidate should inquire about family history of mental illness, illicit substance use and relevant personal history.
   - They should establish the persistent, fluctuating mature of mood, where the individual episodes are mild in nature and that they do not meet the criteria for hypomania/mania or depressive disorder.
   - They should allay patient's anxiety, worries and fears. They should discuss that some individuals with cyclothymia can persist throughout life, may improve for temporarily or develop into bipolar affective disorder. Discuss the genetic vulnerability due to positive family history.
   - They should discuss the overall prognosis and evidence of treatment.

5. **Areas of importance to pass the station:**
   - Eliciting accurate and sufficient information about mood fluctuations, severity of episodes and impact on social life and functioning (50%).
   - Allay patient's anxieties, fears and concerns (30%).
   - Communication (20%).

6. **Equipment checklist:**
   Not applicable

Station 71: Dysthymia: History

Theme: Dysthymia: History taking and discussion

1. **Instructions to candidates:**

   You are asked to see Lily Jenkinson, 52 years of age. She complains of low mood and has tried two antidepressants without much benefit. She has been referred to your clinic for specialist advice.

   Take to her with a view of taking a history and address her fears, anxieties, concerns and expectations.

2. **Instructions to the role player:**

You are 52-year-old Lily Jenkinson, married for 20 years and employed as a cleaner. You have been off sick for few days on several occasions due to tiredness and fatigue. you maintain good eye contact, are cooperative and engaging. Though you say you are depressed you can smile and have normal expression. You give the following information when asked:

- You have depressed mood for the last 20 years. You have tried citalopram and venlafaxine without any benefit.
- You have 'always' felt depressed. There have been few days in the last 20 years when you feel good 'but that is all'.
- You feel tired, fatigued and drained.
- You are unable to concentrate on your job. You do your job just because you have to make ends meet. You don't like being on benefits.
- You find it difficult to cope with work, family and housework. You find it overwhelming.
- You brood and have persistent negative thoughts about your past.
- You have tried citalopram and venlafaxine medications for several months. This had no benefit whatsoever.
- You are happy to consider help but are not hopeful that you will ever get better.
- You continue to go work and do the chores as best as you can even if it is an effort.
- You do not have a history of severe depression, hypomania/mania, hospitalization or any other symptoms of mental illness or physical illness.
- You do not have a history of self-harm/attempted suicide.

You ask:

- **Why me?**
- **Why is the depression medication not working?**
- **I think "I will always stay depressed".**
- **What is dysthymia and how do you treat it?**

3. **Construct:**

This station assesses candidate's knowledge of persistent mood (affective) disorder and ability to elicit history from a woman who has dysthymia.

4. **Expanded construct:**

- The candidate should be able to demonstrate skill in eliciting a history a patient who has dysthymia.
- The candidate should be able to elicit origin, duration, progress, severity and associated factors.
- The candidate should inquire about family history of mental illness, illicit substance use, past psychiatric history/treatment and relevant personal history.
- They should establish the chronic depression of mood, that is lasting for several years and that it is not sufficient enough to meet criteria for recurrent depressive disorder.

- They should allay patient's anxiety, worries and fears.
- They should explain dysthymia, aetiology, prognosis and management to the patient.
- They should discuss the overall prognosis and evidence of treatment.

5. **Areas of importance to pass the station:**
   - Eliciting accurate and sufficient information about chronic nature of mood, severity of episodes and impact on social life and functioning (50%).
   - Allay patient's anxieties, fears and concerns (30%).
   - Communication (20%).

6. **Equipment checklist:**
   Not applicable

Station 72: Bipolar affective disorder, manic episode with psychotic symptoms

Theme: Bipolar affective disorder, manic episode with psychotic symptoms: Take History

1. **Instructions to candidates:**
   You are talking to Dennis Brown, 37-year-old Caucasian man, who has been brought to accident and emergency by his community psychiatric nurse (CPN). Dennis wants to go as he has a flight to board and he has asked if you can keep the interview short. He has a diagnosis of bipolar affective disorder and had been in remission for the past 4 years.
   Take to him with a view of taking a history and do a relevant risk assessment.

2. **Instructions to the role player:**
   You are 37-year-old Dennis Brown. You ask the doctor to call you 'James Bond'. You keep on correcting the doctor if called Dennis Brown. You are elated, happy and extremely cheerful. You are disheveled and have unkempt hair. You become irritable and restless when the doctor does not allow you to leave.
   You give the following information:
   - You have been 'extremely happy' for the past 2 weeks as your services are requested by United Nations (UN).
   - You have to catch a flight so that you can meet the President of UN and discuss the security procedures for the safety of the world.
   - You think you are 'James Bond' and were living in a disguise as a person who has bipolar disorder. But you are a highly skilled spy.
   - You say I need to go now .... My charter flight is waiting for me. It is world security at stake here.
   - You have thousands of ideas of how to keep the world safe, have flight of ideas and talk very fast. You are very difficult to interrupt.

- You try to touch the doctor, CPN to check if they are not carrying any monitoring device. You are slightly disinhibited.
- You don't have time for sleep or food as there is 'lots to do'.
- You think "I am the best in the world and I don't expect you to understand".
- As you are a spy, you can drive a car at 180 miles/hour, carry special gadgets that look like a knife, crew driver and pliers and can be intimate with girls.
- You want to leave so that you can catch your special charter flight from the airport.
- You do not take drugs or smoke, as "I am a spy". You do drink, as "James Bond likes wine".
- You have history of previous similar episode 6 years ago and several depression episodes, last being about 4 years ago.
- You were prescribed Lithium and Depakote. You have stopped taking medications, as you no longer need to be in the role of 'bipolar patient'.

3. **Construct:**

This station assesses candidate's knowledge of bipolar affective disorder and ability to elicit history from a man who is elated, irritable, grandiose and difficult to interview.

4. **Expanded construct:**

- The candidate should be able to demonstrate skill in eliciting a history a patient who has bipolar affective disorder with mania and psychotic symptoms.
- The candidate should be able to elicit duration, progress, severity and associated factors.
- The candidate should establish presence of psychotic symptoms.
- They should be able to control the interview, establish firm boundaries when patient is disinhibited.
- They should carry out a relevant risk assessment and establish risk to self and others.

5. **Areas of importance to pass the station:**

- Eliciting accurate and sufficient information about manic episode with psychosis (40%).
- Risk assessment: Self and others (30%).
- Communication and control of the interview (30%).

6. **Equipment checklist:**

Not applicable.

Station 73: Bipolar affective disorder, hypomanic episode

Theme: Bipolar affective disorder, hypomanic episode: Take history

1. **Instructions to candidates:**

You are doing a prison clinic and asked to see Jonathan Walsh, 42-year-old man in the prison. He has completed 2 months out of his 6 months sentence. The prison warden thinks that he is trying to 'wind them up' as he has nothing else to do.

Talk to him and take a history to arrive at the diagnosis.

2. **Instructions to the role player:**

You are 42-year-old Jonathan Walsh, serving a sentence of 6 months for burglary. You are happy, cheerful and "feel good in myself".

You give the following information:

- You feel 'good' and 'happy' in yourself for the past week. This 'happiness' is more than usual for you.
- You have been involved in most of the activities in prison like basketball, exercising, cleaning and socialising.
- You feel 'full of energy' and display good confidence and self-belief.
- You have been talking more than usual, being friendly with everyone and making him or her laugh with your humour.
- You sleep for about 3 hours and rest of the time you exercise in the cell.
- You have been treated for depression on at least four occasions in past. You have taken fluoxetine for the past 4 years, but stopped after you have come into prison. You never felt 'so good' in yourself in the past.
- You do not have any strange ideas, bizarre/odd or reckless behaviour. You do not think you are 'special' though you are relatively happier than others. You "just want everyone to have fun" and "prison should not be a dull place".
- If you had money you would have bought a drink and lunch for everyone in the prison including the doctor.
- You irritate police officers in the prison by your humour and singing. You think they should have a smile and not be 'grumpy'.

3. **Construct:**

This station assesses candidate's knowledge of bipolar affective disorder and ability to elicit history from a man who has hypomanic symptoms following several depressive episodes.

4. **Expanded construct:**

- The candidate should be able to demonstrate skill in eliciting a history a patient who has bipolar affective disorder with hypomanic symptoms and previous depressive episodes.
- The candidate should be able to elicit origin, duration, progress, severity and associated factors of elated mood.
- The candidate should establish past psychiatric history of depressive episodes and treatment.
- They should carry out a relevant risk assessment and establish risk to self and others.

5. **Areas of importance to pass the station:**

- Eliciting accurate and sufficient information about hypomanic episode and past psychiatric history (60%).

- Risk assessment: Self and others (20%).
- Communication (20%).

6. Equipment checklist: Not applicable.

Station 74: Acute stress reaction

Theme: To understand and recognise the clinical presentation of an acute stress reaction

1. Instructions to candidates:

You are in a mental health assessment unit to review a 22-year-old woman Miss Sheila O'Connor. The A and E mental health liaison nurse admitted her the previous night from the local A and E department following an assessment. Miss O'Connor had taken an overdose of 24 paracetamol tablets. She was discharged from A and E the same day without requiring any further medical treatment.

Take a brief history from this patient to establish what she is most likely to be suffering from.

2. Instructions to the role player:

- You are Miss Sheila O'Connor a 22-year-old woman who was admitted to a mental health assessment unit the night before.
- You had taken an overdose of 24 tablets of paracetamol the day before. Your boyfriend had found you in your flat in a confused state after you had a heated argument with him over the telephone.
- You and your boyfriend have been together for over 4 years. You live together in a flat, and you love you him very much. You also have a 2-year-old daughter. You had recently been talking about getting married.
- You also found out yesterday from one of your girlfriends that your boyfriend had been cheating on you with another one of your girlfriends. This had been a huge shock to you at first and you could not believe that he could have done this to you. You became very tearful and angry.
- You had a heated argument over the telephone with your boyfriend where you ended up breaking up with him. You felt dazed and confused. You then felt scared and began to panic. You experienced palpitations in your chest and felt restless. You suddenly felt quite hopeless imagining the future without your boyfriend and then thought that you would be better off dead. You took the overdose impulsively out of desperation.
- You did not leave a suicide note and you had not planned the overdose. You have never done anything like this before.
- Your boyfriend had called an ambulance.
- You have been well physically and mentally in the past and you have never had contact with psychiatric services. You drink alcohol socially and you do not smoke cigarettes. You do not use illicit substances.

- You are feeling a bit better today having had a good night's sleep and breakfast. Your boyfriend has also been in touch and he is trying to be supportive, though you remain angry with him for what he has done to you.
- You are still feeling panicky at times. Your boyfriend has told you that he regrets what he has done to you. You still feel a little bit confused about what has happened. You also feel embarrassed about having taken an overdose that you now regret.

The doctor will ask you some questions about what has happened to you.

3. **Construct:**

   The station tests the candidate's ability to recognize a clinical presentation of an acute stress reaction.

4. **Expanded construct:**

   The candidate is expected to take a history and recognize an acute stress reaction.

   They should:
   - Elicit the history and clinical features suggestive of an acute stress reaction.
   - Ask a range of questions that demonstrates or excludes psychopathology, e.g., depressive or anxiety disorder.
   - Demonstrates empathy with the patient's experience.
   - Show the ability to focus on the specific problem.

   Interviewing/Communication skills:

   They should:
   - Show an appropriate mix of open and closed questioning.
   - Demonstrate advanced listening skills.
   - Ask questions that are structured, focused and fluent.
   - Be clear and precise using technical language appropriately and with clear understanding.
   - Avoid the use of jargon.

5. **Areas of importance to pass the station:**
   - Ability to elicit the history of an acute stress reaction (40%).
   - Ability to elicit the symptoms of an acute stress reaction (40%).
   - Subsidiary elements are: Interviewing/communication skills (20%).

6. **Equipment checklist:**

   Not applicable

Station 75: Adjustment disorder: Mixed anxiety and depressive reaction

Theme: To understand and recognise the clinical presentation of an adjustment disorder: Mixed anxiety and depressive reaction

1. **Instructions to candidate:**

   A local GP has referred Mr Toby Smith, 36-year-old man complaining of anxiety, low mood, and tiredness and poor concentration. The GP has also told you that Mr Smith and his wife have decided to divorce after 5 years of marriage. Over the past few weeks Mr Smith has noticed that he is finding it difficult to concentrate at work. He is self-employed and owns a construction company but has taken time off work for the past week. You are about to review him in your outpatient clinic.

Take a brief history from this patient to establish what he is most likely to be suffering from.

2. **Instructions to the role player:**
   - You are Mr Toby Smith a 36-year-old gentleman who has been married for 5 years.
   - You also own your own construction company and are self-employed.
   - You have been very busy with work for years and making your company a success.
   - However, this has meant that you have been unable to spend quality time with your wife often coming home late from work.
   - This has led to frequent arguments over the past few years, which have often been quite heated.
   - As a result you have drifted apart and now seem to have quite different goals in life. You both agreed to get a divorce about 3 weeks ago despite the fact that you still love your wife. This has made you feel low in mood and anxious about the future. You are still living together until your jointly owned house can be sold.
   - Your company has been your life. However, your concentration at work has been quite poor at times. You find yourself often worrying about the future without your wife. You also feel more tired than usual and you have noticed that you can be more irritable with work colleagues at times. Your appetite and sleep have been fine. You have not experienced any other problems or symptoms.
   - You have also been drinking more alcohol than usual for the past week though you still feel that it is under control. You have been drinking several pints of lager in the evenings with work colleagues and this seems to be increasing in frequency. You have found it difficult to go back home after work. You smoke 15 cigarettes per day and you very occasionally use cocaine.

   The doctor will ask you some questions about what has been happening to you.

3. **Construct:**

   The station tests the candidate's ability to recognize a clinical presentation of an adjustment disorder, more specifically a mixed anxiety and depressive reaction.

4. **Expanded construct:**

   The candidate is expected to take a history and recognise an adjustment disorder: Mixed anxiety and depressive reaction.

   They should:
   - Elicit the history and clinical features suggestive of an adjustment disorder: Mixed anxiety and depressive reaction.
   - Ask a range of questions that demonstrates or excludes psychopathology, e.g., depressive or anxiety disorder.
   - Demonstrates empathy with the patient's experience.
   - Show the ability to focus on the specific problem.

Interviewing/Communication skills:

They should:

- Show an appropriate mix of open and closed questioning.
- Demonstrate advanced listening skills.
- Ask questions that are structured, focused and fluent.
- Be clear and precise using technical language appropriately and with clear understanding.
- Avoid the use of jargon.

5. **Areas of importance to pass the station:**
   - Ability to elicit the history of an adjustment disorder (40%).
   - Ability to elicit the symptoms of an adjustment disorder: Mixed anxiety and depressive reaction (40%).
   - Subsidiary elements are: Interviewing/communication skills (20%).
6. **Equipment checklist:**
   Not applicable

Station 76: Bereavement versus abnormal grief reaction

Theme: To understand and recognise the clinical presentation of an abnormal grief reaction

1. **Instructions to candidates:**

   Mrs Joan Black is a 61-year-old lady who lost her husband 10 months ago. She has been referred to the Home Treatment Team by her GP as she is low in mood and expressing suicidal ideation. She has not stated a specific plan to end her life. She has been finding it difficult to cope since the sudden death of her husband last year.

   Take a brief history from this patient to establish what she is most likely suffering from.

2. **Instructions to the role player:**
   - You are Mrs Joan Black a 61-year-old lady who was widowed 10 months ago when your husband suddenly died from a heart attack. On the night of his death, you had both gone to bed as usual but your husband had been complaining of shortness of breath.
   - You both thought nothing of it but in the middle of the night you awoke to find your husband choking and clutching his chest. You called an ambulance but paramedics were unable to save him once they attended. Your late husband had been complaining of chest pain in the past week and you had suggested that he went to see his GP. However, he had not taken up your advice and you felt guilty for not having pushed him further to see his GP at the time.
   - You are deeply missing your husband. You ruminate over the plans you had made to enjoy your retirement together by going on world cruises. You are feeling quite hopeless about the future and fearful of being on your own. Your two sons have grown up and have their own respective families and lives. You do not want to burden them.
   - You also occasionally hear your husband's voice; you think that he wants you to join him. You have a plan to end your life on his first death anniversary but you have not yet decided on how you will do this.

- You have been sleeping well but your appetite has decreased over the past few months.
- You have also been drinking more wine than usual since the death of your husband. You sometimes drink a bottle of wine in the evening. Nevertheless you have managed to continue working as a full-time solicitor.
- You do not smoke cigarettes and you do not use illicit substances.
- You have been physically and mentally well in the past and you have never seen a psychiatrist before.

The doctor will ask you some questions about what has been happening to you.

3. **Construct:**

The station tests that candidates understand a normal grief reaction and their ability to recognise a clinical presentation of an abnormal grief reaction.

4. **Expanded construct:**

The candidate is expected to take a history and recognise an abnormal grief reaction.

They should:

- Elicit the history and clinical features suggestive of an abnormal grief reaction.
- Ask a range of questions that demonstrates or excludes psychopathology, e.g., depressive or anxiety disorder.
- Demonstrates empathy with the patient's experience.
- Show the ability to focus on the specific problem.

Interviewing/Communication skills:

They should:

- Show an appropriate mix of open and closed questioning.
- Demonstrate advanced listening skills.
- Ask questions that are structured, focused and fluent.
- Be clear and precise using technical language appropriately and with clear understanding.
- Avoid the use of jargon.

5. **Areas of importance to pass the station:**
- Ability to elicit the history of an abnormal grief reaction (40%).
- Ability to elicit the symptoms of an abnormal grief reaction (40%).
- Subsidiary elements are: Interviewing/communication skills (20%).

6. **Equipment checklist:**

Not applicable

Station 77: Neurasthenia/chronic fatigue syndrome: History taking

Theme: To understand and recognise a clinical presentation of neurasthenia

1. **Instructions to candidates:**

Mrs Sally Molly is a 35-year-old woman who has been feeling low in mood and anxious. She is finding it difficult to cope with daily activities for the past year. Her GP is concerned that she has become bedbound over the past few weeks. She has been experiencing muscular aches and pains all over her body for which she takes several painkillers. You have been asked to perform a domiciliary visit, as Mrs Molly is unable to get out of her house.

Take a brief history from this patient to establish what she is most likely to be suffering from.

2. **Instructions to the role player:**
   - You are Mrs Sally Molly, a 35-year-old woman, who has been suffering from tiredness, low mood, anxiety and pain for the past year.
   - You used to work as a support worker in a local nursing home but found that you were becoming increasingly tired; you have been off work for the past 4 months. You have also found that you are unable to do any housework, as you feel exhausted very quickly.
   - You live with your husband whom has been caring for you at home.
   - You have been experiencing aches and pains all over your body but particularly in your stomach. Your GP has been unable to find any physical cause for your aches and pains. You find it difficult to get out of bed now and this has got worse over the past few weeks. You find it difficult to relax and feel restless. You also have problems with eating and sleeping intermittently. You find it difficult to enjoy anything anymore.
   - You have never been physically unwell in the past and you have never seen a psychiatrist before. You had been visiting your GP more frequently before you became bedbound.
   - He had prescribed you antidepressant medication Prozac 40 mg daily, which you have taken for 4 months but this is not helping.
   - You do not drink alcohol or smoke cigarettes and you do not use illicit substances.

   The doctor will ask you some questions about what has been happening to you.

3. **Construct:**

   The station tests the candidate's ability to recognise a clinical presentation of neurasthenia.

4. **Expanded construct:**

   The candidate is expected to take a history and recognise neurasthenia.

   They should:
   - Elicit the history and clinical features suggestive of neurasthenia.
   - Ask a range of questions that demonstrates or excludes psychopathology, e.g., depressive or anxiety disorder.
   - Demonstrates empathy with the patient's experience.
   - Show the ability to focus on the specific problem.

   Interviewing/Communication skills:

   They should:
   - Show an appropriate mix of open and closed questioning.
   - Demonstrate advanced listening skills.

- Ask questions that are structured, focused and fluent.
- Be clear and precise using technical language appropriately and with clear understanding.
- Avoid the use of jargon.

5. Areas of importance to pass the station:

- Ability to elicit the history of neurasthenia (40%).
- Ability to elicit the symptoms of neurasthenia (40%).
- Subsidiary elements are: Interviewing/communication skills (20%).

6. Equipment checklist:
Not applicable.

Station 78: Depersonalisation–Derealisation syndrome: History

Theme: To understand and recognise a clinical presentation of Depersonalisation–Derealisation syndrome

1. Instructions to candidates:

Ms Joanna Harper is a 23-year-old woman who has been referred to you by her GP. She has been feeling quite strange for several months. She is finding it difficult to feel any emotion and finds this very unpleasant. She does not feel like her usual self and she is worried about what is happening to her. She has been off work for several weeks. Miss Harper has come to see you in your outpatient clinic.

Take a brief history from this patient to establish what she is most likely to be suffering from.

2. Instructions to the role player:

- You are Miss Joanna Harper, a 23-year-old single woman, who has become worried about changes in the way you experience things around you.
- You feel as if you are not really here and you are finding it difficult to feel any emotions. You sometimes feel that the world around you is not real. Everything seems very dull. You are unsure why everything seems different but you do not believe that other people or forces are imposing these changes.
- You are not hearing or seeing any hallucinations.
- You recall the changes started quite suddenly about 3 months ago. You had been to the gym one evening for a good workout. You came back home to relax and then suddenly started to feel as if you were detached from your thoughts and your body. You realised that this was strange and you tried to continue with everyday life. However, you have had to take some time off work for the past week as you have sometimes felt that your workplace is not real. This feeling was unpleasant for you. You are unsure whether you were better off being at work. You are a data inputter for a local company.
- You have never had any physical health problems in the past and you have never seen a psychiatrist before.
- You drink alcohol very occasionally on social occasions and you do not use any illicit substances. You do not smoke cigarettes.

- You are eating and sleeping well. Your concentration and memory are fine. You have occasionally experienced déjà vu where you think you see something that you have already seen before in the past.

The doctor will ask you some questions about what has been happening to you.

3. **Construct:**

   The station tests the candidate's ability to recognise a clinical presentation of depersonalisation–derealisation syndrome.

4. **Expanded construct:**

   The candidate is expected to take a history and recognise depersonalisation–derealisation syndrome. They should:

   - Elicit the history and clinical features suggestive of depersonalisation-derealisation syndrome.
   - Ask a range of questions that demonstrates or excludes psychopathology, e.g., psychotic, depressive or anxiety disorder.
   - Demonstrates empathy with the patient's experience.
   - Show the ability to focus on the specific problem.

   Interviewing/Communication skills:

   They should:

   - Show an appropriate mix of open and closed questioning.
   - Demonstrate advanced listening skills.
   - Ask questions that are structured, focused and fluent.
   - Be clear and precise using technical language appropriately and with clear understanding.
   - Avoid the use of jargon.

5. **Areas of importance to pass the station:**

   - Ability to elicit the history of depersonalisation-derealisation syndrome (40%).
   - Ability to elicit the symptoms of depersonalisation-derealisation syndrome (40%).
   - Subsidiary elements are: Interviewing/communication skills (20%).

6. **Equipment checklist:**

   Not applicable

Station 79: Mixed personality disorder: Collateral information

Theme: Mixed personality disorder (Predominantly Cluster B type): Collateral history

1. **Instructions to candidates:**

   You are meeting the partner of Mr Nigel Cameron who is 28, unemployed and is admitted to your ward. He had presented with an overdose of multiple drugs and alcohol. His GP had diagnosed him with mixed personality disorder, predominantly Cluster B type.

   Take a full history to confirm the diagnosis and address her fears, concerns and expectations.

2. **Instructions to the role player:**

   You are Jane Clegg; partner of Nigel Cameron who would like to talk his psychiatrist about him. You have known him for about 9 months. At times you have felt that you did not whether you were coming or going with him. He had displayed a wide range of emotions. You remember the following features:

   - Callous disregard for your and other people's feelings.
   - He had several girlfriends until you met him.
   - He keeps insulting people without apologizing.
   - He had spent a few months in prison for ABH.
   - He cannot take any criticism without losing his temper.
   - He feels miserable most of the time but clings on you in case you will leave him.
   - He has harmed himself on a number of occasions.
   - He sometimes expresses excessive affection to you and his family.
   - He wants to appear smart and attractive most of the time.

3. **Construct:**

   This station assesses the candidates' ability to distinguish mixed personality disorder. It consists of several personality disorders, but without a predominant set of symptoms that would allow more specific diagnosis.

4. **Expanded construct:**

   The mixed personality disorder consists of features of several personality disorders without a predominant set of symptoms that would not allow a more specific diagnosis. In the given example, the patient presents with a mixed picture suggestive of dissocial, emotionally unstable and histrionic personality disorders (Cluster B).

   - Callous disregard for the feelings of other persons.
   - Incapacity to maintain enduring relationships, though they have no difficulty in establishing them.
   - Incapacity to experience guilt and profit from experience, particularly punishment.
   - Outbursts of violence and threatening behaviour are common in particular response to criticism by others.
   - Chronic feelings of emptiness.
   - Acts of self-harm.
   - Excessive efforts to avoid abandonment.
   - Self-dramatisation, theatricality.
   - Exaggerated expression of emotions.
   - Shallow and labile affectivity.
   - Over concern with physical attractiveness.

5. **Areas of importance to pass the station:**

   - Establish diagnosis of mixed personality (60%).

- Address the fears, concerns and expectation of the patient's partner (20%).
- Communication (20%).

6. **Equipment checklist:**
Not applicable

Station 80: Narcissistic personality disorder: History

Theme: Narcissistic personality disorder: Collateral information from the partner

1. **Instructions to candidates:**
You are meeting Rose Morrish, long-term partner of Eric Dobson who was referred to you by his general practitioner who considers that Mr Dobson might have a narcissistic personality.
Take a full history to confirm the diagnosis, explain the possible aetiological factors and allay her fears, concerns and fears.

2. **Instructions to the role player:**
You are Rose Morrish, long-term partner of Eric Dobson who was referred to mental health service for assessment. You have been concerned about his attitude and excessive for admiration all the time. His general practitioner considers him having a narcissistic personality disorder. You have observed the following features over a long period of time.
   - A pervasive pattern of grandiosity and need for excessive admiration.
   - Lack of empathy.
   - Grandiose sense of self-importance, e.g., exaggerated achievements and talents.
   - Preoccupation with fantasies of unlimited success, power, brilliance and ideal love.
   - He believes that he is 'Special' and 'Unique'.
   - He has a sense of entitlement, especially favourable treatment or automatic compliance with his expectations.
   - He takes advantage of others to achieve his own ends.
   - Lack of empathy.
   - He believes that others are envious of him.

   You are concerned about him want to know what is wrong with him and what might have caused this?

3. **Construct:**
This station assesses the candidates' ability to diagnose narcissistic personality by gathering information from the patient's long-term partner. It is characterised by a pervasive pattern of grandiosity (in fantasy or behaviour), need for admiration and lack of empathy.

4. **Expand construct:**
The candidates are able to elicit accurate history from the patient's partner about narcissistic personality disorder:
   - Its origin, duration and progress.
   - They should be able to elicit possible aetiological factors.

- They should briefly ask about symptoms of possible differential diagnosis or comorbid disorders.
- Grandiose sense of self-importance.
- Preoccupation with fantasies of unlimited success, power, brilliance and ideal love.
- Belief that the patient is 'special' and 'unique'.
- Requires excessive admiration.
- Sense of entitlement of favourable treatment or automatic compliance with his expectations.
- Lack of empathy and often envy of others.
- Often arrogant haughty attitudes.

Aetiology

- No demonstrable factors identified.
- Some aspects of narcissism may be related with inappropriate seeking for excitement and reward, and associated with monoamine function abnormalities at the mesolimbic reward systems.
- Severe frustration with early objects is considered important in the defensive genesis of narcissistic personality disorder.
- Behind the compensatory grandiose self, a hungry and inferior real self resides as the core problem.
- Often high parental expectations and harsh criticism of the child is present in the family.

5. **Areas of importance to pass the station:**
   - Detailed history (60%).
   - Explanation of aetiological factors (20%).
   - Communication (20%).
6. **Equipment checklist:**
   Not applicable

Linked Stations: 81–86

Station 81: Link 1: Sexual dysfunction caused by side effects of antipsychotics: History
Station 82: Link 2: Sexual dysfunction caused by side effects of antipsychotics: Management

Station 81: Link 1: Sexual dysfunction caused by side effects of antipsychotics: History

Theme: Sexual dysfunction caused by antipsychotics: History and investigations

1. **Instructions to candidates:**

   A 25-year-old Alan Dunkerley with complaints of sexual dysfunction is referred to your outpatient clinic. He was diagnosed with first episode psychosis about a year ago. He receives oral antipsychotic drug with beneficial effect but he would like to discuss his sexual problems with you.

   Take detailed history about sexual dysfunction and discuss relevant investigations and mechanisms of his problems.

2. **Instructions to the role player:**

You are 25-year-old Alan Dunkerley with a diagnosis of first episode psychosis about a year ago. You have achieved a great deal of improvement and stability in your condition. However, you have some sexual problems, which have impaired quality of your life and you are thinking of stopping your medication.

- You have lost desire for sex for the 6 months and have limited arousal when you want to make love to your partner.
- You have problems with erection, but whenever you achieve erection you are unable to ejaculate or at time you experience premature ejaculation.
- You have noticed that your breasts have enlarged and you find it a bit embarrassing. You have also noticed a milky discharge from your breasts.
- You want to discuss what investigations about your condition.
- Your doctor will tell you that blood test to find out the levels of prolactin will be arranged. Raised prolactin levels cause lack of libido, amenorrhoea in women, breast enlargement and milky discharge (Galactorrhoea) in both men and women.
- Your doctor should provide you with information on sexual side effects of antipsychotics and its mechanism.
- Doctor should inform you that sedation and weight gain may reduce sexual desire.

All this information should be provided in easy to understand manner without use of medical jargons.

2. **Construct:**

This station assesses the candidates' ability to assess sexual problems in patients taking antipsychotic drugs, explain relevant investigations and mechanisms of the problems experienced by the patients.

3. **Expanded construct:**

- Sexual dysfunction can affect quality of life and compliance with medication. It is one of the major causes of treatment dropouts.
- Measurement of serum prolactin is the first step in investigating this problem.
- Four phases of human sexual response.
- Desire is related to testosterone men, possibly increased by dopamine and decreased by prolactin.
- Arousal is influenced by testosterone in men and oestrogen in women, central dopamine stimulation, peripheral alpha agonism, modulation of cholinergic/adrenergic balance, nitric oxide pathways.
- Orgasm may be related to oxytocin and inhibited by increase in serotonin activity and alpha1 blockade.
- Sexual dysfunction is a side effect of all antipsychotics.
- Individual susceptibility varies and all effects are reversible.
- Anticholinergic effects can cause disturbance of arousal.
- Peripheral alpha1 receptor blockade causes problems with erection and ejaculation in men.

- Both peripheral alpha1 and cholinergic receptors blockade causes priapism.
- Sedation and overweight may reduce sexual desire.

5. **Areas of importance to pass the station:**
   - History suggestive of variety of sexual dysfunction (60%).
   - Explaining relevant investigations and mechanisms of the problems (30%).
   - Communication (10%).
6. **Equipment checklist:**
   Not applicable.

Station 82: Link 2: Sexual dysfunction caused by side effects of antipsychotics: Management

Theme: Sexual dysfunction caused by antipsychotics: Explain management to the patient's partner

1. **Instructions to candidates:**
   You saw Mr Alan Dunkerley in the previous station with multiple sexual dysfunctions. You are now meeting his partner Jane Abbotts who is concerned about him. She is keen to know what is wrong with him and how you are going to help him.
   Explain the management sexual dysfunction to her and allay her fears, anxieties concerns and expectations.
2. **Instructions to the role player:**
   You are Jane Abbotts who is living with Alan Dunkerley for the past 2 years. He has been receiving antipsychotic treatment for his first episode psychosis. Unfortunately, he has developed sexual side effects due to his medication. This causes friction in your relationship for the past 6 months. You have the following questions for the psychiatrists.
   - What is wrong with Alan? We had enjoyed a good sex life until 6 months ago.
   - What is causing this problem?
   - Will you do any investigations?
   - How are you going to treat him?
   - I have heard that the problem may go away without any treatment. Is it possible with Alan?
   - Are there any drugs available to treat this problem as it has been caused by his current drug?
   - Is there any way I can help him?
3. **Construct:**
   This station assesses the candidates' ability to understand the principles of managing drug-induced sexual dysfunction in men.
4. **Expanded construct:**
   Management of drug-induced sexual dysfunction:
   - Spontaneous remissions do occur.
   - *Normal Prolactin levels:* Women 0–25 ng/ml, men 0–20 ng/ml.
   - *First step* to reduce the dose of antipsychotic or discontinue the offending drug if appropriate and involve the partner.

- *Next step:* Switch to a different drug that is less likely to cause the problem.
- If this fails or is not practicable, 'antidote' drug can be tried, e.g., Cyproheptadine (5HT-2 antagonist at doses of 4–16 mg/day) for SSRI induced sexual dysfunction.
- Amantadine, bupropion, buspirone, bethanechol and yohimbine for increasing libido, arousal and orgasm.
- Testosterone patches to increase libido in women.
- Sildenafil, tadalafil or vardenafil for erectile dysfunction.

5. Areas of importance to pass the station:

- Explanation of management of drug-induced sexual dysfunction (70%).
- Communication (30%).

6. Equipment Checklist:

Not applicable.

Linked Stations: 83 and 84

Station 83: Link 1: Gender identity disorder: Transsexualism/male to female: History

Station 84: Link 2: Gender identity disorder: Transsexualism/male to female: Management

Station 83: Link 1: Gender identity disorder: Transsexualism/male to female: History

Theme: Gender identity disorder: Transsexualism/male to female: Take history from the patient

1. Instructions to candidates:

You are meeting Mr Vivien Marshall who is 45 years old, accountant, married with a grown up son wants a gender change as he had always believed to be trapped in wrong sex.

Take a full history to arrive at the diagnosis of gender identity disorder. Take your notes to the next station to discuss his management with his wife.

2. Instructions to the role player:

You are Mr Vivien Marshall who is transgender and wants to live as a woman for your rest of life. You had always believed that you were trapped in a wrong sex as you had regarded yourself as a woman. However, you are married and have a grown up son. Your wife supports you in your decision to change your sex, but she will not be able to live with you any longer. Your son is also supportive of your decision. You may discuss the following with the psychiatrists who would want to know more about you.

- You had a life-long desire to be accepted as a woman and lived with a sense of discomfort with your anatomical/biological sex.
- You want to have hormonal treatment and surgery to make your body as congruent as possible being a woman.

- You have no mental health problems or any genetic or chromosomal abnormality.
- As a school boy, you had preferred to play with girls and your parents had dressed you a girl on many occasions.
- Female dolls were your favourite toys.
- As a boy, you had asserted that your penis and testes were disgusting and wished they disappear.
- You had felt humiliated by teasing and bullying by other boys.
- Your parents had supported you wholeheartedly.
- You had homosexual liaisons with several men before you married.
- You remain preoccupied with the removal of your penis and testes.

3. Construct:

This station assesses the candidates' ability to diagnose gender identity disorder. It is a desire to live and be accepted as a member of the opposite sex, usually accompanied by a sense of discomfort with or inappropriateness of one's anatomical sex. The person wishes to have hormonal and surgical treatment to make one's body as congruent as possible with the preferred sex.

4. Expanded construct:

- The candidates are able to elicit accurate history from the patient to establish a diagnosis of gender identity disorder.
- It is a desire to live and be accepted as a member of the opposite sex, usually accompanied by a sense of discomfort with or inappropriateness of one's anatomical sex.
- The person wishes to have hormonal and surgical treatment to make one's body as congruent as possible with the preferred sex.
- The disorder must be present for at least 2 years and must not be a symptom of another mental disorder, such as schizophrenia or associated with any intersex, genetic or chromosomal abnormality.
- In men, typically it starts to manifest from preschool years, e.g., the boys are preoccupied with types of play and other activities stereotypically associated with girls, preference for dressing in girls or women's clothes, female dolls are often their favourite toys and girls are their regularly preferred playmates.
- As a boy, they assert that their penis or testes are disgusting or will disappear. They experience humiliating teasing or rejection by other boys.
- They get distressed by the conflict with expectations of their family or peers.
- They may have homosexual orientation during or after adolescence.

5. Areas of importance to pass the station:

- Accurate history of gender identity disorder (80%).
- Communication (20%).

6. Equipment Checklist:

Not applicable

Station 84: Link 2: Gender identity disorder: Transsexualism/male to female: Management

Theme: Explain the management of gender identity disorder to the patient's wife and address her fears, concerns and expectations

1. **Instructions to candidates:**

   You are meeting Mrs Alison Marshall, wife of the patient you had seen in the previous station. She would like to know about the management of her husband's condition even though she has decided to divorce him.

   Explain the management plan to Mrs Marshall and address her fears, concerns, anxieties and expectations.

2. **Instructions to the role player:**

   You have supported your husband in his decision to change his sex having been married for 22 years. You will find it very difficult to live with him after the surgery. You have mutually agreed to an amicable divorce. You would want to ask the following questions to the psychiatrists:

   - Why did he marry me and kept me in the dark till our son was 15?
   - Do you think my husband suffers from a psychotic disorder?
   - Was he born like this?
   - How are you going to assess him?
   - What is 'Real Life Experience'? How long it will last and why is it necessary?
   - What does hormonal treatment involve and how does it help his condition?
   - What does the surgical treatment consist of and it is reversible if my husband changes his mind after the operation?
   - What is the likelihood of him adjusting successfully in his new gender?
   - What of the legal issues, such as, change in legal sex, new birth certificate, passport, driving licence, etc.?
   - Do you think our son will turn out to be transgender?

3. **Construct:**

   This station assesses the candidates' ability to discuss management plan of gender identity disorder and address the wife's fears, anxieties, concerns and expectations.

4. **Expanded construct:**

   The management of gender identity disorder includes the following:

   Assessment:

   - Full psychosexual history with emphasis on the onset and development of gender dysphoria, attempts at treatment.
   - Long-term goals.
   - Appreciation of obstacles to be confronted.
   - General psychiatric and medical status.

   Real Life Experience–Reversible procedures

   - Clothing change, name change and cross–gender role socialisation would precede hormonal treatment.

- Living full time for at least a year and preferably 2 years in preferred sex.
- High doses of cross-sex hormones.
- Full time employment in the new role for at least one year.

If he demonstrates that he has successfully negotiated the 'Real Life Experience' and is adjusting well in this role, he can be referred for surgery.

Surgery

- It includes penectomy, orchidectomy and creation of a neovagina. The neovagina may be created from penile skin, perhaps augmented by other skin or from a portion of large intestine.

Outcome

Follow-up reports on operated transsexuals are favourable.

Family matters

- When children are involved, efforts should be made to deal with the feeling of betrayal or abandonment by the patient and reactions by their peers.
- No evidence of gender identity in the children of transsexual patients.

Legal matters

- Gender Recognition Act (2004) in UK allows a new birth certificate and change in legal sex.
- Discrimination in employment is illegal.

5. **Areas of importance to pass the station:**
   - Discussion of management of gender identity disorder (70%).
   - Addressing the patient's wife's fears, concerns and expectations (30%).
6. **Equipment Checklist:**
   Not applicable.

Linked Stations 85 and 86

Station 85: Link 1: Passive – aggressive (negativistic) personality disorder: Collateral history from the mother

Station 86: Link 2: Passive – aggressive (negativistic) personality disorder: Management

Station 85: Link 1: Passive – aggressive (negativistic) personality disorder: Collateral history from the mother

Theme: Passive – aggressive (negativistic) personality disorder: Collateral history from the mother

1. **Instructions to candidates:**

   You are meeting Mrs Pascoe, mother of 25-year-old Alan Pascoe who works as an IT analyst with an international bank. He has had three similar jobs since he left university 4 years ago. She is very worried about her son who has been unsettled for the past 3–4 years. He has been unable to meet demands of his work and social life. He has always been negativistic in his attitude to life.

Take a detailed history from the mother to make a diagnosis of passive – aggressive (Negativistic) personality

Address her fears, anxieties, concerns and expectations about her son.

2. **Instructions to the role player:**

You are meeting the psychiatrist who would like to you about son Alan. You are clearly very worried about him and welcome the opportunity to discuss with the psychiatrist.

- Alan is unable to meet the daily demands of his life, he has always displayed argumentative, oppositional behaviour and defeatist attitude.
- He has a low self-image and unable to find a steady girlfriend.
- He complains of being misunderstood and unappreciated by others.
- He had running's with his university tutors but managed to get 2:1 in his degree.
- He expresses envy and resentment towards his siblings and cousins who he thinks are more fortunate than him.
- He becomes easily irritable and gloomy, alternates with hostile defiance and contrition.
- He attends his GP repeatedly for vague physical symptoms.
- He drinks alcohol excessively, he feels he is a victim of misfortune and his destiny.

You want to know what is wrong with your son, what can be done to help him and if and when he will recover from this condition as they want him to settle down in his life.

3. **Construct:**

This station assesses whether the candidates understand what the passive – aggressive (negativistic) personality disorder means and how it affects those around the person. Its central features are resistance to demands for adequate social and occupational performance and negativistic attitude to life. A pervasive pattern of argumentativeness, oppositional behaviour and defeatist attitudes are typical.

4. **Expanded construct:**

- The candidates are able to elicit accurate history from the patient's mother about passive–aggressive disorder.
- Its origin, duration and progress.
- They should be able to elicit possible aetiological factors.
- They should briefly ask about symptoms of possible differential diagnosis or comorbid disorders.
- The patient passively resists fulfilling routine social and occupational tasks.
- Unreasonably criticise and scorn authority.
- Sullen and argumentative.
- Complain of being misunderstood and unappreciated by others.
- Express envy and resentment toward those apparently more fortunate.
- Voice exaggerated and persistent complaints of personal misfortune, blame others for their own bad luck.
- Alternate between hostile defiance and contrition.

- Prone to diffuse somatic complaints, hypochondriasis, and psychosomatic complaints.
- Prone to alcohol abuse, frequently comorbid with major depression, dysthymic disorder, anxiety and panic disorder.

5. **Areas of importance to pass the station:**
   - Eliciting accurate and sufficient information about passive–aggressive (negativistic) personality disorder (50%).
   - Discussing the mother's fears, anxieties, concerns and expectations (30%).
   - Communication (20%).
6. **Equipment checklist:**
   Not applicable.

Station 86: Link 2: Passive–aggressive (negativistic) personality disorder: Management

Theme: Passive – aggressive (negativistic) personality disorder: Management

1. **Instructions to candidates:**
   You are now meeting Alan's father who wants to know what is wrong with Alan, how his son can be helped and what will happen to him. Use the notes from the previous station.
   Explain management and prognosis to the father of Alan Pascoe.
2. **Instructions to the role player:**
   You are worried about Alan who was a bright student and got a 2:1 degree in IT. He leads an erratic life and abuses alcohol frequently.
   You will ask the following questions to the psychiatrist.
   What is wrong with my son? Has he gone mad?
   What is diagnosis?
   What investigations will you do?
   How are you going to treat him?
   Will he ever get normal?
   Will he be able to hold down a job?
3. **Construct:**
   The station assesses whether candidates are able to discuss biopsychosocial approach to the management of passive–aggressive personality disorder and its prognosis with the patient's father.
4. **Expanded construct:**
   - The candidate is able to demonstrate clear understanding of the comorbid conditions, such as, major depression, dysthymic disorder, hypochondriasis, psychosomatic disorders, anxiety and panic disorders.
   - Discuss biopsychosocial approach to the management of the condition.
   - The goal of the treatment is to help the patient escape from the vicious cycle of self-defeating behaviour and develop mature ways of expressing anger and other feelings.

- *Psychopharmacology:* Treat target symptoms, such as, depression, anxiety and somatic complaints with antidepressants and benzodiazepines.
- Psychotherapy is the treatment of choice. Various modes of therapy are available.
- Supportive psychotherapy.
- Psychodynamic psychotherapy.
- Behavioural assertiveness training.
- Paradoxical approach in group or individual settings.
- *Prognosis:* It will depend on the level of insight, motivation and co-operation with the treatment.

5. Areas of importance to pass the station:

- Explanation of relevant investigations, management and prognosis (60%).
- Address fears, concerns, anxieties and expectations of the father (20%).
- Communication (20%).

6. Equipment checklist:

Not applicable.

Single Stations: 87–89

Station 87: Dissociative amnesia

Theme: Dissociative amnesia: Collateral history from the mother

1. Instructions to candidates:

You are talking to the mother of a 31-year-old man George Pattison who was sent home from the battlefield in Iraq. He was involved in an intense battle with the enemy during which he lost his five colleagues.

Take a history from mother about dissociative amnesia and address her fears, anxieties, concerns and expectations about her son.

2. Instructions to the role player:

- You are the mother of George Pattison, a soldier with British Army who was sent home from Iraq recently.
- He was involved in a fierce and intense battle in which he lost few of his close friends. He became confused, and shell-shocked after returning to his base. You noted the following in your son and are very worried about his condition.
  - He cannot remember being in Iraq, let alone being involved in the battle with the enemy.
  - He is able to remember everything else.
  - He sometimes wanders in the house and in the local areas aimlessly.
  - He generally remains anxious, perplexed, and confused but he has lucid period during which he is his usual self.
  - He seeks repeated reassurances from you but cannot be reassured.

- He is neglecting his personal hygiene.
- He has no previous history of any mental health problems, alcohol or drug abuse.

You want to know what is wrong with him, whether he will ever get better or not and how long it will take him to make full recovery.

3. **Construct:**

This station assess whether the candidates are able to understand whether the memory loss is due to a dissociative disorder or not. In such disorders, it is presumed that the ability to exercise a conscious and selective control over mental function is impaired.

4. **Expanded construct:**

- The candidate should be able to demonstrate skill in eliciting a history from the informant that picks up relevant information about dissociative amnesia.
- Its origin, duration and progress.
- They should be able to elicit possible aetiological factors.
- They should briefly ask about symptoms of possible differential diagnosis or comorbid disorders.
- They need to elicit the informant's fears, anxieties, concerns and expectations and address them appropriately, e.g., Her son's condition is due to intolerable traumatic events in Iraq and he cannot solve it himself. It is a separation of unpleasant emotions and memories from conscious awareness with subsequent disruption to normal life. This is somehow transformed into his current symptoms, which tend to resolve after a few weeks or months.
- Understanding that the amnesia is not due to organic mental disorders and cannot be explained by ordinary forgetfulness or fatigue.
- The amnesia is usually centered on the traumatic events. It may vary from day to day and between investigators.

5. **Areas of importance to pass the station:**

- Eliciting accurate and sufficient information about dissociative amnesia (50%).
- Discussing the mother's fears, anxieties, concerns and expectations (30%).
- Communication (20%).

6. **Equipment checklist:**

Not applicable.

Station 88: Dissociative fugue

Theme: Dissociative fugue: Collateral information from the patient's partner

1. **Instructions to candidates:**

You are talking the partner of 29-year-old calls himself as Barak Obama who presented to your Accident and Emergency department in London. However, in ID card on him indicates that he is John Smith from Edinburgh and works in an NHS hospital as a community mental health nurse. He is unable to tell you anything about him except that he has been depressed following death of his father recently.

Take a history from the informant about dissociative fugue and address her fears, anxieties, concerns and expectations about her partner.

2. **Instructions to the role player:**

You are the partner of John Smith who works as a community mental health nurse in Edinburgh. You live together for the past 2 years. His father died suddenly and unexpectedly about 2 weeks ago. He organised the funeral and conducted himself well until 3 days ago when he left home without informing you.

- You had noticed that he was depressed and had expressed negative thoughts.
- He was due to return to his job yesterday.
- He had never been to London before and wondered how had arrived here.
- He did not carry any luggage with him.
- He was unable to remember how he had arrived in London and called himself as Barrack Obama.
- You are clearly very worried and perturbed by John's behaviour.
- You want to know what is wrong with and whether he will make full recovery from his condition.
- You want to take him home with you.

You want to know what is wrong with him, whether he will ever get better or not and how long it will take him to make full recovery.

3. **Construct:**

This station assess whether the candidates are able to understand whether the memory loss is due to a dissociative disorder or not. In dissociative fugue, there is a purposeful journey away from home or place of work during which self-care is maintained. In such disorders, it is presumed that the ability to exercise a conscious and selective control over mental function is impaired.

4. **Expanded construct:**

- The candidate should be able to demonstrate skill in eliciting a history from the informant that picks up relevant information about dissociative fugue.
- Its origin, duration and progress.
- They should be able to elicit possible aetiological factors.
- They should briefly ask about symptoms of possible differential diagnosis or comorbid disorders.
- Sudden and expected travel away from home or work place with inability to recall one's past, but maintenance of basic self-care.
- In some cases, new identity may be assumed, usually only for a few days, but occasionally for a long time.
- They need to elicit the informant's fears, anxieties, concerns and expectations and address them appropriately, e.g., Her partner's condition is due to intolerable traumatic experience of his

father's unexpected and sudden death. It is a separation of unpleasant emotions and memories from conscious awareness with subsequent disruption to normal life. This is somehow transformed into his current symptoms, which tend to resolve after a few weeks or months.

- Understanding that the fugue is not due to organic mental disorders and cannot be explained by ordinary forgetfulness or fatigue.
- The amnesia is usually centerd on the traumatic events. It may vary from day to day and between investigators.

5. **Areas of importance to pass the station:**
   - Eliciting accurate and sufficient information about dissociative fugue (50%).
   - Discussing the mother's fears, anxieties, concerns and expectations (30%).
   - Communication (20%).
6. **Equipment Checklist:**
   Not applicable.

Station 89: Multiple personality disorder

Theme: Multiple personality disorder: Collateral information from patient's wife

1. **Instructions to candidates:**

   You will meet Mrs Abdulla who is worried about her husband's behaviour for the past 6 months. She believes that he is not the same person she had married 3 years ago. He is acting in completely strange manners. One day, he is Mr Abdul Abdulla and next time, he is Sadam Hussein. When he is Sadam, he acts aggressively, orders people around and will not believe that he is actually Abdul. However, a few days later, he comes down to earth and acts appropriately as my husband. He denies any memories of being Sadam Hussein and will not accept that he had ever claimed to be Sadam. He will then assume the role of a Mr Nasser Ali who is gentle and kind. He will deny ever being Nasser Ali. This has repeated a few times over past 6 months.

   Take a history from the informant about multiple personality disorder and address her fears, anxieties, concerns and expectations about her husband.

2. **Instructions to the role player:**

   You are wife of Abdul Abdulla and have been married for 3 years. You are worried about changes in his behaviour over the 6 months. He was fired from his job as an administrator at the time. He has not been able to find another job. His father became seriously ill 3 months ago. He is the only child of his parents.

   - You believe that he behaves like Jackal and Hyde.
   - When he is Abdul, he is very caring, compassionate and easy going.
   - However, when he believes that he is Sadam Hussein, nothing can persuade him otherwise. He becomes aggressive, and orders his parents and me. He will spend money on things we don't need.
   - After a while, he will be Abdul whom I have known for several years. He will deny being Sadam Hussein and will laugh and tell me not to take mickey out of him.

- He will then assume the role of a Mr Nasser Ali who is gentle and kind. He will deny being Abdul at all.
- When he is Abdul, he will deny being either Sadam Hussein or Nasser Ali at all.
- His two personalities are distinct and separate from each other.
- His memory is normal and does not suffer from any physical or mental illness.
- A recent brain MRI scan and EEG were normal.
- He does not drink alcohol or take illicit drugs.

You want to know what is wrong with your husband, what can be done to help him and if and when he will recover from this condition as they plan to start a family.

3. **Construct:**

This station assesses whether the candidates are able to understand that multiple personality/dissociative identity disorder is a dissociative disorder. Its essential feature is an apparent existence of two or more distinct personalities within an individual, with one of them being evident at a time. Each personality is complete with its own memories, behaviour and preferences.

4. **Expanded construct:**

- The candidates are able to elicit accurate history from the patient's wife about multiple personality disorder/dissociative identity disorder.
- Its origin, duration and progress.
- They should be able to elicit possible aetiological factors.
- They should briefly ask about symptoms of possible differential diagnosis or co-morbid disorders.
- The two personalities are almost always unaware of each other's existence.
- They need to elicit the informant's fears, anxieties, concerns and expectations and address them appropriately, e.g., Her husband's condition is due to intolerable traumatic experience of his sacking and father's unexpected and sudden ill health. It is a separation of unpleasant emotions and memories from conscious awareness with subsequent disruption to normal life. This is somehow transformed into his current symptoms, which tend to resolve after a few weeks or months.
- Understanding that his condition is not due to organic mental disorders, physiological effects of substances and cannot be explained by ordinary forgetfulness or fatigue.
- The candidates should be aware of the double phenomenon, which describes the self-existence of those who feel that there are two different parts of themselves in conflict with each other. They are fully aware both at the same time.

5. **Areas of importance to pass the station:**

- Eliciting accurate and sufficient information about multiple personality disorder (50%).
- Discussing the mother's fears, anxieties, concerns and expectations (30%).
- Communication (20%).

6. **Equipment Checklist:**

Not applicable

2. Alcohol and Substance Misuse

Babu Mani Sandilyan

Stations 90–95

Station 90: Social complications of alcohol dependence

Theme: Assess social complications of alcohol dependence

1. **Instructions to candidates:**

   You are working for the local Alcohol Service. Mr Bottle a 48-year-old male patient was referred to your team by his GP with a history of 'excessive alcohol use'.

   Please make an assessment of his alcohol related problems, specifically focussing on social complications.

2. **Instructions to the role player:**

   - You are 48-year-old and live with your wife Kate in a 3-bedroom house in Bedford. You have two sons, Bob, aged 18 and George, aged 17.
   - You have been drinking alcohol 'throughout your life' but for the last 4 years you have been drinking on a daily basis. You drink anything between 4 and 10 pints of special brew (9%), mostly in the local pub with your work colleagues but also at home. During weekends you additionally drink up to one bottle of vodka, if you can afford it. You sometimes drink upon waking up to steady your nerves. You cannot remember the last time you did not drink at all.
   - Your wife keeps nagging you and wants you to address your alcohol problems. She forced you to go to your GP and ensured you also attended today. She threatened to leave you on a number of occasions. She said she was upset about your drinking but you suspect she may be seeing someone else. Your sons have left home some time ago. You do not get on with them because they are arrogant and disrespectful. You also have problems with your brothers who are nosey and controlling.
   - Your GP did some blood tests and told you that there are problems with your liver. He told you though that it is only a matter of weeks before they get better, when you decide to stop drinking. This shows that there is nothing seriously wrong with your health.
   - You were working as a sales manager for a car dealership but you were fired 2 months ago. You missed some crucial appointments and your manager became very angry. You know though that it was down to the recession and they were looking for an excuse to fire staff any way. You have not yet secured new employment.
   - You have 'some debts' but if necessary, you could sell the family house and downsize. You have not talked to your wife about this plan but the house is in your name anyway.
   - DVLA recently revoked your driving licence. You were involved in 'a few accidents'. You were over the drink-drive limit three times. You lost the company car after you were fired and the family car is old and expensive to maintain. You have been involved in fights in the past, whilst intoxicated but only when provoked. You have been in prison twice for common assault and ABH but this was almost 20 years ago.

- You are bored at home and you have nothing better to do. Going to the pub helps you fill your days and catch up with friends. You would miss all that if you were abstinent. You get annoyed when people criticise your drinking habits but you also feel guilty sometimes.

3. **Construct:**
The station tests the candidate's ability to elicit a comprehensive history of alcohol dependence, specifically focussing on the social complications of excessive alcohol use.

4. **Expanded construct:**
   - Candidate should be able to demonstrate motivational interviewing skills.
   - Candidate should be able to sensitively elicit a history of alcohol harmful use/dependence.
   - Candidate should be able to elicit history of social complications of alcohol dependence.
   - Candidate should be able to establish the impact of alcohol misuse on family, friends and occupation.
   - Candidate should be able to establish the forensic history/legal problems/accidents as a result of alcohol misuse.
   - Candidate should be able to establish physical and psychiatric comorbidity.

5. **Areas of importance to pass the station:**
   - Elicit a comprehensive history of alcohol dependence (20%).
   - Make a holistic and comprehensive assessment of the service user's social circumstances (60%).
   - Advanced communication skills and empathic interviewing (20%).

6. **Equipment checklist:**
Not applicable

Station 91: Alcohol dependence

Theme: Assessment of alcohol dependence

1. **Instructions to candidates:**
You are seeing Mr Best a 55-year-old male patient, in the local Alcohol Service. Mr Best self-referred to your team and is keen to receive treatment for his alcohol-related problems.
Make an assessment for alcohol dependence.

2. **Instructions to the role player:**
   - You are 55-year-old. You are divorced and live on your own in a flat in Bedford.
   - You have been drinking alcohol since your adolescence. After your best friend died from a heart attack 5 years ago, alcohol use became more persistent. You now drink on a daily basis, mostly cider but also spirits or wine. You need at least 3 litres of 7.5% cider daily to keep you from feeling unwell.
   - If no alcohol is available, you become shaky and sweaty, nauseous and anxious. You can only sleep after drinking but even then your sleep is broken and with vivid nightmares. You always keep a bottle next to your bed as this makes you feel safe.

- You used to drink in the local pub but not anymore, as it is too expensive. You buy big bottles of cider from the supermarket. You sometimes find it difficult to control the amounts consumed and you end up emptying all the bottles in the house.
- You feel low in mood and unmotivated. You are unhappy with your life circumstances and you feel lonely and abandoned. You wonder whether you might be better off dead. You have not attempted to end your life and you have no specific plans to do so currently. When you talked to your GP about how you felt, he prescribed an anti-depressant. The local counselling service would not see you whilst you still drink.
- Your energy levels have been affected and you find it hard to concentrate. Your GP told you about significant liver changes and referred to the liver specialists.
- You are a carpenter by trade and you are self-employed. Things are tight financially but you have no major debts.
- You were recently involved in a road traffic accident. A cyclist fell on your car and needed hospital treatment for a fractured leg. Even though you were not responsible, you worry you might end up getting the blame. You were not intoxicated at the time but you know you should not be driving.
- This incident made you eager to deal with your alcohol use. You are happy to accept any treatment recommendations, including hospital treatment if necessary. You find it hard to imagine how life would be without alcohol but you see that there is no option other than abstinence.

3. Construct:

The station tests the candidate's ability to elicit a comprehensive history of alcohol dependence.

4. Expanded construct:

- Candidate should be able to demonstrate motivational interviewing skills.
- Candidate should be able to sensitively elicit a history of alcohol dependence.
- Candidate should be able to establish physical and psychiatric comorbidity.
- Candidate should be able to establish the impact of alcohol misuse on depression.
- Candidate should be able to establish the social circumstances.

Communication

The candidate Should adopt motivational interviewing principles:

- <u>F</u>eedback: Provide feedback on the client's personal circumstances.
- <u>R</u>esponsibility: Emphasise the client's personal responsibility/choice to change.
- <u>A</u>dvice: Offer practical advice regarding alcohol use.
- <u>M</u>enu: Explain possible treatment options and invite the client to decide.
- <u>E</u>mpathy: Avoid confrontation and be supportive.
- <u>S</u>elf-Efficacy: Encourage optimism.

5. Areas of importance to pass the station:

- Establish whether criteria for alcohol dependence are met (30%).
- Establish a comprehensive medical and psychiatric history (30%).
- Establish the client's social circumstances (20%).
- Motivational interviewing/communication skills (20%).

6. Equipment Checklist:

Not applicable.

Station 92: Psychiatric sequelae of alcohol dependence

Theme: Establish patterns of drinking and its effects upon the patient's mood and risk to himself and others

1. **Instructions to candidates:**

   You are working for the local Drugs and Alcohol Team. You are seeing Mr Foster a 43-year-old male, who has a long history of alcohol use and depression. He is attending with his CMHT care coordinator.

   - **Assess Mr Foster for the presence of alcohol misuse, examine the interaction between alcohol misuse and depression and complete a risk assessment.**

2. **Instructions to the role player:**

   - You are Mr Foster. You are 43 years old. You live with your wife and 17-year-old son in Luton.
   - Your regular alcohol use started about 10 years ago. At the time you were suffering from depression and you found that alcohol could help you cope better. You now drink on a daily basis, 20 units on average. You buy bottles of wine from the super market. Your wife is unhappy with your alcohol use and is trying to monitor you. This makes you even more upset.
   - You do not always drink in the morning. You look forward to coming home from work to have your first drink of the day. You get carried away and drink more than originally planned.
   - You were experimenting with illicit substances when younger. You started smoking cannabis aged 14. By the time you finished school, you were a regular user of amphetamines, ecstasy and crack cocaine. You stopped most of these substances about 10 years ago, 'coincidentally' when alcohol use became more problematic.
   - You had your first episode of depression aged 19, after your partner left you. You have a number of hospital admissions and you have tried to take your own life. You are now on anti-depressants, which do not seem to work. You started CBT but treatment had to be postponed after you turned up in an intoxicated state on two occasions.
   - You still feel low in mood and unmotivated. You wonder whether you might be better off dead. Your energy and concentration levels are poor. You have lost interest in sex and you believe that your wife finds you unattractive. You feel guilty for that. You are not jealous of her.
   - You work as an IT manager in a building firm. You had to take time off because of your latest episode of depression.
   - You are still driving but you are 'never drunk' when you are behind the wheel.

3. **Construct:**

   The station tests the candidate's ability to elicit a comprehensive history of alcohol dependence in the context of an affective disorder (dual diagnosis) and make a comprehensive risk assessment.

4. **Expanded construct:**

   - Candidate should be able to demonstrate motivational interviewing skills.
   - Candidate should be able to sensitively elicit a history of alcohol dependence.
   - Candidate should be able to establish physical and psychiatric comorbidity.

- Candidate should be able to elicit history of depression.
- Candidate should be able to establish the impact of alcohol misuse on depression.
- Candidate should be able to do a brief risk assessment of self-harm/suicide.

5. Areas of importance to pass the station:

- Establish whether criteria for alcohol dependence 30%.
- Establish whether criteria for depression 30%.
- Establish the link between alcohol dependence and depression 20%.
- Empathic interviewing/communication skills including motivational interviewing 20%.

6. Equipment checklist:

Not applicable.

Station 93: Methadone withdrawal

Theme: Assessment of a service user with opiate dependence, identification of opiate withdrawal symptoms

1. Instructions to candidates:

You are working for the Liaison Psychiatric Team in the A and E Department of a General Hospital. Your A and E colleagues have asked you to assess Mr John Smith. He self referred to A and E and described a long history of heroin use. He is on a methadone maintenance programme but claims that it is not 'holding him', as he failed to collect today's dose. He is asking for his 'usual daily methadone'.

Assess Mr Smith for presence of opiate withdrawal symptoms.

2. Instructions to the role player:

- Open the station by asking 'give me some methadone'. Show that you are agitated and anxious. If the doctor is not empathic raise your voice and ask 'can't you see, I am clucking?'
- You are a 25-year-old man with a 6-year history of daily heroin use. You used to buy up to 5 bags a day (£50, 1 gm) and used to inject in the arms, legs and groin. You used to share needles with your mates. You started attending the local Drugs and Alcohol Service 3 months ago. You are on 80 ml of methadone, which you consume every day in the local pharmacy. You still smoke heroin, up to 2 bags every other day.
- You do not like going to a pharmacy every day. You would like to collect your methadone once a week. You are asking to have 'your 80 ml of methadone' which you missed today when your car broke down on the way to the pharmacy.
- You smoke crack cocaine 'once in a while' but you do not consider this a problem. You have tried most other substances when you were a teenager but not recently. You smoke 'one joint' of cannabis at night to relax. Your alcohol use has increased recently (4 pint cans of special brew 9%) but you do not see this as a problem.
- You have no previous contact with mental health services but have felt desperate and suicidal in the past. You stopped injecting after you were told you have hepatitis C. You have not been

vaccinated for hepatitis B. You had a number of skin abscesses and your right leg became painful and swollen 6 months ago but you did not tell anyone.

- You had a good childhood but you 'mixed with the wrong crowd' when 15. You live in a bedsit and you do not work. You have friends who are also using substances. You have not been to prison but you have been arrested for shoplifting, assaults and drink driving.

3. **Construct:**

The station tests the candidate's ability to elicit a comprehensive history of opiate dependence, identify the symptoms of opiate dependence and organise appropriate management plans in an A and E setting.

4. **Expanded construct:**
   - Candidate should be able to demonstrate motivational interviewing skills.
   - Candidate should be able to sensitively elicit a history of opiate/multiple substance harmful use/dependence.
   - Candidate should be able to identify symptoms of opiate withdrawal.
   - Candidate should be able to make appropriate management plans.

5. **Areas of importance to pass the station:**
   - Elicit a comprehensive history of opiate dependence; elicit a comprehensive history of other illicit substance harmful use/dependence (40%).
   - Identify symptoms and signs of opiate withdrawal (20%).
   - Make a reasonable initial management plan (20%).
   - Motivational interviewing/communication skills (20%).

6. **Equipment checklist:**

Not applicable.

Station 94: Methadone in pregnancy

Theme: Treatment options for opiate dependence during pregnancy

1. **Instructions to candidates:**

You work in the local Drugs and Alcohol Service. You have been asked to see a 25-year-old Margaret Thompson. She has a history of heroin dependence and for the last 6 months she is on methadone. She just found out she is 8 weeks pregnant and wants to stop taking methadone to safeguard her child's health.

Assess and discuss treatment options for opiate dependence during pregnancy.

2. **Instructions to the role player:**
   - You are 25 years old. You started using heroin 8 years ago. You were initially smoking during weekends with friends. You very quickly ended up using daily. You used to spend up to £50 and there were frequent instances where you ended up injecting. You were only injecting in

the arms. You started attending the local Drugs Service 6 months ago, after your 9-month-old daughter Emma was given up for adoption. You are on methadone 60 ml, which you collect three times a week. You have stayed off heroin most of this period but you still feel vulnerable and on occasions crave heroin.

- You do not use cocaine, amphetamines or other illicit substances. After finding out about the pregnancy, you also stopped drinking alcohol.
- You have no history of medical problems. You have no mental health problems.
- You are in a long-term relationship with Ian. He is also on methadone. You live together in a council flat. You are on benefits. You have no current legal problems.
- You are very pleased with the pregnancy and you want to stop methadone as soon as possible. You have made plans about your baby and you may even use some of the things bought for Emma. Last time you were pregnant, social services intervened and removed your daughter Emma after birth.
- You say you want to stop methadone to ensure that your baby will not withdraw after birth. You have seen some awful videos of babies withdrawing after birth, whose mothers were on methadone during pregnancy.
- You admit, if asked, that you really only want to stop methadone because you believe that this is the only way to convince social services to let you keep your baby.
- Your midwife has already been in contact with social services and John Smith; Social Worker will visit you in 2 weeks.

3. **Construct:**

The station tests the candidate's ability to discuss treatment options for opiate dependence in a pregnant service user in a sensitive but thorough way.

4. **Expanded construct:**

- Candidate should be able to demonstrate motivational interviewing skills.
- Candidate should be able to sensitively elicit a history of opiate/multiple substance harmful use/dependence.
- Candidate should be able to assess pregnancy: Progression, social and psychological circumstances, supports networks.
- Candidate should be able to obtain information regarding current treatment arrangements.
- Candidate should be able to discuss the treatment options for opiate dependence in pregnancy.
- Candidate should be able to engage with service user in a collaborative treatment plan.

5. **Areas of importance to pass the station:**

- Elicit a comprehensive history of opiate dependence/other illicit substance harmful use/ dependence (10%).
- Establish the circumstances of pregnancy (20%).
- Discuss the treatment options of opiate dependence in pregnant service users (40%).
- Establish the service user's capacity and facilitate an informed treatment choice (10%).
- Empathic interviewing/communication skills (20%).

6. **Equipment checklist:**

Not applicable.

Station 95: Opiate dependence

Theme: Assessment of a patient with opioid dependence

1. **Instructions to candidates:**

   You are working in the local Drugs and Alcohol Team. Mr John Taylor has self-referred to the team. He described a long history of heroin use. He is requesting treatment for his 'addiction'.

   Assess Mr Taylor for the presence of opioid dependence.

2. **Instructions to the role player:**

   - You are a 25-year-old man who lives with a friend. You first tried heroin aged 17. Daily heroin use started 5 years ago. You are now buying up to 5 bags of heroin a day (£10 per bag). You prefer to smoke it. You used to inject in the arms, legs and groin. You used to share needles with your mates. You last used heroin this morning before coming to your appointment. When you cannot find heroin, you buy methadone, subutex, DFs or diazepam but 'it is not the same'.
   - You smoke crack cocaine every other day. You spend up to £200 on occasions. You do not consider this a big problem. You started smoking cannabis when you were 14. You still smoke 'one joint' at night to relax. Your alcohol use is intermittent but there are periods you drink 8–10 cans of special brew.
   - You have not seen a psychiatrist before. You have felt desperate and suicidal in the past. Your GP prescribes an antidepressant, diazepam and a sleeping tablet. You would be lost without them.
   - You have not been tested for hepatitis or HIV and it is one of your worries. You had a number of skin abscesses and your right leg became painful and swollen 6 months ago but you did not tell anyone.
   - You have not been to prison but you have been arrested numerous times for shoplifting and begging.
   - You have friends who are also using substances. Two of them recently died from 'accidental overdoses' but you believe they may have committed suicide. You now want to escape from this lifestyle.

3. **Construct:**

   The station tests the candidate's ability to establish a diagnosis of opioid dependence.

4. **Expanded construct:**

   - Candidate should be able to take a history of opioid use and establish the presence of dependence.
   - Candidate should be able to take a history of other substance harmful use/dependence.
   - Candidate should be able to take a comprehensive medical and psychiatric history, developmental history and review current social circumstances and motivation to effect change.
   - Candidate should be able to consider risks to self and others, including the impact of substance use to family and friends.

5. **Areas of importance to pass the station:**
   - Take a history of opioid use and establish the presence of dependence (30%).
   - Take a history of other substance harmful use/dependence (20%).
   - Take a comprehensive medical and psychiatric history, developmental history and review current social circumstances and motivation to effect change (20%).
   - Consider risks to self and others, including the impact of substance use to family and friends (10%).
   - Empathic interviewing/communication skills (20%).
6. **Equipment checklist:**
   Not applicable.

3. Forensic Psychiatry

Nuruz Zaman and Shazada Hussain Shah

Linked Stations: 96–99

Station 96: Link 1: Assess: Fitness to plead
Station 97: Link 2: Discuss: Fitness to plead

Station 96: Link 1: Assess: Fitness to plead

Theme: To demonstrate understanding and ability to assess a patient's fitness to plead

1. **Instructions to candidates:**
   Patient's name: Michael Evans
   You are a junior doctor who is looking after Michael Evans who was recently diagnosed with paranoid schizophrenia. He is currently treated in medium security unit. He is charged for Actual Bodily Harm and awaiting a trial. You have been asked to assess Mr Evans' fitness to plead at his court case.
   - **Assess his fitness to plead.**
   - **Do not perform a mental state examination.**
2. **Instructions to the role player:**
   - You are Michael Evans, a 19-year-old admitted to a medium security unit after transfer from remand in prison. You were arrested at a local shopping mall after injuring a man by causing a superficial laceration with a knife.
   - You know that a cult of devil worshippers have moved to the local area. You have been instructed by God to eradicate these devil worshippers. You believe the man you wounded was a devil worshipper. He had made eye contact at a shop and then you knew he was going to hurt you, so you had to take action.

- You believe you are not guilty of the charge made against you. You know that guilty means you did the crime and that you could be imprisoned for some time. You also accept you could be detained indefinitely in hospital for treatment.
- You generally hear God's voice giving you a commentary of your life as it progresses and occasionally you are told that certain people are devil worshippers and as a result you are suspicious towards them.
- You, a university student, who studied physics course 2 years ago and since you have been on a secret mission as an agent for the MI5. You are not on any medication.
- You are visibly angry and agitated by the circumstances you find yourself in.
- You know that a court is comprised a jury of 12 members of the public. You know that a Judge keeps order in a court and will direct the jury on interpreting the law. You know that there is a prosecution solicitor and a solicitor who will help you to defend you in court. You know you will instruct the solicitor on the facts of the case as you see it. You know that evidence in the form of witness statements will be presented in court. You know you can question the evidence and challenge a member of the jury, should you know them and feel your case may be biased as a result. You know that at the completion of evidence and judge's summary of the case, the jury will be giving their verdict.
- You are co-operative generally with the doctor but appear angry, agitated and irritable at times.

3. **Construct:**

The station tests the candidate's ability to assess a patient's fitness to plead in court. It tests a candidate's ability to convey information and work towards building rapport with an angry and agitated patient.

4. **Expanded construct:**

- The candidate should be able to assess the patient's fitness to plead in a focussed, fluent and empathetic manner.
- The candidate should elicit the patient's ability to express his plea and understanding of pleading guilty or not guilty.
- The candidate should enquire about the patient's understanding of court proceedings and evidence.
- The candidate should enquire about the patient's understanding of instructing a solicitor and challenging a juror.
- The candidate should elicit symptoms of paranoia and degree which this conviction is held.
- Candidates should be able to demonstrate advanced communication and management skills with an acutely agitated and angry patient.
- The candidate should be able to ask questions that are structured, focused and fluent.
- The candidate should be able to demonstrate diplomacy and empathy with the patient.
- The candidate should be able to use language, i.e., simple and understandable and avoid jargon.

5. **Areas of importance to pass the station:**

- Ability to elicit and explore the criteria (60%).

- Subsidiary elements are: Interviewing/communication skills (20%).
- Ability to manage an acutely agitated and angry patient (20%).

6. **Equipment checklist:**
   Not applicable.

Station 97: Link 2: Discuss: Fitness to plead

Theme: Discuss patient's fitness to plead with his legal representative

1. **Instructions to candidates:**

   Patient's name: Michael Evans

   You are a junior doctor looking after Michael Evans, who has recently been diagnosed with paranoid schizophrenia. You saw him in the previous station. You will now discuss your findings with his legal representative.

   - **Discuss his fitness to plead his case.**
   - **Address the legal representative's views, expectations and concerns.**

2. **Instructions to the role player:**
   - You are Tim Terry, the legal representative for Michael Evans.
   - Michael Evans a 19-year-old admitted was to a medium security unit after transfer from remand in prison. He was arrested at a local shopping mall after injuring a man by causing a superficial laceration with a knife.
   - Michael suffers from paranoid schizophrenia. He believes that a cult of devil worshippers have moved to the local area. He has been instructed by God to eradicate these devil worshippers. He believed the man he wounded was a devil worshipper.
   - He hears God's voice giving him a commentary of his life as it progresses and occasionally he is told that certain people are devil worshippers and as a result he is suspicious towards them.

   You ask the following questions:
   - **Is he fit to plead?**
   - **Why do you believe he is fit or not fit to plead?**
   - **How does his psychosis affect his fitness to plead?**
   - **Is there anything that shall help him to enter a plea in court?**
   - **What alternatives to tablets are available?**

3. **Construct:**
   The station tests the candidate's ability to explain fitness to plead to a solicitor.

4. **Expanded construct:**
   - The candidate should be able to explain the patient's fitness to plead.
   - The candidate should be able to give a coherent explanation of the reasons whether the patient is fit or not to plead.
   - The candidate should be able to demonstrate advanced listening skills.

- The candidate should be able to use language, i.e., simple and understandable and avoid jargon.
- The candidate should be able to avoid a didactic pseudo-academic lecture.

5. **Areas of importance to pass the station:**
   - Ability to explain the fitness to plead (40%).
   - Communication skills (30%).
   - Ability to respond appropriately to the questions posed (30%).
6. **Equipment checklist:**
   Not applicable.

Linked Stations: 98 and 99

Station 98: Link 1: Assess: Risk of violence
Station 99: Link 2: Discuss: Risk assessment

Station 98: Link 1: Assess: Risk of violence

Theme: Assess the risk of violence in a patient with psychosis

1. **Instructions to candidates:**
   Patient's name: John Fitzgerald
   You are a junior doctor looking after John Fitzgerald. You are due to see him on the ward. He has been admitted after transfer from a police station.
   - **Assess his risk of violence.**
2. **Instructions to the role player:**
   - You are John Fitzgerald, a 26-year-old man, brought to ward after transfer from a police station and are formally detained. You were found outside a shopping center talking to yourself. Staff had called the police and you brandished a knife, which lead to a police officer being hurt seriously.
   - You believe that you are a world famous gangster rap artist. You have been given special messages hidden in rap music to release the people from Capitalistic oppression. You were on a special mission to bring down the big high street names.
   - You wanted to kill the managers of the shops at the shopping center by stabbing them.
   - You were sacked from a job at the age of 16 because you swore at your manager after 1 day in the job. He had pressurised you into working long hours. The longest you have had a job is 3 days. You generally get into a fight with a manager.
   - You are very angry that the police and doctors don't understand that you are on a special mission and that they are holding you back from your job. Initially you are pleasant with the doctor. As time progresses you receive messages into your secret ear microphone, that you are urgently needed back at the shopping mall. You are distressed by the fact both the police and doctors don't understand despite your clear explanation.

- You generally hear voices telling you a commentary of your life as it progresses and you are suspicious towards all shop managers.
- You are co-operative generally with the doctor because you want them to know about your injustice and how you were going to correct it.
- You were scholastically backward at young age.
- Your father physically, sexually and verbally abused your mother. He left the family when you were 6-year-old.
- You were brought up by a step-father who used to burn his cigarettes on you.
- You were not good with your studies at school and often got into fights. You were expelled on three occasions for fighting and abusing teachers.
- You used to enjoy burning frogs with a cigarette lighter at the local park.
- You have irregularly smoked cannabis. In the last 3 weeks, you have also begun to smoke crack and heroine. You have financed your habit by robbery and theft.
- You have spent in total 30 months in prison for various charges including assault and grievous bodily harm a few years ago. You attacked a night club bouncer on one occasion, using a baseball bat.
- You are currently on a probation order and have a probation officer.
- You live alone and have no family or friends. You enjoy your gangster rap and spend most of your time making special CDs.
- You are not on any medication. You have never been seen by a psychiatrist before. You don't feel you need any help and you need to get on with completing your task. You are visibly angry and agitated by the circumstances you find yourself in.

3. **Construct:**

The station tests the candidate's ability to assess the risk. It tests a candidate's ability to convey information and work towards building rapport with an angry and agitated patient.

4. **Expanded construct:**

- The candidate should be able to assess factors important in a risk assessment of violence. It should be focussed, fluent and empathetic.
- The candidate should be able to seek to understand what is happening and elicit symptoms of paranoid schizophrenia, substance misuse and dissocial personality.
- Candidates should be able to demonstrate advanced communication and management skills with an acutely agitated and angry patient.
- The candidate should be able to show an appropriate mix of open and closed questioning.
- The candidate should be able to demonstrate advanced listening skills.
- The candidate should be able to diplomacy and empathy with the patient.

5. **Areas of importance to pass the station:**

- Ability to assess risk of violence (60%).
- Communication skills (40%).

6. **Equipment checklist:**

Not applicable.

Station 99: Link 2: Discuss: Risk assessment

Theme: Discuss the risk assessment with the probation officer

1. **Instructions to candidates:**

   Probation officer's name: Derek Thompson

   You are a junior doctor looking after John Fitzgerald, who has recently been admitted after stabbing a police officer whilst he was psychotic. You have seen him in the previous station. You are due to discuss his case with the probation officer.

   - **Discuss the current and future risk of violence.**
   - **Explain reasons for your findings.**
   - **Address his views, expectations and concerns.**

2. **Instructions to the role player:**

   - You are Derek Thompson, the probation officer for John Fitzgerald. He has been recently admitted to hospital after stabbing a police officer.

   You ask the following questions:

   - **What are current risks he is posing and why?**
   - **What is the likelihood of further risk of violence in future?**
   - **What would the doctor like to do to manage the risk of further violence?**
   - **What treatment would they like to offer the patient?**
   - **Is he safe in the hospital?**
   - **Are other people safe?**
   - **What should be done to reduce the risk of violence in the future?**
   - **What are the alternatives to him being in hospital?**

3. **Construct:**

   The station tests the candidate's ability to explain the initial and long-term management of violent patients.

4. **Expanded construct:**

   - The candidate should be able to explain the risk factors of violence.
   - The candidate should be able to give a coherent explanation of management of violence risk.
   - The candidate should be able to explain the need for secure environment.
   - The candidate should be able to explain the need for monitoring on a regular basis and considerations for non-compliance.
   - The candidate should be able to demonstrate advanced listening skills.
   - The candidate should be able to use language, i.e., simple and understandable and avoid jargon.
   - The candidate should be able to avoid a didactic pseudo-academic lecture.

5. **Areas of importance to pass the station:**
   - Ability to explain the acute management of violence (40%).
   - Communication skills (40%).
   - Ability to respond appropriately to the questions posed (20%).
6. **Equipment checklist:**
   Not applicable.

Single Station

Station 100: Discuss the management of paedophilia

Theme: Discussion of management with a person convicted of paedophilia

1. **Instructions to candidates:**

   You are meeting a 35-year-old Justine Caudwell who was convicted of paedophilia 5 years ago. The Ministry of Justice has ordered him to receive treatment for his condition as a condition of early release from the prison.

   You have assessed him before and now will discuss the management with him.

2. **Instructions to the role player:**

   You are 35-year-old Justine Caudwell who was recently released on license after serving 5 years in prison. You are obliged to consider treatment for your condition. You are indeed pleased to know that long last you will receive treatment.

   You want to know the following:
   - **To understand why he was attracted to children.**
   - **To understand how he can help himself.**
   - **What are the treatment options available for him?**
   - **How can he find work?**
   - **How can he normalize his life?**
   - **Is there any hope for him in future?**

3. **Construct:**

   This station assesses the candidates' understanding of principles of managing patients with paedophilia.

4. **Expanded construct:**

   Paedophilia is a sexual preference for children usually of pre-pubertal or early pubertal age. Some paedophiles are attracted only to girls, some only to boys and others are interested in both sexes. It is rarely identified in women. Some men who retain a preference for adult sexual partners but as they are chronically frustrated in achieving appropriate contacts, habitually turn to children as substitutes. Men who molest their own pre-pubertal children occasionally approach other children as well, but in either case, their behaviour is indicative of paedophilia.

- General principles:
  - Paedophiles are typically in crisis when they present for treatment.
  - Identify why the patient is seeking treatment now.
  - Sexual urges are controllable and the sexual acts are the person's responsibility.
  - It is important to assist in establishing and maintaining a healthy social support system.
  - Group therapy is particularly helpful in assisting to confront cognitive distortions and learning from other paedophiles who have improved.
  - Advice about appropriate work, finding work and ways to spend leisure time in constructive and pro-social ways.
  - Facilitate disclosure.
  - Avoid one-sided treatment plans.
  - Intervene quickly, be persistent, inclusive with treatment and optimistic.
- Medication:
  - Selective serotonin reuptake inhibitors to decrease sexual anxiety and impulsivity.
  - Antiandrogens to moderate sex drive.
  - Gonadotrophin–releasing hormone (GNRH) analogues, such as, triptorelin to eliminate sex drive.

5. **Areas of importance to pass the station:**
   - Explain the treatment options (70%).
   - Communication (30%).

6. **Equipment checklist:**
   Not applicable.

4. Old Age Psychiatry

Ajaya Upadhyaya and Vishalle Kamath

Old Age Psychiatry

Linked Stations: 101–128

Station 101: Link 1: Dementia and Psychosis: History taking and risk assessment

Station 102: Link 2: Dementia and Psychosis: Discuss management

Station 101: Link 1: Dementia and Psychosis: History taking and risk assessment

Theme: History taking and risk assessment in dementia

1. **Instructions to candidates:**
   You are asked to see Mr John Barton, a 76-year-old gentleman, in the A and E, who is quite confused,

answering your questions with irrelevant answers. He is accompanied by his daughter. Mr Barton has a longstanding history of dementia in Alzheimer's disease, which is now of severe degree. Mr Barton was assessed in the Memory Assessment service and was taken off his Acetylcholinesterase Inhibitors, due to the severity of his illness. The A and E staffs have ruled out any acute treatable medical condition. He was found by police wandering the street. He was wearing an alert bracelet; hence, the police were able to get in touch with his daughter after bringing him to A and E.

- **Your role is to take and assess the risks that Mr Barton presents.**
- **You should assume that the history above is accurate.**

Keep your notes for the following station, where you will discuss long-term management with the daughter.

2. **Instructions to the role player (Patient's daughter Jean Barton):**

You are a 37-year-old teacher. Your father lives by himself. He has had carers coming in four times a day. He was diagnosed with Dementia in Alzheimer's disease 4 years ago. This has progressively become worse. Your father has begun self-neglecting, refusing to wash. When the carers come in, he is usually already dressed, without washing, in dirty clothes. On most occasions, he refuses to have a wash or change into clean clothes. He has on occasion become verbally abusive to the carers, when they encourage him to change his clothes. You have the Power of Attorney to look after his affairs, which was registered about 18 months ago. His cooker was disconnected about a year ago, as he had on several occasions left it on, with an empty pan on it. He once placed a pair of his pants on the heater to dry, which caught fire. He put it out himself, by stamping on it. He has on many occasions left his front door open. He has also on several occasions been brought back by his neighbours after wandering out in the village, then forgetting how to get back home. He has had assisted technology in his house, which alerts him when he leaves the house. He has now begun to stop recognizing these warnings. He has on occasions refused to take his medication from the carers. The duty psychiatrist will ask you some questions.

3. **Construct:**

The core task at this station is to complete a detailed risk assessment in the context of a dementia.

4. **Expanded construct:**

They should:

- Ask about demographic risk factors, including if the person lives alone.
- Assess what level of care he is already receiving, which may include the use of assistive technology.
- Take a history of possible risks associated with dementia.
- Ask about risks of fire, including use of the cooker, oven or occasions of accidental fires setting.
- Ask about risk of flooding, including whether they have left taps on any occasion.
- Ask about risk of wandering.
- Ask about risk of aggression or agitation, including resistance to care.
- Ask about risk of financial exploitation and abuse.
- Ask about self-neglect and self-harm.

Interview/Communication skills:

- Appropriate mix of open and closed questions.
- Demonstrate advanced listening skills.
- Elicit history of risky behaviour whilst being empathic to the patient's daughter.

5. **Areas of importance to pass the station:**

The core task at this station is to complete a detailed risk assessment for a patient with dementia, and the following elements should contribute to the bulk of the marks (% relative weighting).

- Interview/communication skills (40%).
- Ability to elicit history of risks in a patient with dementia, including risks of fire, flood, wandering, self-neglect, financial exploitation and abuse, harm to self or others (60%).

Station 102: Link 2: Dementia and Psychosis: Discuss management

Theme: Discuss your findings and management with the patient's daughter

1. **Instructions to the candidates:**

You have ascertained the possible risks that Mr Barton presents in the context of his dementia. You are aware of his history.

Please feedback to his daughter based on the information you elicited in the previous station, what the likely long-term management for this patient might be.

2. **Instructions to the role player:**

The duty psychiatrist will now tell you what they think is the best possible long-term management of your father. Listen carefully, questioning why he has come to this conclusion. It is likely that the duty psychiatrist will suggest permanent care in a dementia care home, given that the risk your father presents are too high to let him to live at home. You should become emotional, stating that you never wanted your father to be put into a home. Ask if there is anything else that can be done to enable him to remain at home. If the duty psychiatrist suggests that he returns home, explain that you are very worried about his safety at home and do not feel that is a feasible option.

3. **Construct:**

The core task at this station is to talk about the long-term management for this patient, based on the risk assessment.

4. **Expanded construct:**

The candidate is expected to:

- Summarise the risks assessed in the previous station.
- Explain that given the degree of risk, it is unsafe for the patient to return home.
- He has both a care package and assistive technology, which are now no longer able to contain these risks.
- There is no other intervention that can be put in the community.
- Allow time for the daughter to register what he/she is saying.

- Ask the daughter to stop/clarify issues as they go along.
- Show empathy towards the daughter, particularly with regards to making a decision about permanent care.

6. **Areas of importance to pass the station:**
   - Communication skills (80%).
   - Summarise risk in a succinct and clear manner (20%).

Station 103: Link 1: Dementia with Lewy Bodies: Assess and discuss Dopamine Transporter/DAT scan

Station 104: Link 2: Dementia with Lewy Bodies: Explain management plan to a carer

Station 103: Link 1: Dementia with Lewy Bodies: Assess and discuss DAT scan

Theme: Assess Dementia with Lewy Bodies and discuss DAT scan with the patient

1. **Instructions to candidates:**

   You are seeing Mrs Briggs in the Memory Assessment service to gain a collateral history, while the psychologist is carrying out a neuropsychometric battery on her husband.

   Elicit a history of Dementia with Lewy Bodies and explain to her relevant investigations, including DAT scan.

2. **Instructions to the role player:**

   You are Mrs Briggs. Your husband is a 69-year-old ex-merchant navy officer. Over last 18 months he has developed multiple problems, which are becoming progressively worse. These include him thinking that there are naval seamen in your house. He has been having falls and last year sustained a fracture of his wrist after falling in the town. His memory appeared to be relatively good, until very recently, when he appears to be having periods when he thinks he is back in the merchant navy again. He has become more irritable and short with you, which is quite out of character for him. He was an avid fisherman, which he has completely stopped. He has always taken care of the bills and finances, but you are finding you have to do more these days. You have noticed that there are few scratches and little bangs on the car. When you have enquired about these with him, he does not appear to be aware that anything has happened. You feel slightly unsafe when sitting in the car with him, as he appears to be unaware of the distance of oncoming traffic.

3. **Construct:**

   This station sets out to ascertain the candidate's knowledge of symptomatology of Dementia with Lewy Bodies and the role of DAT scan in this condition.

4. **Expanded Construct:**
   - Take a history.
   - Explain details of a DAT scan, including its purpose and process.

   The candidate should:
   - Gain history of fluctuating cognitive impairment, visual hallucinations or other psychotic phenomenon, parkinsonian features with some functional decline.

- Be empathetic.
- Explain DAT scan: This scan gives a picture with valuable information about function of the brain. It can help diagnose Parkinson's disease. It can also aid in differentiating Lewy Body Dementia (LBD) from non-LBD, including the most common cause of dementia, i.e., Alzheimer's disease.

5. **Areas of importance to pass the station:**

   Core elements that need to be demonstrated in this station are ability to elicit a clear and comprehensive history, whilst being empathetic to the carer (40%).

   - The candidate should demonstrate good communication skills, whilst listening carefully and allowing the carer to speak (20%).
   - The candidate should be able to explain clearly what a DAT Scan is and its relevance in confirming a diagnosis of Dementia with Lewy Bodies (40%).

Station 104: Link 2: Dementia with Lewy Bodies: Explain management plan to a carer

Theme: To explain the management of Dementia with Lewy Bodies to a carer

1. **Instructions to candidates:**

   Explain to Mrs Briggs the management of Dementia with Lewy Bodies.

   Assume that all investigations have been completed. You are not expected to take a history.

2. **Instructions to the role player:**

   The candidate will explain to you the management of Lewy Body Dementia, which your husband has been diagnosed with. Ask about the role of Donepezil, that you heard of on the news, i.e., used to treat dementia. Ensure you ask if this can be offered him and what is his prognosis. Ask the candidate how his visual hallucinations will be treated and is the treatment similar to that used in illnesses like schizophrenia. Ask the candidate if things like 'brain games' are of any value. Be sure to ask about the role of talking therapies.

3. **Construct:**

   The candidate should be able to discuss the management of Lewy Body Dementia comprehensively.

4. **Expanded construct:**

   The candidate should be able to discuss the management of Lewy Body Dementia in detail.

   - It is essential that the candidate explain that this is a progressive illness, i.e., irreversible.
   - Discuss all elements of management, including from a biopsychosocial point of view.
   - This includes the role of medication; although there is some evidence to suggest that there may be some role of Acetylcholinesterase inhibitors, this is, however, not supported by NICE.
   - It is important for the candidate to explain that for the visual hallucinations or other psychotic symptoms, there is a limited role for antipsychotic medications, as the patient is likely to be extremely sensitive to antipsychotics.
   - It is important that the candidate give the carer information with regards to driving and the importance of informing the DVLA of the diagnosis.

- Give the carer information with regards to Lasting and Enduring Power of Attorney.
- The possible role of cognitive stimulation therapy which is recommended by NICE,
- Consider alternative therapies, included in the NICE guidelines; music therapy, reminiscence therapy.

5. **Areas of importance to pass the station:**

The core elements to be attained by the candidate are a clear and comprehensive management of Dementia with Lewy Bodies. The candidate should be empathetic communicate using simple language and allowing the carer to take the information on board.

Important elements:

- Communication skills (40%).
- Comprehensive management plan (60%).

Station 105: Link 1: Dementia: Assessment of testamentary capacity

Station 106: Link 2: Dementia: Discuss testamentary capacity

Station 105: Link 1: Dementia: Assessment of testamentary capacity

Theme: Assessment of testamentary capacity to write a valid will

1. **Instructions to candidates:**

You are asked to see a 71-year-old gentleman with a history of dementia in Alzheimer's disease. Mr Tanner has recently been started on galantamine in the memory clinic. He continues to function at a reasonable level.

Mr Tanner's solicitor has asked if you could assess his testamentary capacity as Mr Tanner would like to prepare a will. Please keep your notes for the following station.

2. **Instructions to the role player:**

You are a 71-year-old gentleman. You were recently assessed at your local memory clinic. A part of the advice given to you at the feedback at the memory clinic was to ensure that all your affairs were in order, including preparing an enduring power of attorney and a will. You recently contacted your solicitor to prepare a will following this appointment. You are well-versed with the extent of your assets. You have decided to whom you would like these to be distributed to following your death. You feel no pressure from any of your family members or friends about being beneficiaries. Your solicitor was concerned that given your recent diagnosis, you need to have your capacity assessed by a psychiatrist to determine if you are able to complete making a will. You continue to function at a very high level, able to carry out your activities as you have always been able to do.

3. **Construct:**

The core task at this station is to assess testamentary capacity.

4. **Expanded construct:**

The candidate is expected to elicit relevant facts to complete an assessment of testamentary capacity.

The candidate should:

- Establish any existing mental disorder.
- Establish if the patient understands what a valid will is?
- Understand the nature and extent of his assets.
- Know who the beneficiaries are and establish that he is under no duress from anybody.
- Understand which assets he would like to give to whom.

5. **Areas of importance to pass the station:**

The core task at this station is to assess the patient's testamentary capacity.

- Ability to elicit all elements of testamentary capacity which includes, being able to understand the extent of his assets, who the beneficiaries will be and how he would like his assets distributed, with no duress from anybody (60%).
- Interview/communication skills (40%).

They should:

- Show an appropriate mix of open and closed questioning.
- Demonstrate advanced listening skills.
- Elucidate the way in which a patient with early psychosis may present.
- Focus on this individual's experience of the disorder.

Station 106: Link 2: Dementia: Discuss testamentary capacity

Theme: Discuss testamentary capacity to write a will with the legal representative

1. **Instructions to candidates:**

You will now speak to Mr Eamon Hugh, patient's legal representative over the telephone. He has called asking about your assessment of Mr Tanner's testamentary capacity in the previous station. **Please give a feedback the details of your assessment and your conclusion with regards to Mr Tanner's testamentary capacity.**

2. **Instructions to the role player:**

You are the legal representative of Mr Tanner. He had come to you to complete a will. He told you that he has recently been diagnosed with dementia in Alzheimer's disease. You are concerned that his dementia may have impacted on his capacity to prepare a will. You have asked a psychiatrist to assess his testamentary capacity. You call the psychiatrist following his assessment for feedback.

3. **Construct:**

The candidate should be able to feedback all elements of the testamentary capacity assessment to Mr Tanner's solicitor.

4. **Expanded construct:**
   - The candidate is expected to give feedback to Mr Tanner's solicitor.
   - The candidate should explain all elements of the testamentary capacity assessment and address any concerns.

5. **Areas of importance to pass the station:**
   - The core elements are the components of a testamentary capacity assessment (60%).
   - The candidate should be able to communicate this information clearly and succinctly (40%).

Station 107: Link 1: Assess: Causative factors of Behavioural and Psychological Symptoms of Dementia (BPSD)

Station 108: Link 2: Discuss: Role of antipsychotics in dementia

Station 107: Link 1: Assess: Causative factors of Behavioural and Psychological Symptoms of Dementia (BPSD)

Theme: Assess causative factors of Behavioural and Psychological Symptoms of Dementia (BPSD)

1. **Instructions to candidates:**

   Carer's name: Jean Fannigan

   You are asked to speak with a carer in a care home, who is looking after Mr John Hugh. He is an 82-year-old gentleman with a history of dementia in Alzheimer's disease. He was placed in the home about 6 months ago. You are asked to see him as an emergency due to emergent behavioural difficulties.

   Take a history to identify the particular difficulties, as well as to establish possible aetiological factors. Please keep your notes for the next station.

2. **Instructions to the role player:**

   You are the carer in a residential home. Mr Hugh is a resident at the home. He has been living there for the past 6 months. Mr Hugh has a diagnosis of dementia in Alzheimer's disease, which is severe in degree. His wife was unable to cope with him at home as he was wandering and needed more supervision than could be provided for at home. He seemed to settle, but over the last week has become very agitated. He is resistive to care and constantly pacing up and down. He has also begun interfering with other residents. He has not been eating as well and is not sleeping at night. He does not appear to have a fever. You were asked by the GP to collect a urine sample, but were unable to do so. He is incontinent of his urine. There have been no recent stressors or changes in the home.

3. **Construct:**

   The core task is for the candidate to ascertain the symptoms of BPSD and possible aetiological factors.

4. **Expanded construct:**

   The candidate can be expected to:
   - Take a collateral history.

They should:

- Elicit the history of the behavioural and psychological symptoms of dementia.
- Ask a range of questions that demonstrates knowledge of the various symptoms of BPSD in dementia including agitation, resistance, aggression, restlessness, changes in eating or sleeping, refusal of care or medications.
- Ask about possible aetiological factors, including changes in physical health, recent falls or trauma, changes in the environment or staff or other residents. Any recent stressors.

5. **Areas of importance to pass the station:**

   The core task at this station is to elicit a coherent history, and the following elements should contribute to the bulk of the marks (% relative weighting):

   - Interview/communication skills (40%).
   - Ability to elicit behavioural and psychological symptoms of dementia (40%).
   - Ability to explore underlying causes of BPSD (20%).

Station 108: Link 2: Discuss: Role of antipsychotics in dementia

Theme: Talk to the daughter of the above man and explain your findings. Discuss the role of antipsychotics in dementia. Address her views, concerns and expectations

1. **Instructions to candidates:**

   Please speak with the daughter of Mr Hugh. You had spoken with the carer in the previous station. Please explain to the daughter the context of his current behaviour as well as possible causes.
   Discuss management options with her.

   The GP started him on haloperidol for his behaviour. Discuss the implications of this treatment with the daughter.

2. **Instructions to the role player:**

   You are the daughter of Mr Hugh, who is a gentleman with severe dementia in Alzheimer's disease. He has recently been presenting with a variety of behavioural problems, making it very difficult for the carers at the care home to continue looking after him. He was recently started on some medication by his GP, which in your view has appeared to help with this behaviour. You feel he should be put on some medication to help with the behaviour or else he will be asked to leave the care home. You worry that you will be asked to take him home. You are very worried about what is going to happen.

3. **Construct:**

   The core task is to explain the elements of BPSD to the daughter of Mr Hugh.

4. **Expanded construct:**

   The candidate can be expected to:

   - Explain to the daughters what BPSD is in the context of dementia.

   They should:

   - Explain the possible aetiology of BPSD and the pattern of behaviour her father presented with.

- Address concerns about the use of medications, particularly the role of antipsychotic medications, including their increased vascular risk factors associated with anti-psychotics in dementia, possibly making mention of the Banerjee Report. *(http://www.rcpsych.ac.uk/pdf/Antipsychotics/Bannerjee Report).*

5. **Areas of importance to pass the station:**

The core task at this station is to explain that the current symptoms of BPSD in dementia and the side effects of antipsychotic medications and the following elements should contribute to the bulk of the marks (% relative weighting).

- Interview/communication skills (40%).

They should:

- Demonstrate advanced listening skills.
- Elucidate the way in which a patient with early psychosis may present.
- Focus on this individual's experience.
- Ability to be empathetic to the daughter, reassuring her (20%).
- Explain the possible aetiology of BPSD and management, including the side-effects of anti-psychotic medications (40%).

Station 109: Link 1: Cognitive assessment and risk assessment of a wandering patient with dementia

Station 110: Link 2: Discussion with her daughter

Station 109: Link 1: Cognitive assessment and risk assessment of a wandering patient with dementia

Theme: Cognitive and risk assessment of a wandering patient with dementia

1. **Instructions to candidates:**

Mrs Eileen Parker was picked up by police for her own safety, when she was spotted walking on a busy dual carriage way in the early hours of the morning. The police have found out that she is 80-year-old and lives alone in the nearby village. She has been spotted previously wandering in odd hours by the villagers, who had managed to persuade her to return to her house without much resistance or any incident. According to her GP, she is generally physically fit and rarely attends the surgery. She does not smell of alcohol and has no obvious injury.

Describe your clinical approach to this problem with Emphasis on:

1. **Mental state examination in order to arrive at a diagnosis.**
2. **Risk assessment.**

2. **Instructions to the role player:**

You, Mrs Eileen Parker, are an 80-year-old woman and you have lived alone in the nearby village for most of your life. You cannot remember how and under what circumstances the police found you. You also cannot remember who brought you here. You feel fine and have no worries at all.

So you are puzzled about the fuss over you and repeatedly ask as to what is going on. You also repeatedly ask why you are brought to a hospital as you have no injury or illness.

You remember your younger days but not sure of what had happened more recently. You did odd jobs in your younger years. Your husband died many years ago and you have been living alone since. You have a daughter who lives many miles away and visits you periodically. You are not sure how you get by but if probed further you say that your friends and neighbours help you out. In particular Jean, one of your friends has been very helpful in shopping and other daily chores.

When specifically asked about the day/date/month/season/year, you say you are not sure, also that you do not need all this, but if asked again give wrong answers (thus showing that you do not know the correct date/day, etc.). When asked about the name of the place, you say that you are in a hospital but have no clue about its name or location. Similarly, if asked about your own address, you give the name of your village and nothing else. If pressed further, you get irritable.

When given three objects to repeat/remember, you repeat them correctly but after a lapse of time when asked to recall, you draw a blank. If asked to spell WORLD backwards or to subtract serially 7 from 100, you give wrong answers (such as 93, 78, then ask "what do you want me to do next?" struggle to answer and hesitantly give 'DRLD'. If asked to copy a drawing, scribble something. If asked to draw a clock face/show time on a clock face, you become irritable and refuse to co-operate. If pressed further, you say it is getting silly and you should get back to your walk.

3. **Construct:**

The candidate is able to do a mental state examination, with particular emphasis on cognitive examination.

The candidate is able to make a working diagnosis or draw a list of differential diagnoses as the basis for further investigations and management plan.

4. **Expanded construct:**

- To elicit absence of significant psychopathology in areas other than the cognitive domain.
- To elicit global cognitive deficits by doing a structured cognitive test, such as, Mini-Mental State Examination (MMSE).
- To elicit cognitive deficits through questioning in a sensitive manner thus avoiding upsetting the patient and losing her co-operation.

5. **Areas of importance to pass the station:**

- Accurate observation of the patient's behaviour, relative absence of psychopathology but for cognitive deficits (60%).
- Sensitive style of questioning to allow completion of part of the MMSE/cognitive testing (40%).

  In order to pass this station, the candidate should be able to elicit most of the cognitive deficits to enable a diagnosis of dementia and form an opinion on the risks arising out of her wandering.

6. **Equipment checklist:**

Pencil and paper.

Station 110: Link 2: Discussion with her daughter

Theme: Discussion of the diagnosis and risk assessment with family/carer of patient with dementia

1. **Instructions to candidates:**

   From your interview, you think the most likely diagnosis is dementia, which needs further investigations to establish the likely aetiology of her dementia. She is, however, completely lacking in insight into her deficits and unaware of the dangers arising out of her wandering. Her daughter, who lives far away but who visits her periodically, has arrived in the meantime and wants to speak with you about her mother's condition.

   Discuss how you would convey to her daughter:

   1. **Diagnosis.**
   2. **Risk assessment.**

2. **Instructions to the role player:**

   You are the daughter of the 82-year-old Mrs Parker. You live about a 100 miles away and can afford to visit her only about twice a month. You have noticed your mother becoming forgetful over past 3 years. She is, however, physically fit and does not suffer from any medical condition and she has no complaints. She is temperamentally placid but a rather a strong-willed person, who always prided on her independence. She does not realise her memory has become poor and tends to minimise this by attributing it to her age. She has also been neglecting her diet and lately her personal hygiene has also declined. Your attempts to draw her attention to all these have been met with indifference or even denial. However, over last 6 months, you have been sufficiently concerned about her condition to arrange her friend/neighbour, Jean to visit her at least once a day to ensure that she has enough to eat. Jean also does her shopping once a week. This has been an informal but satisfactory arrangement so far as she has reluctantly accepted this intrusion.

   She loves to go for walks in the country side, which is her favourite past time. She has done this all her life and despite the recent concerns about her memory, appears to have a reasonable road sense. She has never got lost nor come to any harm. If any concerns over her safety arising out of her walks are discussed, she becomes dismissive. If pressed further she says she would rather be dead than stop her walks.

   You are worried about her general decline and suspect that something is seriously wrong with her. You have heard of senile dementia and Alzheimer's disease but you are not sure of the difference between these and whether your mother suffers from one or the other condition. You would like to know the exact nature of your mother's diagnosis and what treatment is available for her.

   Although you are concerned about her safety, whilst walking, you are also inclined to give in to her demands for going on walks as you are certain that if she is prevented from walking she would be absolutely miserable.

3. **Construct:**

   The candidate is able to communicate the diagnosis and convey the risks arising out of her wandering.

4. **Expanded construct:**

   - Able to communicate in non-technical language, the nature of dementia including the underlying neurological diagnosis

- Able to discuss the difficulties in making the decision in a professional manner without being dogmatic in style or patronising in tone.

5. **Areas of importance to pass the station:**
   - Eliciting informant history for a patient with dementia and corroborating/confirming the collateral history obtained from other sources (30%).
   - Communication of the diagnosis and explanation of the nature of brain disease in non-technical language (40%).
   - Discussion of risks/ethical dilemma in managing risks associated with her walks (30%).

   In order to pass this station, the candidate should be able to gather sufficient collateral history to narrow the list of diagnosis, be in a position to give a provisional diagnosis and its most likely aetiology, and discuss the dilemma in management of risks arising out of her walks/wandering.

6. **Equipment checklist:**
   Not applicable.

Station 111: Link 1: Assess: Behavioural and psychological symptoms of dementia (BPSD)

Station 112: Link 2: Discuss: Risk management and treatment with family

Station 111: Link 1: Assess: Behavioural and psychological symptoms of dementia (BPSD)

Theme: Assessment of behavioural and psychological symptoms of dementia (BPSD)

1. **Instructions to candidates:**

   A 76-year-old man has been referred by his GP with a 6 months history of wandering at odd hours. He was diagnosed with dementia a year ago and is supported by carers who visit him twice a day. The carers have reported lately that when they turn up they find him out of the house, clutching wads of money, walking aimlessly. On one occasion, they found him offering money to a taxi driver for driving him to London.

   Do a mental state examination with a view to assessing:

   1. **The psychopathology (do not do a full MMSE).**
   2. **Risk assessment.**
   3. **Management plan.**

2. **Instructions to the role player:**

   You are a 76-year-old retired postman and live alone in your own house. You have been told that you have become forgetful and that you need supervision and assistance in managing your life. Although you do not fully agree with this you have reluctantly accepted strangers into your house to give you a helping hand in your daily routine. You do not drink alcohol and you have no serious health problem.

Recently, you have been concerned about intruders in your house; they turn up in odd hours and go through your belongings. You think they are after your money as you hear them talking about money. You have started hiding your money to keep them out of their reach but you feel you have failed as the money has gone missing anyway. You have, therefore, decided to carry the money on your person. The intruders, at the same time have stepped up their action and are planning to snatch your money off you. So, you have lately tried to escape from your house and get back to London where you think you and your money will be safe. You have approached local taxidrivers to take you to London but are puzzled at their reluctance despite being offered large sums of money.

You can clearly hear and at times see the intruders. You do not recognise them but you are sure they are up to some mischief by the look on their face. You are not sure how else to protect you and your money from them. Eventually you have come up with a plan to face them head on. You have considered attacking them with a hammer when you see them next. So you now keep a hammer near the front door of your house.

If asked by the candidate to give day/date/month/season/year or your address or repeat three objects, decline to engage in testing saying this is not important. If pressed give wrong answers (to show that you do not know the answers).

3. **Construct:**

The candidate is able to do a psychiatric assessment with focus on non-cognitive symptoms or problem behaviour in a patient with dementia.

4. **Expanded construct:**

The candidate is able to:

- Elicit the form/content of patient's psychotic experiences.
- Incorporate this into his background problem of dementia, already diagnosed assess risk of accidental harm or financial exploitation.

5. **Areas of importance to pass the station:**

- Eliciting the nature of psychotic experience (60%).
- Linking these to his impaired cognitive status (given his diagnosis of dementia) (20%).
- Assessing the risks of accidental harm to self, financial exploitation and assault on others (20%).

A passing performance for this station must include eliciting the core psychotic symptom and appreciating the serious risk of physical violence/assault on others.

6. **Equipment checklist:**

Pencil and paper.

Station 112: Link 2: Discuss: Risk management and treatment with family

Discussion of risk management and treatment with family

Theme: Discussion of risk management and treatment of BPSD with carer/family of patient with dementia

1. **Instructions to candidates:**

The daughter of the above patient wants to speak with you about his management. She has heard and read in the news about the dangers of prescribing antipsychotic drugs to older persons with dementia.

Discuss how you will address:

1. **The presenting problems and the risk assessment.**
2. **Role of antipsychotic in its management.**

2. **Instructions to the role player:**

You are the daughter of the retired postman who was diagnosed with dementia about 2 years ago. He is otherwise well, physically fit and mobile. But he needs supervision and prompting in his personal care, medication management. With the help of the local specialist mental health team, he has been on donepezil and a care package in form of a visit by personal carers twice a day. The carers have reported that when they arrive sometimes he is out, at times, with the front door unlocked and occasionally wide open.

You have been concerned about the reports of his wandering with thousands of pounds on his person and him offering large sums of money to taxi drivers asking them to take him to London where he lived almost four decades ago. On questioning, he maintains that he has to protect himself and his money from the intruders and that he has been left with no choice but to get away from them. He is frustrated by the lack of co-operation from the local taxi drivers and has lately been talking about doing "whatever it takes to protect himself and his money". You find a hammer near the front door of the house and he has talked of using it when he next faces the intruders.

You have heard of dangers of using antipsychotic drugs in older dementia patients. It has been reported on radio, TV and in newspapers that it causes unnecessary death from strokes. You have also heard of doctors in the NHS opting for drug therapy for patients mainly for convenience rather than using talking therapy, which is more expensive and not easily available. So, you would like an assurance that your father must be given a chance to talk to a 'therapist' as he might be confusing at times the carers as intruders or even responding to something he has dreamt. In your mind, if medication is necessary a sleeping pill or a sedative would be a safer option than an antipsychotic for your father.

3. **Construct:**

- The candidate is able to communicate the nature of BPSD in dementia and the associated risks.
- He is able to discuss the management plan, including the option of using antipsychotic drugs.

4. **Expanded construct:**

- Communicate the severity and seriousness of psychotic experience (delusion, hallucination and their contents).
- Able to identify this as the main target symptom and the associated behaviour (of wandering and thought of using a weapon against intruders).
- Able to discuss risk/benefit analysis of antipsychotic drug use.

5. **Areas of importance to pass the station:**

- Communicating the nature and seriousness of psychotic experience (30%).

- Communication of risks associated (40%).
- Discussion of risk/benefit analysis of antipsychotic drug use in dementia (30%).

In order to pass this station, the candidate should be able to convey the abnormal belief and the potentially dangerous behaviour leading to the justification for anti-psychotic medication.

6. **Equipment checklist:**
   Not applicable.

Station 113: Link 1: Assess: Psychotic symptoms in Parkinson's disease
Station 114: Link 2: Discuss: Management plan with the patient's general practitioner

Station 113: Link 1: Assess: Psychotic symptoms in Parkinson's disease

Theme: Assessment of psychotic symptoms in Parkinson's disease

1. **Instructions to candidates:**

   A 78-year-old Mr Paul Smith is referred by his GP for a psychiatric assessment. He has a diagnosis of Parkinson's disease and is on co-careldopa. Following a recent neurology review the dose of co-careldopa has been increased. He has for the past 6 months been seeing immigrants in his garden, who he believes are out to steal his possessions. He implores his wife to call the police but as she sees no basis in reality and questions him he becomes aggressive and even threatening in his manner.

   Carry out a mental state examination (do not need to conduct a full Mini-Mental State Examination).

2. **Instructions to the role player:**

   You are Mr Smith, a 78-year-old man, living at home with your wife. You have seen a specialist in the last 2 years for shuffling gait, tremor, and slow movements. You have been taking tablets for these symptoms and recently the dose has been increased which has improved your mobility.

   You are most concerned to have spotted coloured people in the garden trying to hide behind the trees. You believe them to be illegal immigrants who are hiding from the authorities. You have seen some of them inside your house and you think they are out to steal from your house. You see them clearly in broad day light and hear them talking in foreign tongues. So you do not know what they are talking about. However, some expensive pieces of jewellery have recently gone missing from the house and you are convinced that they have stolen these items. You want the police to apprehend them and bring them to justice. However, your wife does not believe you and refuses to call the police. She 'fobs' your account off as your imagination. You find this frustrating and this has led to several arguments. You know that your memory may not be perfect but there is nothing wrong with your mind otherwise.

   If the candidate asks you questions about day, date, month, season and year, you should answer the month, season and year correctly but give wrong day and date (narrow mistakes by one day/date). If asked about orientation to place, answer them correctly. If given three items to repeat and recall, do repeat them correctly and on recall give two of the three items. If asked to do serial subtractions or spell WORLD backwards, spell WORLD backwards correctly but make two mistakes on serial sevens; i.e., 93, 85, 78, 71, 63. On three steps command make one mistake; i.e., fold the paper twice instead of once. Name the pen and watch correctly. Do the reading, writing and repetition item correctly but in the intersecting pentagons, make one of the figures four-sided and the intersection a triangle rather than a diamond.

3. **Construct:**

The candidate is able to assess the nature and seriousness of psychotic symptoms in a patient with Parkinson's disease.

4. **Expanded construct:**

The candidate is able to:

- Carry out a mental state examination to elicit the nature and contents of psychotic experiences; and
- Consider aetiology of such symptoms.

5. **Areas of importance to pass the station:**

- Detailed mental state examination with some elements of cognitive examination (not the full MMSE) (50%).
- Establishing the details of psychotic experience (50%).

A passing performance for this station must include a satisfactory mental state examination, thus eliciting the relatively mild cognitive impairment but clear psychotic symptom.

6. **Equipment checklist:**

Pencil and paper.

Station 114: Link 2: Discuss: Management plan with the patient's general practitioner

Theme: Discussion of the management plan with the patient's general practitioner

1. **Instructions to candidates:**

Mr Paul Smith's GP is keen to meet with you to discuss his:

1. **Diagnosis.**
2. **Management plan.**

2. **Instructions to the role player:**

You are the Mr Smith's general practitioner. He presented 2 years ago with tremor, slow movements and a shuffling gait. A neurology opinion, obtained a year ago, confirmed the diagnosis of Parkinson's disease and upon commencing him on co-careldopa his mobility improved. The dose of co-careldopa was increased about 3 months ago. Around this time, his wife has called the surgery on several occasions with reports of strange behaviour, talking about coloured immigrants in the garden and in the house who are stealing their jewellery. On examination, his parkinsonian symptoms had improved since the increase in the dose of co-careldopa. On cognitive examination, his score on MMSE was 23/30, with loss of two points each for orientation and serial 7's and one point each for recall, three steps command and visuo-spatial functioning.

You wonder if his diagnosis is a dementia of Lewy bodies type rather than simple Parkinson's disease. On the other hand, you also are unsure if the emergent psychotic symptoms are a side effect of anti-parkinsonian drug. You are seeking a psychiatric opinion on the best management strategy; i.e., whether to reduce the anti-parkinsonian drug or to treat him with an antipsychotic drug. If so, you are not sure of the exact drug and its dosage. You also want to know if a further neurology review would be required.

3. **Construct:**

The candidate is able to discuss the pathological significance of psychotic symptoms, the underlying aetiology and treatment options.

4. **Expanded construct:**

- Discuss the nature and seriousness of psychotic experiences.
- Discus the differential diagnosis of these symptoms (which includes side effect of anti-parkinsonian medications).
- Discuss the management plan including danger of sensitivity to antipsychotic drugs in Lewy Bodies dementia and the role of cholinesterase inhibitor in managing such symptoms.

5. **Areas of importance to pass the station:**

- Discussion of the differential diagnosis of the underlying cause of psychotic symptoms in a patient with Parkinson's disease: 50%.
- Discussion of treatment approach of this presentation: 50%.

A passing performance in this station must include the possible causes of his psychotic experience, appreciation of the dilemma in management of psychotic symptoms in a patient of Parkinson's disease, and a cautious approach to the use of antipsychotic drug.

6. **Equipment checklist:**

Not applicable.

Station 115: Link 1: Assess: 'Depressive pseudodementia'

Station 116: Link 2: Discuss: Differential diagnosis and management plan

Station 115: Link 1: Assess: 'Depressive pseudodementia'

Theme: Assessment of patients presenting with features of depression and dementia ('Depressive pseudodementia')

1. **Instructions to candidates:**

A 72-year-old Mrs Jones has been referred by his GP for an assessment in the OP Clinic. She has a history of low mood, loss of interest, social withdrawal and slow activities over previous 3 months. Lately she has been sitting around a lot and hardly engages in any meaningful activities or hobbies. Over the last week, she is neglecting her personal hygiene, which has prompted the family to arrange an urgent assessment.

Carry out a mental state examination.

2. **Instructions to the role player:**

   You are a 72-year-old housewife and live at home with your husband. You have no past history of mental health problems and you do not drink or smoke. Your medical history is significant for controlled hypertension, raised cholesterol and rheumatoid arthritis. Your husband was recently hospitalised for a heart attack. He made a reasonable recovery and returned home after 2 weeks. However, you have been worried about your future as you are generally dependent on him for most decisions and you are not sure how you would manage your affairs if he were to die from a heart attack. You have lost interest and all energy to do any housework. You feel your memory has gone down and you feel you are going to lose your mind. Lately you do not bother to change your clothes for days at a time and you have become incontinent of urine.

   When the doctor enquires about your main problem, you tell him that your memory is bad. You answer his questions slowly and with long latencies. When he asks you questions about day, date, month and year, you answer them correctly but only after long pauses. When he asks you to remember certain items, your first response should be that your memory has become weak and you will not be able to remember anything. However, when you are asked to recall three objects as a part of your memory test, you answer them correctly but hesitantly. If asked to copy drawings or draw a clock face, etc. your first response should be your mind does not work and you won't be able to do anything. However, if insisted upon, you should do everything slowly but correctly. If asked questions on general knowledge, your initial response should be 'I don't know' but if pressed you answer them correctly but in a hesitant and non-confident tone. If asked about why you do not change clothes or about your incontinence, your answer should be 'I don't know' or 'my brain does not work'.

3. **Construct:**

   The candidate is able to:

   - Elicit both depressive features and cognitive deficits, which are severe enough to suggest a dementing illness; and
   - Gauge their relative significance to arrive at a working diagnosis.

4. **Expanded construct:**

   The candidate should be able to:

   - Elicit relevant symptoms and signs for a diagnosis of a severe depressive disorder.
   - Allow for the patient's slow responses and conduct the mental state examination at an appropriate pace.
   - Assess the temporal sequence of psychopathology and relative significance of the affective and cognitive symptoms in discussing differential diagnosis.

5. **Areas of importance to pass the station:**

   - Sensitive but confident conduct of MSE in a reassuring and comforting manner (20%).
   - Eliciting features of depressive illness (40%).
   - Eliciting cognitive deficits (40%).

   A passing performance in this station must include a careful consideration of temporal sequence of events and appreciation of qualitative aspect of cognitive impairment suggestive of an affective disorder rather than a primary dementia.

6. **Equipment checklist:**
   Pencil and paper.

Station 116: Link 2: Discuss: Differential diagnosis and management plan

Theme: Discussion of differential diagnosis and management plan with the consultant

1. **Instructions to candidates:**
   You are to present your findings to your consultant with a view to:
   1. **Discussing the differential diagnosis; and**
   2. **Discussion of the management plan.**
2. **Instructions to the role player:**
   Ask the doctor to present the salient features of the case in terms of history, findings of mental state examination and then his/her differential diagnosis or working diagnosis. In history, look for the duration and chronology of symptoms, pace of onset and the development of symptoms. In the MSE, look for comments on the qualitative features of the patient's cognitive deficits viz., 'I don't know' responses, slow response and generally correct responses in contrast with an initial negative outlook.
   Also look for a conservative approach to making a working diagnosis. In particular, the obvious benefit of treating this as a primary depressive disorder in the first instance before considering dementia as a diagnostic possibility must be demonstrated by the candidate.
3. **Construct:**
   The candidate is able to:
   (i) Discuss differential diagnosis; and
   (ii) Management plan for a patient presenting with depression and dementia.
4. **Expanded construct:**
   The candidate is able to:
   - Approach the presentation of mixed depressive features and cognitive deficits in a methodical way.
   - Able to differentiate severe depression and primary dementia by history and examination findings.
5. **Areas of importance to pass the station:**
   Lucid presentation of history (20%) and Mental state examination findings (30%).
   Discussion of differential diagnosis (30%).
   Brief management Plan (20%).
   A passing performance in this station must include appreciation of distinguishing features of 'pseudo dementia' and the conservative approach to diagnosis in such a presentation.
6. **Equipment checklist:**
   Not applicable.

Station 117: Link 1: Assess: Psychosis in older adults ('paraphraenia')

Station 118: Link 2: Discuss: Management with a relative

Station 117: Link 1: Assess: Psychosis in older adults ('paraphraenia')

Theme: Assessment of psychosis in older adults ('paraphraenia')

1. **Instructions to candidates:**

   Miss Mary Little, a 76-year-old retired book keeper who lives alone in the first floor of a block of flats, has been referred by her GP for a psychiatric assessment. She tells you that her neighbour is running a brothel and also uses her flat for such activities whilst she is out. She is convinced of this because she hears strange but suggestive noises through the walls at night and she can find tell-tale signs of interference and sexual activities in her flat. She is annoyed that despite repeated complaints to the police no action has been taken.

   Carry out a mental state examination with a view to arriving at a diagnosis.

2. **Instructions to role player:**

   You are a 76-year-old retired book keeper and you live alone. You never married and your only close relative is a niece who lives far away and your contact with her is only through occasional phone calls. You have no past psychiatric history and you do not drink or smoke. You are a rather solitary person and have few friends. You rarely engage in social activities and your favourite pastime is reading books and magazines.

   You have been gravely concerned about recent developments in your block of flats. You see many young women getting into and leaving the block of flats at all hours of the day and night. You also hear noises, suggestive of sexual activities, through your walls at night. You are suspicious of their movements and your worst fears are confirmed when you notice lately that your flat has been interfered with and you discover tell-tale signs of sexual activity on your bed upon returning from your trips to shops and local library. You are now convinced that your neighbour is running a brothel and is using your room for the same purpose whilst you are out. You have tried to alert the police, who do not believe you and they have taken no action.

   You get quite angry when the candidate suggests that you might be imagining all this. You repeatedly ask him if he believes you or not. If he quizzes you more about your beliefs, you get increasingly angry, saying "you seem to be on their side". You also ask the candidate if he is going to do something about this and express amazement and despair if the candidate implies that no action was required. If any treatment is implied, you openly state that you do not need any and perhaps the people next door should be approached instead.

3. **Construct:**

   Eliciting the nature and significance of onset psychotic symptoms in older adults.

4. **Expanded construct:**

   The candidate is able to:

   - Elicit onset psychotic symptoms through sensitive questioning and a sympathetic approach.
   - Establish absence of cognitive deficit on mental state examination.

5. **Areas of importance to pass the station:**
   - Eliciting psychotic symptoms (60%).
   - Sensitive questioning to maintain her engagement in interview (20%).
   - Eliciting other psychopathology, i.e., comorbid minor depression (20%).

   A passing performance in this station must include a sensitive and non-judgmental approach in interviewing the patient in order to elicit the clear psychotic symptomatology and avoid taking sides or alienating the patient through a diplomatic style of interview.

6. **Equipment checklist:**

   Pencil and paper.

Station 118: Link 2: Discuss: Management with a relative

Theme: Discussion with patient's daughter regarding the management plan

1. **Instructions to candidates:**

   Miss Little's niece, her only relative, wants to speak with you regarding her aunt's condition.

   Discuss how:

   1. **You will convey the diagnosis; and**
   2. **The management plan.**

2. **Instructions to the role player:**

   You are the niece of Miss Little and want to understand the nature of your aunt's condition. From your conversations with her, she appears upset and angry. You think that as your aunt is otherwise lucid and level-headed; her complaints should be taken seriously and investigated thoroughly. Unlike many women of her age, her memory is sharp and she is otherwise independent in her daily life. You think dismissing her complaints without a thorough investigation is unfair.

   If the candidate mentions paraphraenia, schizophrenia or delusional disorder you question the nature of this and if offered an explanation in terms of a psychotic illness, you question about other possibilities, such as, depressive illness. As she appears sad and at times tearful, you question if she has got muddled about the happenings in her flat because of depression.

   You question the candidate about the process of confirmation of the working diagnosis. You specifically enquire about blood tests and brain scans and if the candidate mentions these tests, ask what changes are expected.

   You also enquire what treatment is available for her and specifically enquire about an antidepressant as she appears depressed. If the doctor mentions an antipsychotic, mention your concerns about side effects.

   You also specifically enquire if her moving away from her flat would solve her problem and whether this is a better option than treating her with potentially dangerous drugs.

3. **Construct:**

   The candidate is able to:

(i) Communicate possible diagnoses and the most likely diagnosis.

(ii) Outline management plan to patient's family.

4. **Expanded construct:**

The candidate is able to communicate in non-technical language the nature of paraphraenia, its differential diagnosis, likely course and management plan.

5. **Areas of importance to pass the station:**

- Communication of the nature of paraphraenia in non-technical language (40%).
- Discussion of diagnostic possibilities and the basis for the most likely diagnosis of paraphraenia (30%).
- Discussion of investigations and management plan (30%).

A passing performance in this station must include a confident discussion of the nature of 'paraphraenia' and its comorbidity, prognosis and management plan.

6. **Equipment checklist:**

Not applicable.

Station 119: Link 1: Assess: Severely depressed patient under Mental Health Act
Station 120: Link 2: Discuss: Your findings with a colleague

Station 119: Link 1: Assess: Severely depressed patient under Mental Health Act

Theme: Assessment of patient for possible detention under Mental Health Act

1. **Instructions to candidates:**

Mrs Harris, a 75-year-old woman with a past history of bipolar disorder, presents with a 2 months history of progressively worsening low mood. She lives on her own in her two bedroom bungalow. She has been treated with sertraline up to a dose of 200 mg/day for 6 weeks with little improvement. Lately she has been eating little with weight loss of about 10 lbs in 2 weeks. She explains her poor food intake by her conviction of her bowels having disintegrated as she finds it hard to open her bowels. Her family is extremely concerned about her health and would like her to be admitted to hospital for treatment but she refuses to comply saying she is beyond help.

Carry out a mental state examination with a view to:

1. **Demonstrating her main psychopathology.**
2. **Arriving at a working diagnosis.**

2. **Instructions to the role player:**

You are Mrs Harris, a 75-year-old woman who has been feeling unwell for 3 months. You can't open your bowels and are convinced that your bowels are disintegrating. Hence, you do not eat much. Lately, you are restricting fluids as well for the same reason. You have taken tablets prescribed by your doctor but you are not keen to continue with this treatment any more as you believe you are beyond help.

At interview you answer the candidate's questions slowly with long latencies. Your responses are also hesitant with long silences. If asked to explain the reason for your slowness, you are dismissive saying there is no point talking about it now, as it is too late.

When hospital admission is broached your response is again hesitant and slow. You may remain silent and when asked again you respond by saying you are beyond help and the candidate should not waste his time by talking to you further. When the concerns of her family are mentioned, you say that you are a burden on them and they would be better off if you died.

3. **Construct:**
   The candidate is able to:
   - Assess the severity of the depressive disorder and elicit psychotic features.
   - Consider the need for compulsory hospital admission.

4. **Expanded construct:**
   The candidate is able to:
   - Assimilate historical data and findings on mental state examination.
   - Elicit severity of depressive illness and establish the severity of psychosis.
   - Make a risk assessment with regards to the need for urgent medical treatment in the hospital.

5. **Areas of importance to pass the station:**
   - Eliciting features of severe depression with psychotic features and suicidal ideation (70%).
   - Sensitive style of interview (30%).

   In order to pass this station, the candidate should be able to elicit the features of severe depression with psychotic features and passive suicidal ideation.

6. **Equipment Checklist:**
   Not applicable.

Station 120: Link 2: Discuss: Your findings with a colleague

Theme: Discussion with the Approved Mental Health Professional (AMHP) or equivalent personal regarding justification for detention under the Mental Health Act

1. **Instructions to candidates:**
   You conclude from your examination that she is suffering from a depressive disorder with psychotic symptoms. In view of the risks from her worsening physical and mental health you consider an admission to a mental health unit necessary. With this in mind, you have contacted an AMHP.

   Discuss with the AMHP how and why a compulsory admission is justified.

2. **Instructions to the role player:**
   You are the duty AMHP and have been contacted by the candidate for an assessment of Mrs Harris

for possible detention under the Mental Health Act. You question the candidate about the degree and nature of her mental disorder. You also question the candidate on the risks to patient's own health, own safety or danger to others. The candidate is expected to know the key principles underpinning the application of the Mental Health, viz, autonomy, respect, purpose, participation, effectiveness efficiency, equity and least restrictive option in treating her condition. As the patient seems to lack capacity to decide about treatment, discussion of whether the Mental Capacity Act (MCA) or Mental Health Act (MHA) is appropriate may be relevant for this discussion.

3. **Construct:**

   The candidate is able to communicate the severity of the illness and the justification for compulsory hospital admission to an AMHP.

4. **Expanded construct:**

   The candidate is able to convey:

   - The salient features of severe depressive disorder and the nature and severity of psychotic features.
   - The potential dangers to the patient's health arising out of her poor oral intake.
   - High risk to her own safety.
   - Necessity to review her diagnosis and treatment in hospital.
   - The practical difficulties of treatment in the community because of her reluctance to take medication.
   - The necessity to investigate her physical health and activities of daily living.

5. **Areas of importance to pass the station:**

   - Understanding of the basic principles of compulsory hospital admission under MHA (20%).
   - Establishing the degree and nature of mental disorder (30%).
   - Establishing the degree of risk to justify compulsory hospital admission (30%).
   - Choice of MCA vs. MHA (20%).

   A passing performance in this station must include justification of compulsory admission in light of the severity of the depressive disorder, psychotic nature of the illness, loss of insight and risks of untreated illness in the community. A superior candidate may elaborate the legal aspects of detention under the MHA vs. the MCA.

6. **Equipment checklist:**

   Not applicable.

Station 121: Link 1: Assess: Severe refractory depression

Station 122: Link 2: Discuss: Role of ECT with a relative

Station 121: Link 1: Assess: Severe refractory depression

Theme: Assessment of severe refractory depression

1. **Instructions to candidates:**

   Mrs Joan Mulligan, a 72-year-old woman is referred by her GP for assessment and management of her depression. She gives a 6 months history of low mood, loss of interest, anergia, poor sleep and feelings of being a burden on her family. The treatment with fluoxetine at a dose of 40 mg/day for 6 weeks, followed by venlafaxine in therapeutic dose for 6 weeks and lately a combination of sertraline and mirtazapine for 6 weeks has made little difference. Over the last month, she has been talking of her feelings of life being not worth living.

   Carry out a mental state examination with a view to:

   1. **Establishing a working diagnosis.**
   2. **Risk assessment.**

2. **Instructions to the role player:**

   You live alone in your own home and take pride in your independence. Over the past 6 months, you have not felt right although if asked you are unable to pinpoint your problem. On specific enquiry, you admit that you feel low in your mood and do not enjoy life as much as before. You also sleep badly and lack your customary energy to do your usual chores. You have so far gone along with your doctor and taken the medications prescribed. However, you do not feel much better and wonder if you would ever feel well again.

   At interview, you are slow in your response to the questions put to you by the candidate. You feel you will never recover from this and would be a burden on your family. You, therefore, feel that you would be better off dead. But you feel you are a coward and would not be able to kill yourself easily. You, therefore, ask the candidate if she could give you a lethal dose of morphine to help you sleep so that you would never wake up.

3. **Construct:**

   The candidate is able to gauge the severity of depressive disorder and be familiar with the concept of refractory depression.

4. **Expanded construct:**

   The candidate is able to:

   - Elicit the features of severe depression; and
   - Establish that the depressive disorder is refractory to treatment with a number of pharmacological treatment strategies.
   - Risk to her own health and safety.

5. **Areas of importance to pass the station:**

   - Eliciting features of severe depression (30%).
   - Establishing suicide risk (30%).
   - Familiarity with concept of refractory depression (20%).
   - Role of ECT in treatment of refractory depression (20%).

   A passing performance in this station must include eliciting key features of severe depression with high suicide risk.

6. **Equipment checklist:**

   Not applicable.

Station 122: Link 2: Discuss: Role of ECT with a relative

Theme: Discussion of role of ECT with the patient's daughter

1. **Instructions to candidates:**

   After your examination you conclude that patient is in need of ECT on grounds of high suicide risk. The patient says she can't decide about ECT and asks you to speak with her daughter regarding ECT.

   Discuss ECT with the daughter.

2. **Instructions to the role player:**

   You are the daughter of Mrs Mulligan and a journalist by profession. You are concerned about your mother's condition but you feel she would benefit from talking therapy. She had a deprived childhood and has had very low self-esteem throughout her life. You firmly believe that if she could talk about her feelings she could get over her death wish.

   You have also heard of horrible stories about ECT and would like to stop the doctors from giving ECT to your mother. You have done some research on ECT and discover to your horror that the mechanism of action ECT is unknown. You also find that some psychiatrists are opposed to ECT as a treatment. Some believe ECT amounts to torture and you believe that ECT seems to work by obliterating memory. You also have, through your research, found out that there are other methods of treating refractory depression including Transcranial Magnetic Stimulation (TMS) but you suspect they are not easily available in the NHS because of their cost.

   You question the candidate about how ECT works and if he sounds diffident, tell him that the mechanism of action of ECT is unknown. You also tell him that your research into ECT has shown several side effects of ECT, including permanent memory loss.

3. **Construct:**

   Understand and communicate the role of ECT in treating refractory depression.

4. **Expanded construct:**

   The candidate is able to:

   - Demonstrate her understanding of the risk benefit analysis of ECT.
   - Explain the efficacy of ECT in treatment of refractory depression.

5. **Areas of importance to pass the station:**

   - Understanding concept of severe depression as an illness distinct from unhappiness (30%).
   - Role of ECT in treatment of refractory depression (30%).
   - Risk benefit analysis of ECT (40%).

   In order to pass this station, the candidate must show appreciation of refractoriness of patient's depressive disorder and the role of ECT with its risk benefit analysis in patient's management.

6. **Equipment checklist:**

   Not applicable.

Station 123: Link 1: Assess: Frontotemporal dementia

Station 124: Link 2: Discuss: Differential diagnoses and management

Station 123: Link 1: Assess: Frontotemporal dementia

Theme: Assessment of Frontotemporal dementia

1. **Instructions to candidates:**
A 53-year-old successful business executive with impeccable character and no past psychiatric history is referred for a psychiatric assessment. He has a 12 months history of gradual decline in his social grace and grooming noticed by his associates. More recently concerns were raised at his work because of his sexually disinhibited behaviour towards a young intern who started working in the firm 2 weeks ago. His score on the Mini-Mental State Examination (MMSE) was 29/30 with loss of 1 point for recall.
Do a mental state examination with dementia as a possible diagnosis (do not perform an MMSE).
Do the appropriate additional examination to aid in confirming the likely type of dementia (The number of tests may be specified).

2. **Instructions to the role player:**
You are a 53-year-old business executive. You run a successful and established business. You are happily married with two grown-up children. You have no previous psychiatric history and no history of problem drinking. During the interview you are somewhat over familiar with the candidate and ask if you could call him by his first name. If the candidate enquires about the recent changes in your behaviour noted by your business associates, you dismiss this as sheer nonsense. The candidate also enquires about your flirtatious behaviour towards the young female intern. You minimise the concern expressed by your colleagues saying they are jealous of your sexual attractiveness. You also defend your conduct by saying there is nothing wrong with a sexual fling as long as it is consensual. When questioned about its impact on your wife and marriage, you dismiss this as 19th century prudery and narrow thinking. If the candidate implies that this as morally wrong you suggest that he needs to be sexually liberated. If the candidate continues in this vein, you start asking him personal questions about his marriage and extramarital activities.
When the candidate examines you for frontal lobe tests, you deliberately make mistakes to show that your frontal lobe functioning is impaired.

3. **Construct:**
The candidate is able to:
Assimilate history and mental state examination in a patient of frontotemporal dementia.

4. **Expanded construct:**
The candidate is able to:
   - Sensitively conduct a mental state examination and elicit abnormalities in judgment, social and sexual disinhibition.
   - Assimilate these findings with the history to make a working diagnosis.

5. **Areas of importance to pass the station:**
   - Eliciting disturbance in judgment and evidence of sexual disinhibition (50%).
   - Frontal lobe testing (50%).

   Bedside frontal lobe tests, otherwise also known as tests for Frontal Executive Function are broadly of two types: cognitive tests and neurological tests.

   The cognitive tests consist of verbal fluency tests, such as letter fluency (F, A, S) and category fluency and tests of abstraction, such as, proverb interpretation, similarities test and cognitive estimates test.

   The other type of frontal lobe tests, which can be done by bedside, tests the ability to shift from one cognitive set to another and to inhibit inappropriate responses. This group consists of Alternating Sequences Test, Go-No-Go Test and Motoring Sequencing Test, such as, the Luria Three-step-Test and Alternating Hand Movements Test.

   A passing performance in this station must include appreciation of special features of fronto-temporal dementia (disturbance in judgment and social behaviour rather than cognitive deficits) and accurate demonstration of some bedside frontal lobe tests.

6. **Equipment checklist:**

   Paper and pencil.

Station 124: Link 2: Discuss: Differential diagnoses and management

Theme: Discussion with your consultant differential diagnosis and management of frontotemporal dementia

1. **Instructions to candidates:**

   You have to present your findings on this patient to your consultant with a view to finalising his diagnosis and associated investigations and management plan.

   Discuss with your consultant.

2. **Instructions to the role player:**

   You are Dr Emil Brown, Consultant Psychiatrist, who is the clinical supervisor for the candidate. He is going to present the work up on the above patient to you. You ask him to present the salient features of the case in about 4 minutes. You then ask for a list of differential diagnosis or a diagnosis. You then ask for the list of investigations needed for confirming the diagnosis. Finally, ask for a management plan, which should have a biopsychosocial approach. It should include the relatively minor role for psychotropic drugs but the predominantly practical approach to ease the burden of his care on his family. It should also include plans for lasting power of attorney (LPA), respite care and possible residential care as the dementia advances.

3. **Construct:**

   The candidate is able to make a working diagnosis and plan investigations to confirm the diagnosis and his management.

4. **Expanded construct:**

   The candidate is able to:

- Assimilate the historical information, findings from mental state examination, and focussed neurological examination to make a working diagnosis.
- Produce a list of differential diagnosis.
- Plan investigations and management.

5. **Areas of importance to pass the station:**
   - Presentation of the history, mental state and focussed neurological examination (30%).
   - Differential diagnoses (20%).
   - Investigations (20%).
   - Management plan (biopsychosocial approach) (30%).

   In order to pass this station, the candidate must make a lucid presentation of key features in history and examination supporting a diagnosis of frontotemporal dementia, discuss a minimum of investigations to confirm clinically the degenerative nature of the disease and focus on psychosocial aspects of management in absence of specific pharmacological treatment.

6. **Equipment checklist:**
   Not applicable.

Station 125: Link 1: Assess: Behavioural and psychological symptoms (BPSD) and mental capacity

Station 126: Link 2: Discuss: Management of BPSD and mental capacity

Station 125: Link 1: Assess: Behavioural and psychological symptoms (BPSD) and mental capacity

Theme: Assessment of behavioural and psychological symptoms (BPSD) and mental capacity for discharge in patient with dementia in a general hospital ward

1. **Instructions to candidates:**

   You are assessing a 75-year-old man, a retired bus driver, admitted to a general hospital medical unit for chronic confusion and fall. He lives alone since the death of his wife a year ago, but his daughter who lives nearby and visits him regularly reports a gradual decline in his memory, general grasp of his situation and management of his affairs.

   In the hospital, he intrudes into other patient's spaces, and disrupts nursing activities. When directed to return and stay in his bed area he becomes aggressive. He then wants to leave the hospital. As the staff have doubts his capacity to live safely in the community, they prevent him from discharging himself from hospital and this makes him increasingly aggressive and hostile.

   Do a mental state examination with a view to:

   1. **Arriving at a psychiatric diagnosis.**
   2. **Assessment of his capacity to decide about his discharge.**

2. **Instructions to the role player:**

   You are a 75-year-old man and you live alone since the death of your wife. You are told that you had to go into the hospital because you were confused and had a fall. You do not believe there is anything seriously wrong with you. On specific questioning, you believe that you would be fine at home and would have no problems managing your affairs. You are not sure how you got into hospital but you do not think you need any help or treatment. Therefore, you insist on discharge from hospital to return home and are genuinely puzzled as to why the staff is stopping you from leaving the hospital.

When enquired about day/date/month/season/year, you give the correct year and season but the wrong day, date and month. On enquiry about your address, you give the correct address but you are not sure what the address of the hospital is. You register three objects correctly but when asked to recall you recall only one object. On spelling WORLD backwards you give DROW and on serial 7 subtractions, you give 93, 76, 67, 60 and 53. You answer all the other questions correctly on cognitive testing except you draw the intersecting pentagons wrong by drawing one pentagon with 4 sides and making the intersection a triangle rather than a diamond. When asked to write a sentence you write your name. If asked to draw a clock and show the time, you put the number unevenly and if asked to show the time at 10 past 11, show the hands at 10 and 11.

If asked about the risks at home and when the risk of fall is identified as a source of concern by the staff, you claim that anybody could have a fall and that is not a good enough reason against discharge. If asked about how you would summon help, you claim that you have excellent neighbours to help you. If asked further about their details or how you would contact them you get irritable and attempt to walk away saying you would rather be home.

3. **Construct:**

   Candidate is able to assimilate history and MSE findings for a patient with dementia who presents with BPS on a medical unit.

4. **Expanded construct:**
   - Candidate is able to combine information from many sources with findings on mental state examination.
   - Assessment of mental capacity for discharge from hospital.

5. **Areas of importance to pass the station:**
   - Mental state examination, including cognitive examination (60%).
   - Assessment of his understanding of risks and his capacity to decide about his discharge (40%).

   In order to pass this station, the candidate must carry out a satisfactory mental state examination to elicit global cognitive deficits and assess the patient's capacity to decide about his discharge/future accommodation.

6. **Equipment checklist:**

   Pencil and paper.

Station 126: Link 2: Discuss: Management of BPSD and mental capacity

Theme: Discussion with the medical team regarding management of BPSD and assessment of mental capacity regarding discharge against medical advice from hospital

1. **Instructions to candidates:**

   Following this assessment, you are going to meet the medical staff on the ward, who would like to discuss with you about how best to manage his disruptive behaviour. They also believe that as his diagnosis is dementia, he must be incapable of living safely in the community and hence, he lacks capacity. However, the team social worker disagrees with this view and hence, they request your opinion on his capacity to discharge himself against medical advice.

   Discuss his management and capacity assessment.

2. **Instructions to the role player:**

   You are the junior trainee doctor of the medical ward in the general hospital. You are also the only doctor available to meet with the psychiatrist to discuss management of this patient. You believe that he scores about 21/30 on MMSE and he has little insight into his cognitive deficits. His diagnosis is dementia and his behaviour on the ward is not acceptable. He is also putting other patients at risk by interfering with their treatment. He needs to be sedated frequently and also by the quickest means available. You ask which drug and what dose would be ideal.

   You also argue that as he has already had falls and he is unsafe to live in the community, he must not be allowed to discharge against medical advice and should be transferred to a residential home. If the candidate talks about the Mental Capacity Act and the decision-specific nature of capacity assessment you ask him about the steps of capacity assessment.

3. **Construct:**

   Candidate is able to communicate the overall approach of managing disruptive behaviour on a medical ward and assessment of mental capacity to the medical staff.

4. **Expanded construct:**

   The candidate is able to:

   - Communicate the steps for analysing the basis of disruptive behaviour, and managing this through environmental modification if possible and the option of psychopharmacology only if absolutely required.
   - Discuss the principles of assessing mental capacity and its application to the specific decision for the patient.
   - Discuss whether the patient has mental capacity to discharge against medical advice.

5. **Areas of importance to pass the station:**

   - Discussion of management of his disruptive behaviour on the ward (50%).
   - Assessment of his mental capacity to discharge against medical advice (50%).

   A passing performance in this station must include a systematic approach to managing his disruptive behaviour on the medical ward, including environmental modification to nursing interventions and judicious use of psychotropic drugs if necessary. An understanding of assessment of capacity and underlying principles, quite distinct from diagnosing his condition as dementia, is also necessary.

6. **Equipment checklist:**

   Not applicable.

Station 127: Link 1: Assess: Delirium in a general hospital setting

Station 128: Link 2: Discuss: Management of delirium

Station 127: Link 1: Assess: Delirium in a general hospital setting

Theme: Assessment of delirium in older patient in a general hospital setting

1. **Instructions to candidates:**

   Mr James Jones, an 80-year-old gentleman, admitted to hospital with a history of memory problems following a collapse at home. On the medical ward, he is observed by the nurse to be muddled and 'confused'. You are asked to see the patient on a liaison consultation. At interview he is distractible and dosing off to sleep during the interview. On waking him up, he talks of people walking round his garden and he appears apprehensive talking about them as he is not sure of what they are up to. **Carry out a diagnostic assessment with a view to arriving at a diagnosis.**

2. **Instructions to the role player:**

   You are an 80-year-old gentleman, Mr Jones. You are being interviewed by the candidate in the hospital. You cannot remember how or why you got into the hospital. You feel sleepy and dose off during the interview for a few seconds and on waking up talk about people in the garden in a disjointed manner. You also start picking at your bed clothes as if you are looking for crawling insects on your bed.

   If asked about day/date/address etc., you give completely wrong answers or do not answer at all. If asked to repeat three objects or spell WORLD backwards or recall three objects you give wrong or no answers at all. If asked to continue with this testing, you sit there blankly or dose off. During interview you suddenly get off the bed/chair and try to hide behind the chair as if you are trying to escape from some danger. If asked why you are frightened, you mention the snakes crawling towards you.

3. **Construct:**

   Candidate is able to diagnose delirium and demonstrate how it differs from dementia.

4. **Expanded construct:**

   The candidate is able to:

   - Elicit features of delirium.
   - Show understanding of the distinguishing features of delirium from dementia.

5. **Areas of importance to pass the station:**

   - Eliciting features of delirium on mental state examination (70%).
   - Managing the patient's behaviour in a calm and reassuring manner (30%).

   A passing performance in this station includes eliciting features of delirium despite the patient's distracting behaviour as a result of delirium.

6. **Equipment checklist:**

   Pencil and paper.

Station 128: Link 2: Discuss: Management of delirium

Theme: Discussion management of delirious patient with the medical team

1. **Instructions to candidates:**

   After your assessment you are meeting with the nursing staff who seeks your advice on management of the problem. Unfortunately only the most junior nurse on the ward is available to talk to you. She has little understanding of the interplay between delirium and dementia and shows surprise when the diagnosis of delirium is mentioned. She was told by the doctor at the time of admission of the patient that he had dementia.

   Discuss the diagnostic possibilities and management plan.

2. **Instructions to the role player:**

   You are the most junior nurse available on ward B2 where this patient is being admitted. When he was admitted, the ward doctor told you that his diagnosis was dementia. The ward doctor has done some blood tests and he is awaiting results of his brain scans and other tests. He has in the meantime been treated with an antibiotic. However, his behaviour in the meantime has become more and more muddled.

   When the candidate mentions delirium as the most likely diagnosis, you question him as your ward doctor's diagnosis for Mr Jones was dementia. You wonder who is right and ask for clarification. You also know that delirium is commonly caused by infection and the patient has already been treated with an antibiotic so the delirium should no longer be an issue. You understand from your earlier discussion with the ward doctor that the patient should be transferred to the mental health unit for further management. If the candidate expresses reservations you seek advice on how best to manage this behaviour on the medical ward.

3. **Construct:**
   - Able to discuss the interplay of delirium and dementia with nursing staff.
   - Able to discuss the management plan with the medical staff.

4. **Expanded construct:**

   The candidate is able to:
   - Demonstrate knowledge of the common causes of delirium.
   - Distinguish delirium from dementia and their relationship.
   - Offer advice on management of delirium on a medical ward.

5. **Areas of importance to pass the station:**
   - Discussion of delirium, its causes and its interplay with dementia (70%).
   - Management of delirium on the Medical ward (30%).

   In order to pass this station, the candidate must be able to discuss the nature, aetiology of delirium, its overlap with dementia, and basic principles of managing a delirious patient on a Medical ward.

6. **Equipment checklist:**
   Not applicable.

Single Station

Station 129: Explain: Management of Alzheimer's disease to the relative

Theme: Explain diagnosis and management of Alzheimer's disease to the relative

1. **Instructions to candidates:**

   You are meeting with son of 68-years-old patient Sandy Smith who is currently an inpatient in your ward for last 4 weeks. She was brought in by police who found her wandering on a busy road. She has been diagnosed with Alzheimer's dementia.

   The son is very concerned about her mother's discharge back home and wants to discuss her diagnosis and management.

   Explain the diagnosis and its management.

   Address ideas, concerns and expectations.

2. **Instructions to the role player:**

   You are Jason Smith, son of 68-year-old patient Sandy Smith who is in hospital for last 4 weeks. She was admitted to hospital after she was found wandering on a busy road by the police. She was well until 3 years ago when she developed problems with her memory. Because of her increasing forgetfulness, you changed the gas cooker in her house to electric. As you are increasingly concerned about her safety, lately you visit her every day. She manages her blood pressure tablets in a dosett box. She lives alone and you are concerned about her discharge back to home.

   The doctor is going to explain her diagnosis and management.

   When the doctor tells you, your mum suffers from dementia you appear shocked and say "I can't believe."

   You ask the doctor the following questions:

   What is wrong with my mum?

   Did she have any tests?

   What treatment she is on?

   What other type of treatments are available?

   I have read in newspaper about tablets which cure dementia. Can she have them?

   If she is discharged home what support is available for carers like me?

   Will I get dementia?

   Will she be allowed to drive?

   Will she be able to look after her finances?

How can the family support her?

How long she will live?

3. Construct:

The core task at this station is to check the ability of the candidate to explain about immediate/short term and post-discharge management of dementia.

4. Expanded construct:

- To develop rapport with a concerned relative.
- To explain management plan using biopsychosocial model.

Candidate is expected to know ICD-10 criteria for different dementias and be able to explain difference between normal aging and dementia.

The candidate should:

- Explain to the relative with information in the language he understands.
- Address the concerns with empathetic responses.
- Explain dementia screening and neuropsychological tests, occupational therapist assessment and assessment of social needs of both the patient and the carer(s) as part of her management plan.
- Explain medical management, i.e., use of acetylcholinesterase inhibitors, treatment of behavioural and psychological symptoms of dementia.
- Explain non-pharmacological management, i.e., reminiscence, reality orientation, validation therapy, cognitive stimulation therapy, art, music and aroma therapy and multisensory approaches.
- Explain social management, i.e., home care visits, meals-on-wheels, day center, respite care, and long-term placement in care homes.
- Provide information about voluntary agencies, i.e., Alzheimer's society, Age concern and Advocacy Services.
- Give information about financial and legal matters or guide them to appropriate agencies.

Interview/Communication skills:

They should include:

- Demonstration of Advance listening skills.
- Diplomacy and empathy with the relative.
- Use language, i.e., simple and avoid jargon.

5. Areas of importance to pass the station:

The following elements should contribute to the bulk of the marks (% relative weighting).

- Ability to discuss about assessment and management plan with concerned relative (30%).
- Diagnosis explained fluently and succinctly (10%).

- Interview and communication skills (40%).
- Inform carer about voluntary agencies and support groups and their role (20%).

6. **Equipment checklist:**
Not applicable.

5. Child and Adolescent Psychiatry

Linked Stations: 130–135

Station 130: Link 1: Assess: Childhood depression

Station 131: Link 2: Discuss: Management of childhood depression

Station 130: Link 1: Assess: Childhood depression

Theme: Assessment of childhood depression

1. **Instructions to candidates:**
Eight-year-old Miss Casey Jones has been referred to the child psychiatry department by her GP after concerns were raised in school. There are reports that Casey has been missing school and when she does attend school complains of headaches. You are asked to speak to her mother, Ms Sarah Jones.
Take a history from her mother to arrive at a diagnosis. You may wish to take notes to discuss the case with your consultant in the next station.

2. **Instructions to the role player:**
You are Ms Sarah Jones, 36-year-old, a housewife, who has been separated from her husband Tim Jones 4 years ago. You live with your two children Sally, 12 years old and Casey, 8 years old. There are no concerns about Sally.
   - Casey was born 2 weeks premature via normal delivery. There were no concerns during infancy. She attained developmental milestones in a timely fashion. She settled well in nursery and there were no concerns during her initial school years.
   - In the last 6 months, she has become increasing irritable and has started to refuse to attend school.
   - She makes vague complaints that you do not feel she is actually experiencing because she settles with no interventions when she gets her way by staying at home. Casey does not play with her favourite toys anymore. She has become more withdrawn and does not play with her friends anymore.
   - There is no history of bullying.
   - She has trouble sleeping recently, frequently waking throughout the night. She does not want to eat and is frequently forced to do so.

- Her performance in school has been affected in the last 4 months, progressively becoming worse.
- She has not harmed herself or voiced thoughts of doing so.
- There is a family history of mental illness on your side with your mother and sister who suffer from depression.

3. **Construct:**
This station assesses candidate's ability to take a corroborative history to elucidate evidence for depression in childhood.

4. **Expanded construct:**
   - They should elicit the history and clinical features suggestive of childhood depression.
   - The candidate should ask a range of questions that demonstrates knowledge of the changes in behaviour and signs that may present in a child who is depressed.
   - They should ask about the mood changes, irritability, somatic complaints, sleep and appetite disturbances, school performance, and changes in social behaviour and self-harm.
   - They should ask briefly about earlier development.
   - They should demonstrate an understanding of presentation of childhood.
   - They should conduct a focused and fluent corroborative history which demonstrates empathy with the patient's mother.

5. **Areas of importance to pass the station:**
   - Eliciting behavioural and mood symptoms suggestive of childhood depression. These should include details of the earlier development (40%).
   - Exploration of impact on home and school life (20%).
   - Communication (20%).

Station 131: Link 2: Discuss: Management of childhood depression

Theme: Discuss management plan of childhood depression with your consultant

1. **Instructions to candidates:**
You have gathered collateral history from Ms Sarah Jones, mother of Casey Jones.
Discuss your findings and management plan with your consultant.

2. **Instructions to the role player:**
You are a Consultant Psychiatrist. In discussion with the candidate you would like to know the following:
   - Presentation of the child at home and school.
   - Notable triggers for, e.g., bullying and change in family circumstances.
   - Developmental history.
   - Immediate and long-term management.
   - Risks to self and others.

- Prognosis.
- Knowledge of national guidelines, such as, NICE.

You must ask the doctor how they arrived at the management plan and whether any other information is still required.

3. **Construct:**

This station assesses the candidate's ability to present the key clinical findings of depression in a child, knowledge of assessment in children and collateral history as well as management of childhood depression.

4. **Expanded construct:**
   - They should show the ability to focus on the problem and nature, presenting the scenario in a systematic fashion to arrive at the diagnosis.
   - They should demonstrate an insight into the principles of the assessment of children and use of the collateral history from other sources such as school.
   - They should demonstrate the knowledge of management of childhood depression, in particular, the role of psychological and pharmacological intervention.
   - They should be able to present their findings succinctly highlighting key features of childhood depression.
   - Present the management in a structured, focused and fluent fashion.
   - Use language, i.e., appropriate to the discussion with a senior medical colleague.
5. **Areas of importance to pass the station:**
   - Ability to describe the clinical presentation of childhood depression (40%).
   - Ability to explain the management (40%).
   - Communication (20%).

Station 132: Link 1: ADHD: History from a parent

Station 133: Link 2: ADHD: Discuss management

Station 132: Link 1: ADHD: History from a parent

Theme: ADHD: History from a parent

1. **Instructions to candidates:**

You are in the outpatient clinic where a general practitioner has referred Kevin Brown to you following concerns raised in school about his behaviour.

Speak to his father Mr Jason Brown and take a relevant history to reach a diagnosis.

The candidate is not expected to share the diagnosis or discuss management in this station.

2. **Instructions to the role player:**

You are Jason Brown and you live with your wife, Kelly Brown. You have one son Kevin, who is 9 years old.

- Kevin has been recently excluded from school following concerns about his behaviour. The teachers say that he does not sit still, is constantly moving and leaves his seat.
- He is easily distractible, fails to pay attention and subsequently does not complete his work. He is very active, constantly running and jumping often injuring himself.
- He has always been an active child since you can remember and appears to be 'driven by a motor'.
- There are no concerns about his early development.
- He got excluded after destroying the computers in class. This appears to be an impulsive act.
- Overall he is performing poorly in school. His difficulties with attention, concentration and impulsivity are present in home and school environment.

3. **Construct:**

This station assesses the candidate's ability to explore the symptoms and signs of ADHD in a child by taking a collateral history from a parent.

4. **Expanded construct:**

- The candidate should take a relevant history and explore key diagnostic features of ADHD.
- They should carry out an assessment, i.e., focused, fluent and demonstrate empathy with the patient's experience.
- They should show an ability to focus on the specific problem and the nature of it by following a systematic approach to questioning.
- They should demonstrate knowledge of childhood developmental disorders and their presentation.
- They should demonstrate skill of using an appropriate mix of closed and open questions.
- They should demonstrate advanced listening skills and ask questions that are focused, structured and relevant.
- They should use language, i.e., simple and understandable and avoid jargon.

5. **Areas of importance to pass the station:**

- Ability to illicit and explore the symptoms and signs of ADHD (40%).
- Ability to illicit the nature and pervasiveness of the disorder, present at least in two different environment with onset before the age of 6 years (20%).
- Ability to exclude other developmental disorder like autism, learning disability (20%).
- Communication (20%).

Station 133: Link 2: ADHD: Discuss management

Theme: ADHD: Discuss management plan with patient's parent or teacher, explain ADHD and address their concerns, views and expectations

1. **Instructions to candidates:**

   You have just taken a collateral history from Kevin's father.

   Discuss your findings and management plan with Kevin's mother Kelly Brown. Address her concerns, views and expectations.

2. **Instructions to the role player:**

   You are Kelly Brown and your only son Kevin has recently been excluded from school. You are concerned about him and want to know the following:

   - What is wrong with Kevin?
   - Why Kevin?
   - Can you help him return to school?
   - Is it treatable?
   - If we have more children, will they also be affected?
   - Did I do something to cause it?
   - Will he always have it?
   - What should I do to help him?

3. **Construct:**

   This station assesses an ability to explain the diagnosis and management to a parent of a child with ADHD.

4. **Expanded construct:**

   - The candidate should discuss the clinical features suggestive of ADHD.
   - They should demonstrate knowledge of the aetiology and management of ADHD, address any concerns and expectations of a parent with a child with ADHD.
   - They should demonstrate empathy and sensitivity.
   - They should demonstrate advanced listening skills.
   - They should use language, i.e., simple and understandable, avoiding jargon.

5. **Areas of importance to pass the station:**

   - Ability to explain the diagnosis and clinical presentation of ADHD (20%).
   - Ability to discuss the aetiology and prognosis of ADHD (20%).
   - Ability to explain the management of ADHD (40%).
   - Interview and communication skills (20%).

Station 134: Link 1. Assess: Child sexual abuse

Station 135: Link 2. Discuss: Management of child sexual abuse

Station 134: Link 1. Assess: Child sexual abuse

Theme: Assessment of child sexual abuse

1. **Instructions to candidates:**

   You are in the outpatient clinic where a paediatrician has referred 13-year-old Sally Jacob to you for an assessment following concerns raised by her mother and school. Sally has become more withdrawn and suddenly lost interest in activities around her.

Explore reasons why this change of behaviour has occurred.

2. **Instructions to the role player:**

Your parents have been separated since you were 2 years old. You are the only child. There are no concerns at school.

- You are a 13-year-old adolescent girl who appears quiet and scared during the interview. You are reluctant to share information unless the candidate is sensitive and reassuring.
- You are finding it hard to concentrate and feeling stressed and anxious.
- If so, you disclose the following:

"All is not well at home" as your mother's partner of 1 year has been sexually abusing you by coming into your room for a month, at night, whilst your mother is asleep. He touches you in places you feel are not right. Two weeks ago, he has raped you. He has told you not to tell anyone or he will hurt your mother and that no one will believe you.

He has also blamed you that it is your fault and you have 'seduced' him. You are afraid and don't want to go home. You do not want the candidate to tell this to anyone.

3. **Construct:**

This station assesses the candidate's ability to explore possible reasons for a change in an adolescent behaviour and in particular to sensitively assess for any possibility of child abuse.

4. **Expanded construct:**

- The candidate should demonstrate empathy with the patients experience.
- The candidate should show an ability to focus on the specific problem.
- They should demonstrate use of an appropriate mix of open and closed questions.
- They should demonstrate advanced listening skills.

5. **Areas of importance to pass the station:**

- Interview, communication skills (40%).
- Ability to elicit details about the specific problem without contamination of evidence (50%).
- Exploration of other reasons for change in adolescent behaviour (10%).

Station 135: Link 2. Discuss: Management of child sexual abuse

Theme: Discuss management of child sexual abuse with a parent

1. **Instructions to candidates:**

You have seen Sally Jacob in the previous station.

Talk to her mother Alice who is waiting to see you. Discuss your findings and management plan with her. Address her concerns and expectations.

2. **Instructions to the role player:**

You are Alice Jacob, a housewife and live with your daughter Sally Jacob.

- Your partner of 1 year has been spending increasing amounts of time at your house in the past 2 months.
- You are depressed and see your GP who has prescribed medications for past 5 years.
- You are concerned about the change in your daughter's behaviour and want to understand what has caused this change. You ask the doctor "Is she depressed like me?"
- When the doctor shares with you the outcome of the assessment, you are initially in disbelief and then blame yourself. You ask the doctor about the next steps and want to call the police.

You ask the following questions:

- What's going to happen now?
- My partner has come with me today. What shall I do?
- Will I lose Sally?

2. **Construct:**

This station assesses the candidate's ability to deal with a child protection concern following a disclosure of child abuse to a parent.

3. **Expanded construct:**

- The candidate is expected to discuss management plan and address parent's concern in a sensitive manner.
- They should demonstrate knowledge of managing disclosure of child abuse.
- They should share information with a concerned parent whilst avoiding contamination of evidence.

Interview/Communication skills:

- Be empathic.
- Demonstrate advanced listening skills.
- Share information in a fluent and focused manner.
- Avoid jargon.

5. **Areas of importance to pass the station:**

- Ability to recognize involvement of children service and the immediacy of situation given the partner's whereabouts. This includes contacting children services, carrying out relevant physical examination, need to interview avoiding contamination of evidence and risk assessment (40%).
- Reassurance of a distressed parent and addressing concerns, e.g., genetic predisposition to depression (20%).
- Communication (40%).

Single Stations: 136–139

Station 136: Explain: Borderline personality disorder to the mother of a 15-year-old girl

Theme: Explanation of borderline personality disorder to the mother of a 15-year old girl

1. **Instructions to candidates:**

   You are about to see Mrs Katie Hamilton who is worried about her daughter Lucy Hamilton. Lucy is 15 years old, attends mainstream school and has been cutting herself using scissors at school since the past 4 months. Lucy generally cuts herself when she is stressed. Mrs Hamilton is concerned that Lucy may have a borderline personality disorder as you have recently seen a television programme about it.

   Discuss with Mrs Hamilton about borderline personality disorder.

   Address her fears, concerns and expectations.

2. **Instructions to the role player:**

   You are Mrs Katie Hamilton and married to David Hamilton. You have two children, Lucy and Bob. There are no concerns about Bob.

   - You have discovered that Lucy has been cutting herself as you noticed scars on her arms.
   - You are worried that she may be suffering from borderline personality disorder.
   - You saw a programme on the television, a month ago, about a girl who has the disorder.

   You ask following questions:

   - **What is a personality disorder?**
   - **Does Lucy have borderline personality disorder?**
   - **Why does she cut herself?**
   - **Can it be cured?**
   - **How do I help her?**
   - **How do you treat it?**

3. **Construct:**

   This station assesses the candidate's ability to explain about borderline personality disorder to a distraught mother.

4. **Expanded construct:**

   - The candidate can be expected to explain borderline personality disorder and address concerns and expectations.
   - They should explain the symptoms and presentation of borderline personality disorder in a fluent and focused manner.
   - They should explain the disorder in a simple and understandable language, avoiding jargons.
   - They should demonstrate advanced listening skills.
   - They should demonstrate appropriate empathy.

5. **Areas of importance to pass the station:**
   - Ability to discuss the diagnosis including knowledge of presentation, aetiology and management (40%).
   - Interview and communication skills (40%).
   - Ability to address specific concerns of self-harm in an adolescent (20%).

Station 137: Assess: Overdose in an adolescent girl

Theme: Assessment of overdose in an adolescent girl

1. **Instructions to candidates:**

   You are about to see 13-year-old Sarah Parker on the paediatric ward following an overdose last night.

   Talk to her by asking a relevant history. Do an appropriate risk assessment.

2. **Instructions to the role player:**
   - You are 13-year-old girl in a mainstream school and live with your family.
   - You took an unplanned, impulsive overdose yesterday after a fight with your boyfriend.
   - You were angry at the time and wanted to teach him a lesson.
   - You took four paracetamol tablets and immediately sent him and your mother a text telling them what you had done.
   - You regret the act.
   - You have not tried to hurt or kill yourself before.
   - The fight was about a trivial matter and now you have made up with him since.
   - You feel well in yourself.
   - There are no concerns at home or in school.

3. **Construct:**

   This station assesses the candidate's ability to take a relevant history of an overdose and carry out a risk assessment.

4. **Expanded construct:**
   - The candidate is expected to take a relevant history and do a risk assessment.
   - They should carry out a fluent and focused history of an overdose.
   - They should focus on the risk and the nature of it by following a systematic approach to questioning.
   - They should demonstrate appropriate mix of open and closed questions.
   - They should ask questions that are structured, focused and fluent.
   - They should demonstrate advanced listening skills.
   - They should use language, i.e., simple, understandable and avoid jargons.

5. **Areas of importance to pass the station:**
   - Ability to elicit and explore the history following an overdose (40%).
   - Ability to do a relevant risk assessment (40%).
   - Interview and communication skills (20%).

Station 138: Conduct disorder: Collateral history

Theme: Conduct disorder: Collateral history

1. **Instructions to candidates:**

   Hayden Burns has been referred by his GP to your clinic since he is getting mood swings for some time. His mother Rachel Burns is finding hard to manage him at home. The referral letter states that Hayden has always been an 'angry little boy' but Mum has managed to cope so far. But, now his aggressive behaviour is putting others at risk and she is seeking help.

   Explore Rachel's concerns to get an understanding of the possible diagnosis of Hayden.

2. **Instructions to the role player:**

   You are 37 years old, Rachel Burns living with your husband Mark Burns and son Hayden. Hayden is your only son and he is 12 years old. He attends St Mary's secondary school and is in year 8.
   - Hayden has always been an 'angry little boy'. As a baby he was hard to console and would often cry for hours despite all efforts. As a toddler, he would often throw things and have temper tantrums. These were noticeable at home and various other places, e.g., supermarkets, parks, school, friends' homes etc.
   - Neighbours stopped inviting Hayden to parties and get-togethers because of his behaviour.
   - The staff at the nursery school which he had attended had expressed concerns regarding Hayden. In the school, he would hit, bite, spit and push other children. At times, he would throw things at staff members and you were called to pick him up since his behaviour was uncontrollable.
   - Similar anger outbursts were seen at his primary school and now in secondary school. There would be no apparent trigger for his outbursts.
   - As a child you have seen him to be cruel to insects. On two occasions, you had to take your pet dog to the vet because he had hit the dog hard and the dog was bleeding from the nose. At that time he has a smirk on his face and did not seem to feel sorry.
   - He has been a bully ever since he went to nursery. He would often initiate fights and hit others without any provocation.
   - Since he has grown up, he has stolen money a few times. He has also been caught stealing from neighbour's house on two occasions. He has also been caught shoplifting four times from the local supermarket. He has run away from house about half a dozen times in the last year and you have had to contact the police because of this. The local police are aware of his bad behaviours since he has been cautioned on numerous occasions for throwing stones at other people's houses, windows and cars.
   - He has been involved in truancy, arson, theft and burglary with his 'gang'.

- You seem to have lost all control over him and feel scared at times due to his behaviour. You fear that if his behaviour continues he may end up going to prison as an adult. This is something the local police officers have also informed you.
- To the best of your knowledge he does not take illicit drugs. He is a happy child especially when he is with his mates. His milestones were fine and he is an average child in school in terms of his work. There are no other concerns.

3. **Construct:**

   This station assesses the ability of the candidate elicit a detailed and systematic comorbid history of conduct disorder including comorbidities.

4. **Expanded construct:**
   - The candidate should demonstrate knowledge and understanding of conduct disorder and its criteria for diagnosis according to ICD-10 classification system.
   - According to ICD-10, Conduct disorder is present when there is a repetitive and persistent pattern of dissocial, aggressive, or defiant behaviours.
   - Such behaviours should amount to major violations of age-appropriate social expectations. It should hence be more severe than ordinary childish mischief or adolescent rebelliousness and should imply an enduring pattern of behaviour, i.e., 6 months or longer. Examples of the behaviours on which the diagnosis is based include excessive levels of fighting or bullying, cruelty to other people or animals, severe destructiveness to property which may be own home or other people's property, fire-setting, stealing, repeated lying, truancy from school and running away from home, unusually frequent and severe temper tantrums, and disobedience. Any one of these behaviours, if marked, is sufficient for the diagnosis, but isolated dissocial acts are not.

5. **Areas of importance to pass the station:**
   - Eliciting collateral history, range and depth of problems to reach a diagnosis of conduct disorder according to ICD-10 classification system (50%).
   - Rule out comorbid disorders and assess risks (30%).
   - Communication (20%).

Station 139: School refusal: Collateral history

Theme: School refusal: Collateral history

1. **Instructions to the candidates:**

   Mrs Smith is attending your CAMHS clinic today regarding Ryan Smith who is 8 years old. Ryan is refusing to go to school for the past 3 months. They have tried numerous techniques to get him to school but none of them seem to be working.

   Talk to Mrs Smith and gather information on reasons for Ryan's non-attendance at school.

2. **Instructions to the role player:**

   You are Mrs Smith, 35-year-old, live with your husband Matthew Smith who is an IT professional.

You do not volunteer any information unless asked or if the doctor is understanding and demonstrates sensitivity to your needs.

- Your son Ryan has started to refuse to go to school for the past 3 months or so. Initially, he was reluctant to go to school but with the passage of time he has become more and more resistive and has completely stopped going to school. On most days, he would cry and get angry in the mornings when you go and try and get him ready to go to school. Sometimes, he will complain of headaches.
- Several attempts by teachers and parents to encourage and reward him for going to school have failed.
- Interestingly, he stops crying and being upset by later in the morning or around noon time.
- Ryan is your eldest child and was born at full-term. His milestones were at normal times, had no problems in nursery and primary school. He normally plays with other children and seems happy. There are no triggers that you could identify, such as, financial, relationship, marital problems, etc.
- Following a fertility treatment you have recently given birth to a girl who is now 5 months of age. You had been trying to have another child for the last few years. You feel drained taking care of her and Ryan being at home, it adds to your pressure to your domestic chores. The baby girl was born prematurely and has suffered from various ailments and required frequent visits to the local hospital.
- If the doctor asks you about the possibility that your daughter's birth may have a bearing on Ryan's school refusal, you say you don't know. If the doctor attempts to make a connection, you agree with what he is suggesting and reflect upon his formulation.
- You have also noticed that Ryan is expecting increased attention and has been demanding.

3. **Construct:**

This station assesses the candidate's ability to explore reasons for school refusal in a child and establish sibling jealousy/rivalry as one of the possible precipitating factor.

4. **Expanded construct:**

- The candidate should use a good mix of open and closed questions.
- They should explore premorbid functioning and behaviour.
- They should explore and identify triggers to school refusal. These may be:
  - Family problems.
  - Birth or death of somebody in the family.
  - Sibling jealousy/rivalry.
  - Illness of the child in question, or anyone in the family (fear of dying while he at school).
  - Problems at school: Educational difficulties, bullying at school.
- They should explore and rule out psychiatric/developmental difficulties, such as, depression, autistic spectrum disorder, oppositional defiant disorder, ADHD, learning disabilities, separation anxieties and organic illnesses. He may suggest that Ryan may be feeling left out since all your attention may have deviated to your daughter.

5. Areas of importance to pass the station:

- Eliciting history and precipitating factors for school refusal (40%).
- Elicit premorbid functioning and rule out other comorbid disorders (30%).
- Communication (30%).

6. Learning Disability

Linked Stations : 140–145

Station 140: Link 1. Assess: Risks with a man with mild learning disability

Station 141: Link 2. Discuss: Your findings and opinion with the above patient's mother

Station 140: Link 1. Assess: Risks with a man with mild learning disability

Theme: Assessing risks and discussing management plans in learning disability

1. Instructions to candidates:

Patients name: Stephen Fallon

You are an ST4 in learning disabilities team. Assess risks and discuss management plan with a man with mild learning disability whose girlfriend also suffers from mild learning disability and is 6 months pregnant. He was convicted of indecent exposure about 18 months ago. The social services have informed that their child will be taken into care soon after birth.

- **Elicit his views, concerns and expectations and discuss management options.**

2. Instructions to the role player:

- You are a 25 years old man with a mild learning disability. Your level of functioning is equal to that of a 13 years old boy. You behave as an adult when speaking to adults. You can be easily persuaded by others but can be stubborn on certain aspects. You are cross with the whole world (and the doctor) that social services will be taking the child away. You start off with expressing your frustration and dissatisfaction but if the doctor engages you in conversation with empathy and sensitivity, then you mellow down.
- You are supported in the community by the local LD team, social services, your mother Elizabeth (Liz) Fallon. You are on Disability Living Allowance (DLA) and other benefits and need help in managing your finances. You had exposed yourself last year because at that time you were going through a period of stress and had a fallout with your girlfriend. That was not the first time you had done that. You feel better when you expose yourself and see no harm in chilling out when stressed. You have exposed to teenagers close to your house who you consider 'mates' and see that as a 'cheeky' behaviour. Last year you exposed yourself to a girl who complained to her parents and police was involved. You have a probation officer Mark who you have seen twice in the last 8 months. He lectures you and you don't like him.

- Your girl friend, Melanie is currently 6 months pregnant. This is an unplanned pregnancy since you did not use contraception. You met her at the clinic few years ago and have been in relationship with her for the last 3 years. You live in supported accommodation with her. Joanne from social services has informed Melanie that the baby will be taken into care once the baby is born. Melanie wishes to have the baby and fears losing her baby. You are okay for the baby to be adopted, however, you are upset and angry because the situation is upsetting Melanie.
- Because of this stress you feel like exposing yourself again to others around the neighbourhood. You do not want to do this, but feel helpless. You want the doctor to listen to your worries and circumstances and assure you that the baby will not be taken away from Melanie after the baby is born.
- If the doctor appears to be empathetic and offering you a ear, you ease down and smile at him. If he checks with you regarding the intentions of exposing yourself, you assure him that you won't do that when he gives you an assurance that he/she will look into it, discuss this with social services and that social services will not take the baby away immediately after birth. The doctor should be able to tell you that people with difficulties that you and your girlfriend have equal rights to others as long as there are no risks. The doctor should be able to inform you that social services should be doing an assessment when the baby is born to check if/how would you and Melanie cope with parenthood. If the doctor is controlling or lacks empathy in his/her demeanour, you get agitated, irrational and stubborn until the doctor takes an empathetic stand.
- You use simple words and phrases. Start off with vague statements such as "I feel stressed doctor", "I think I will do it again (expose myself)", etc. Let the doctor explore these further. Don't tell the story until the doctor has asked you to clarify these vague statements. If the doctor is using any difficult words or phrases, you ask the doctor what does he/she means. Remember your brain development is equivalent to a 13 years old.

3. Construct:

The station tests the ability of the doctor to:

- Assess a patient with learning disability.
- Empathetic listening.
- Provide reassurance.
- Assess risks of exposure.
- Offer hope and information but only, i.e., legally correct.

4. Expanded Construct:

Key points to cover:

- Ensure you allow the patient to express himself first.
- Explore his concerns with open questions followed by closed questions.
- Try and understand his predicaments and circumstances.
- Be empathetic to his and his girlfriends difficulties and distress.
- Explore risks of indecent exposure-frequency, last time he did it, current thoughts, police being aware of these, receiving any work/counselling regarding this.
- Use language, i.e., simple and easy. Do not use jargons. The language should be such that could be used for a 12–13 years old boy.

- Reassure the patient.
- Child will not be taken away immediately after birth.
- Further assessment of their needs and the baby's needs will be done by social services after the baby is born.
- People with disabilities have equal rights to those who do not have disabilities.

5. **Areas of importance to pass the station:**
- Ability to show an understanding of learning disability (30%).
- Elicit relevant risks involved (40%).
- Reassurance and communication skills (30%).

6. **Equipment checklist:**
Not applicable.

Station 141: Link 2. Discuss: Your findings and opinion with the above patient's mother

Theme: Discussing a patient with learning disabilities with their relative

1. **Instructions to candidates:**
Discuss your findings and opinion with the above patient's mother Elizabeth Fallon who is angry and agitated about the situation. She blames doctors for not sterilising her son and putting him in this situation.

2. **Instructions to the role player:**
You have raised your son Stephen, as a single mother with a lot of difficulty. You never received adequate support while bringing him up. You believe that your son was always disliked and rejected by society. Initially, he struggled in school then he could not work and now the NHS and social services have let him down.
You believe that Stephen should have been sterilised even before he formed a relationship. It was the doctor's responsibility to offer him sterilisation and that would have then prevented from all these problems from happening. You tell the doctor (since you believe firmly) that Stephen is going to have a child with learning disabilities since Stephen and his partner both suffer from it. You fear that history is repeating itself and that you will be eventually left to care for this disabled child on your own without any support. While telling all this you become tearful and angry at the same time. You hence say that it will be beneficial for all for social services to take away the child at the time of birth. However, you also acknowledge feeling guilty about thinking this way.
You have supported Stephen ever since he moved out in supported accommodation. You visit him regularly where he lives with his girlfriend Melanie. You work as a barmaid in the evenings. Bringing up your son and providing ongoing support to your son has made you emotionally drained.
What you want from the doctor is to listen to you and understand your difficulties. The doctor should try and explore your difficulties so that you can tell the doctor how hard it has been bringing up Stephen to continue to support him on a daily basis. You start with being frustrated and disappointed with the services and blame doctors for not sterilising your son in the first place. You then ask the doctor to get him sterilised as soon as possible so that he cannot father a child again. You should

continue to press on this point until the doctor makes it clear that people with learning disabilities have rights like others and cannot be compulsorily sterilised.

If the doctor is able to listen to you with sensitivity and appears to show empathy, you calm down. You relax even further if the doctor is able to suggest ways how services can help you and your son. Accept any help the doctor offers you. If the doctor is unable to allow you to express your difficulties, you continue to blame the services for letting you and your son down. Also stick to the need for getting your son sterilised if he appears to be lecturing you or interrupting you while you explain your difficulties.

3. **Construct:**

The station tests the doctors ability to:

- Allow and encourage the mother to express her concerns.
- Show empathy.
- Be aware that people with learning disabilities cannot be compulsorily sterilised.

4. **Expanded construct:**

Key points to consider:

- Allow the mother to express himself first.
- Encourage her to tell you more using open and then closed questions.
- Try and understand her predicaments and circumstances.
- Be empathetic to her difficulties.
- Inform her of the support networks available including yours and social services.
- Inform her that people with disabilities have equal rights to those who do not have disabilities and cannot be compulsorily sterilised.

5. **Areas of importance to pass the station:**

- Ability to express empathy and advanced communication skills 40%.
- Knowledge of support services for people suffering from learning difficulties including the role of social services 40%.
- Knowledge of rights of people with learning disabilities 20%.

6. **Equipment checklist:**

Not applicable.

Station 142: Link 1. Asperger's syndrome: History from a parent

Station 143: Link 2. Asperger's syndrome: Discuss management with a residential care home manager

Station 142: Link 1. Asperger's syndrome: History from a parent

Theme: Asperger's syndrome–Assessment of change in behaviour (collateral history)

1. **Instructions to the candidates:**

Mrs Leslie Bolton has attended your outpatient department with concerns regarding her son Adam

Bolton, who is 25 years old and lives in a residential care home. He was diagnosed with Asperger's syndrome when he was 13 years old. She and the residential care home staff have noticed sudden change in his behaviour and he has become increasingly agitated.

Talk to Mrs Bolton and explore her concerns in order to understand why Adam's behaviour has changed.

2. **Instructions to the role player:**

You are Leslie Bolton, mother to Adam Bolton who is 25-year-old and is currently living in a residential care home in Manchester for the last 4 years.

- You visit Adam on a daily basis; however, there are times when you cannot because of your own health and work commitments. You have a chronic back problem and are on painkillers for this.
- You work as a teacher in secondary school. You live alone and have been divorced for last 20 years. Adam's father has no contact with Adam for the last 10 years or so and even before that he was minimally involved in his care.
- He was diagnosed by local CAMHS services with Asperger's syndrome when he was 13 years old. You have struggled to take care of him because of lack of support, poor health and his worsening symptoms.
- Adam has started to become increasingly agitated for the last 2 months. He is throwing things at the care home staff, swearing at them, and becomes verbally hostile very easily. At times staff is able to contain his behaviour and at other times they find it very hard. In the last week, he has been physically aggressive to the staff as well on couple of occasions. On both occasions, the staff required some first aid but did not need to go to the hospital. The staff do not intend to bring charges of assault but you fear that if his behaviour continues to worsen, he may be eventually charged for assaulting others soon.
- You answer the following only when the doctor specifically asks: there has been no change in the care home environment, the staff have not changed–no new staff or staff retiring/resigning, his diet has not changed either. He has been physically fine, no pains anywhere in the body, and no changes in bowel movements, sleep, appetite or self-care from before. None of the other residents in the care home have moved, no new ones joining or any others leaving. He used to have difficult behaviours in the past but not so intense (hitting out) and for this long (2 months now).
- You have decided to move house and live in Cardiff where your mother and sisters reside. You have also been offered a place at a local secondary school as a teacher.
- You have been thinking of moving to Cardiff for the last 1 year but finally decided regarding this a couple of months ago. You have discussed this with the residential care home staff and also with Adam.
- Adam does not think that you should move to Cardiff. He has not discussed your plans to move with the care home staff and neither has the staff attempted to discuss this any further with him.

3. **Construct:**

This station assesses candidate's ability to listen to a distressed mother, gather relevant information to understand reasons for change in behaviour of a patient with Asperger's syndrome.

4. **Expanded construct:**
   - The candidate should demonstrate empathy, sensitivity and allow mother to express her views, concerns and expectations.
   - They should consider symptoms of Asperger's syndrome and possible precipitating factors for challenging, disturbed behaviour.
   - They should explore risk to self and others.
   - They should explore for any changes in patients lifestyle, habits and environment or even expected changes that he may be uncomfortable accepting for, e.g., mother moving to Cardiff.
5. **Areas of importance to pass the station:**
   - Eliciting collateral information to identify the trigger/precipitating factor for a change in behaviour of a patient with Asperger's syndrome (50%).
   - Ability to show an understanding of Asperger's syndrome and discuss it with the mother (30%).
   - Elicit relevant risks involved (20%).
6. **Equipment checklist:**
   Not applicable.

Station 143: Link 2. Asperger's syndrome: Discuss management with a residential care home manager

Theme: Asperger's syndrome: Discuss management and prognosis with a residential care home manager

1. **Instructions to the candidates:**

   You have seen Adam Bolton's mother in the clinic. She has informed you of Adam's challenging behaviour in the residential care home. The care home manager is struggling to manage Adam and would like to discuss with you.

   Talk to the care home manager; discuss your findings and management plan.
2. **Instructions to the role player:**

   You are Joanne Ward, manager at a residential care home for learning disability. You are concerned about Adam's challenging behaviour.
   - You tell the doctor that staff at the care home is scared of Adam. He is a big lad and he can be very intimidating to others when he is angry.
   - You have known Adam for the last 5 years and this is the worst you have ever seen him. He would kick off for no apparent reason, start shouting and swearing at staff on a daily basis. His behaviour is getting worse. He has assaulted staff on two occasions and it has been unprovoked.
   - You got your GP involved and he has done some blood tests and they have come out to be normal.
   - You tell the doctor nothing has changed: Environment is same, food is same, staff have not changed, other residents have not changed, his mother Leslie Bolton, comes often to see him,

although there are the odd days she can't make it because of her own health problems and work schedule.

- Discuss the following only if the doctor checks with you. You acknowledge the fact that Adam's mother Leslie is planning to move to Cardiff and that means that she will be seeing Adam less often. You have had a discussion with Leslie and she has been planning to move in the last 1 year. She has finally decided on this a couple of months ago and has informed you and Adam about her decision to move. You or your staff has not discussed this matter with Adam; however, Leslie did tell you that she has discussed this with Adam. If the doctor asks, you then reflect and tell them that in hindsight may be this is having an impact on Adam's behaviour. Adam does not like changes in his routine. He is very close to his mother. If Leslie moves, she will see Adam less and he is aware of this. He must be fearing that he will not see her mother as much as he does now.

You ask the doctor:

- What should we do at care home?
- What are the possible reasons for his behaviour change?
- Can you give him some tablets?
- I am worried about staff safety. What do you suggest?
- Does he need admission?

3. Construct:

This station assesses candidate's ability to discuss management options with the care home manager while giving some space to listen to the manager concerns as well.

4. Expanded construct:

- The candidate should explore care manager's concern and agenda for the meeting and address them appropriately.
- The candidate should discuss the possible precipitants for the challenging behaviour including mother moving to Cardiff.
- The candidate should discuss solutions of managing challenging behaviour, such as:
  - o Leslie and a staff with whom Adam is most comfortable–sit with Adam and discuss the matter sensitively.
  - o Encourage Adam to see why Leslie needs to move to Cardiff.
  - o Attempt to identify how often would Leslie be able to meet Adam.
  - o Consider the option of moving Adam to Cardiff but remember people with Asperger's often find change difficult. It would be beneficial if Leslie moves and checks if she is willing to stay in Cardiff and only then consider moving Adam.
  - o Consider medication option but that would be the last resort.
  - o Try and find out what calms Adam down and use those techniques more to contain the risks. Advise staff on the ABC chart–antecedents, behaviours and consequences.

5. Areas of importance to pass the station:

- Discussion of management options based on the information gathered in the earlier station and also information provided by the care home manager (50%).

- Assess risk to patient and others and suggest appropriate management strategy (20%).
- Address care managers concerns, ideas and expectations appropriately (30%).

6. **Equipment checklist:**
   Not applicable.

Station 144: Link 1. Collateral history from a mother about her autistic child

Station 145: Link 2. Discussion of management and prognosis of an autistic child with a school teacher/relative/student nurse/consultant psychiatrist

Station 144: Link 1. Collateral history from a mother about her autistic child

Theme: Childhood autism: Collateral history from mother

1. **Instructions to candidates:**

   You are a specialty registrar year 4 in Child and Adolescent Psychiatry. Mrs Victoria Morgan has come to your clinic regarding her 12-year-old son Andrew Morgan who was diagnosed with autism a year ago. He has been exhibiting worsening aggressive behaviour for the past year.

   Talk to Mrs Victoria Morgan regarding Andrew to understand the problem(s).

2. **Instructions to the role player:**

   You are 40-year-old Mrs Victoria (Vicky) Morgan and live with your 43-year-old husband Steve Morgan and only child Andrew. Do not volunteer any information unless asked and doctor takes a keen interest in knowing your problems.

   - Andrew has become increasingly violent and aggressive for the past 1 year. If the doctor asks then you provide the remaining information.
   - It started in September last year when he became verbally aggressive, irritable and started throwing and breaking things. In January this year, Andrew for the very first time punched Steve out of blue which came as a shock to everyone.
   - Three weeks ago he pushed you and you needed first aid for a cut on forehead but did not need to go to the hospital for any treatment of your injury. Few hours later, Andrew was apologetic to you.
   - You are not sure what is going on with him. You want to seek help. You and your husband are obviously concerned about Andrew and you have started to feel scared of him when he is in a 'mood'.
   - Andrew was born with the help of fertility treatments after you and Steve had tried for a number of years to have a baby.
   - He was noted to be 'different' from other children when he went to nursery. Initially, you thought he was a shy boy but later others also started expressing concerns regarding his solitary play, being in his own world, odd habits, such as, lining things and getting upset if somebody altered his play. He could not make any friends in primary school except a girl who was also shy like him. He would take things literally, would not share items with others and would not

join in any groups of children. The local CAMHS got involved and after assessing him, diagnosed him with autism when he was 9 years old.

- Intellectually, he is fine and has been an average pupil in a mainstream school. He was liked by his teachers and was never a problem in the class.
- Andrew has been struggling to sleep at nights, has poor appetite and reduced weight. He has become socially withdrawn, does not enjoy his X box, had become increasingly tearful and irritable. You have heard him say that family will be better off without him. He has never self-harmed or attempted suicide.
- His environment has remained the same residence, room, X-box, family members. He has moved to a secondary school from a primary school. If the doctor asks–only then tell him/her that when he joined school in September last year, he was bullied at school–verbally and physically. Within the first week of starting school, he came back home with a bandage on his forehead since he was hit by another pupil. The bullying has since been taken care of since then. If the doctor attempts to find a connection between his bullying and initiation of symptoms, you would agree with the doctor and reflect upon this. It is likely that he was bullied at school, he is still being bullied and being a shy boy he doesn't express his distress easily. You accept the support offered.

3. Construct:

This station assesses the ability of the candidate to gather information from a mother of a child with autism. The candidate should be able to identify a trigger and also pick on some symptoms of depression.

4. Expanded construct:

- The doctor should demonstrate advanced listening skills, be empathetic towards mother while she is sharing her concerns, fears and anxieties.
- The candidate should be able to gather detailed and systematic collateral history of autism from mother.
- They should be able to identify possible trigger for Andrews' disturbed behaviour.
- They should elicit symptoms of depression, risks involved to self and others.
- They should offer help to mother in terms of further assessment, liaison with school and reviewing Andrew yourself.
- You are not expected to form a diagnosis of depression in the station. The examiner will be satisfied if you are able to elicit sufficient symptoms of depression from mother.

5. Areas of importance to pass the station:

- Ability to identify precipitating/triggering factors for behavioural problems (40%).
- Explore the possibility of comorbid psychiatric conditions (30%).
- Communication (30%).

6. Equipment checklist:

Not applicable.

Station 145: Link 2. Discussion of management and prognosis of an autistic child with a school teacher/relative/student nurse/consultant psychiatrist

Theme: Autism: Discussion of management and prognosis with a professional (teacher/nurse/consultant psychiatrist)

1. **Instructions to the candidates:**

   You have seen the mother of a child who has been diagnosed with autism. He is showing signs of agitation and aggression at home since he started secondary school. Mother has informed you that he is gradually getting worse and that he was bullied in school when he first started last September. The mother has also given you some symptoms in the boy that are suggestive of depression.

   Discuss your management plan and prognosis with the head teacher of the boy's secondary school. You have permission from his mother to share the information.

2. **Instructions to the role player:**

   You are Mrs Brown, head teacher of Smithy bridge High School in Derby.

   - Andrew came to your school last year and is currently in year 7. Since he has joined school, he has been irritable with others and has often got into fights. There have been times when he had to be physically removed from the scene to avoid further escalation of the situation.
   - You are aware that he is getting aggressive, verbally and physically at home as well.
   - If the doctor asks you about the episodes of bullying, you acknowledge, although you play it down and say that it is not uncommon for children to struggle in secondary schools and despite all efforts by staff, bullying does happen in school, even if it at a very subtle level. If the doctor informs you that bullying in any form should not happen, you agree with the doctor. If the doctor asks you, you confirm that you have an anti-bullying policy in your school and you follow it very strictly.
   - If the doctor asks you about Andrew's mood symptoms, you tell them that Andrew does appear sad compared to other children. He doesn't enjoy any activity in school and keeps to himself. He gets stressed easily and you have seen him scratching himself hard on a few occasions when he got very worked up.
   - If the doctor asks, you would arrange for doctor to do a school observation on Andrew. You would be willing to provide a report on his Educational abilities so far. You have also asked the Special Education Needs Co-ordinator to help Andrew with his studies.

   You ask the following questions:

   - What is wrong with Andrew?
   - What is the cause for this disruptive behaviour?
   - Can you give him a tablet to calm down?
   - Will he get better or cured?
   - Should he change school?
   - What should I do to help him?

3. Construct:

This station assesses the ability of the candidate to discuss autism, precipitating factors for difficult behaviour in autism, prognosis and management options with another professional (in this case the head teacher).

4. Expanded construct:

- The candidate should allow the teacher to express her views first.
- The candidate should demonstrate an awareness of the symptoms/signs of autism, that it is a developmental disorder and that there is no cure for the disorder. Main areas of difficulties are social communication, interactions and restricted interests.
- The candidate should offer hope to the teacher (not false hope though) and inform her of various support networks and agencies, such as, National Autistic Society and special school.
- The candidate should not offer medication at the outset. Focus on the concept of ongoing assessment. However, you may add that you would consider medication if this is required once the assessment is completed.
- The candidate should not sound patronising to the teacher even though the teacher may play down bullying in school. They should use this opportunity for psychoeducation and inform her about the impact of bullying is/may be having on Andrew.

5. Areas of importance to pass the station:

- Discussing nature, signs/symptoms/difficulties in autism, long-term prognosis and management options with the head teacher (any other professional) (30%).
- Ability to address the teacher's concerns and questions (30%).
- Offer hope to the teacher, discuss bullying and provide psychoeducation (20%).
- Communication (20%).

6. Equipment checklist:

Not applicable.

Single Stations: 146–148

Station 146: Collateral history of Down's syndrome from the his mother

Theme: To collect collateral history from a mother regarding a young man with learning disabilities

1. Instructions to the candidate:

You are an ST4 in learning disability. Mrs Jemma Harris is attending your clinic to discuss her 35 years old son Joshua Harris who suffers from Down's syndrome. Joshua has gradually become socially isolated and his appetite has also reduced. He gets easily wound-up and irritable and becomes verbally hostile towards his mum.

Gather information from mother to understand the problem.

2. Instructions to the role player:

You are Mrs Jemma Harris, 58 years old mother to Joshua who suffers from Down's syndrome. You live with your husband Mark Harris who is 60 years old. You and your husband have gradually become concerned about Joshua for the past 6 months or so since he has become more and more socially isolated. He has stopped going out of the house and has become completely housebound for the last 4 months. He has also stopped talking to his friends on the phone. He often appears at edge and irritable. If you or your husband suggests something, he tends to lash out at you and your husband if he is in his 'mood'. You have started to feel scared of Joshua if he is in a bad mood. Last week when you suggested that he should try and go out shopping with Mark, he became very agitated and started hitting his head on the wall. He had never done this ever before. You just don't know what to do and have come here to seek help.

If the doctor asks, only then provide the following information. Joshua has always been a good lad. He was always very loving and caring. He has made friends locally and attends a group every week in Birmingham Town Centre for people with learning difficulties. He has been attending this group for the last 10 years and used to enjoy going there up until 6 months ago. You do not know why he has become socially isolated. There has been no change in the family circumstances, no changes in his routines, recent routine health check up and blood tests did not reveal any abnormalities. There have been no bereavements in the family and as far as you know he has not had any fallouts with any of his friends.

Inform the doctor the following only if specifically asked: He is not eating well for the last 4–5 months and has lost some weight. He does not seem to enjoy his favourite programmes on tele–he used to enjoy Simpsons and Futurama. He used to go out and play football every alternate day with his mates in the local park which has not done for the past 3 months. You have spoken to one of his friends who came home the other day to invite him to play football. His friends informed you that there have been no falling out with Joshua to his knowledge. He also used to go out to the local supermarket with Mark and you but he has not done that for at least a few months. He has also stopped speaking to his cousins on the phone which he used to enjoy before. He has never expressed suicidal ideation, however, the other day he told you that the family would be better off without him. At that time he was agitated about the meal. He has never taken any overdoses or made attempts to harm himself except for that day when he deliberately hit his head on the wall. He has never assaulted anyone within the family or outside. You are not aware of Joshua 'hearing voices' (when nobody is around) or 'seeing things' (which others cannot see). His memory appears fine although his concentration has reduced a little. His sleep patterns have also become erratic and he does not seem to be sleeping as well as he used to. He does not smoke cigarettes, drink alcohol or take illicit drugs.

3. Construct:

The station tests a candidate's ability to gather information about a young man with learning disabilities from his mother.

4. Expanded construct:

Key points to remember:

- Start with open ended questions and then use closed questions.

- Be sensitive and empathetic towards the mother.
- Remember to check for precipitating factors, duration of the problem and its impact on the patient and others around the patient.
- Remember to rule out the following causes for his behaviour:
  - Environmental changes
  - Organic causes
  - Psychiatric illnesses.
- Check for premorbid personality and functioning.
- Check for risks to the patient and others around him. You may wish to discuss risk management strategies depending on the risk assessment.
- You may wish to touch upon your formulation but add that your assessment is ongoing and that you would like to see him as well. You are not expected to make a diagnosis in the station but are expected to ask for relevant symptoms.

5. **Areas of importance to pass the station:**
   - Communication skills 20%.
   - Formulating a biopsychosocial approach 40%.
   - Assessing premorbid functioning 40%.
6. **Equipment checklist:**
   None required.

Station 147: Collateral history: Dementia in a patient with moderate learning disability

Theme: Collateral history: Dementia in a patient with moderate learning disability

1. **Instructions to the candidates:**
   Mr Travis Tatton, 54-year-old man who has moderate learning disability and Down's syndrome has been referred to your clinic by his GP due to deteriorating level of functioning. He has not turned up for the appointment but his 75-year-old mother Shirley Tatton has agreed to provide you with necessary information.
   Talk to Shirley Tatton and gather a collateral history of Travis Tatton's problems.
2. **Instructions to the role player:**
   You are Mrs Shirley Tatton, mother to Travis Tatton who is 54 years old. Travis has moderate learning disability due to Down's syndrome. The doctor should also ask about how he was functioning before. If they forget to ask, you do not provide this information.
   - Over the last 2–3 years you have noticed a change in Travis.
   - He seems to be increasingly forgetful. Now, he is struggling to remember events, such as, what he did last weekend, items from the list that is to be bought from the local off-licence (which is what he was able to do a few years ago). Initially, his memory was worse for recent events. However, it seems his long-term memory is getting affected as well.

- His friends have also noticed a change in him. They say that he does not appear as enthusiastic as before and has become forgetful. He has at times forgotten where he had put his keys, and once he forgot to switch off the electric plate which led to burning the pan. He seems to be 'losing track of time' and unaware of whether it is day or night.
- Three days ago, one of the neighbours found him in early hours of morning in a local park. He was in a confused state and the neighbour brought him home. Since then you have started locking the front door and keep the keys with you at night.
- He has become increasingly dependent with regards to his day-to-day activities. He tends to spend increasing amounts of time in his room.
- There is no concern with regards to his appetite and self-care. His mood is low on occasions but he is able to enjoy activities and have a laugh. He enjoys watching television and chatting to his cousins and other family members. He has no problems with his attention and concentration.
- As a child, he was assessed for his abilities and diagnosed with moderate learning disability. He attended a specialist school till the age of 18 years and then took a part time job in a local off license shop. He has been working at this shop for 20 years. The shop owner has noticed that he has become forgetful not remembering schedules, where items are or regular customer's name which he was good at.
- He is affectionate, likeable and much loved in the community.
- He has no thoughts of hurting self or others. He does not hear voices or see things.
- He was recently seen by his GP and had some bloods done which came out to be normal.
- There is no family history of any psychiatric disorder or dementia.

3. **Construct:**
The station assesses the candidates' ability to gather collateral information from a relative of a moderately learning disabled man with signs of dementing illness.

4. **Expanded construct:**
   - The candidate should allow mother to express her concerns, fears and expectations and address them in an empathetic and sensitive manner.
   - The candidate should use good mix of open and closed questions.
   - The candidate should explore patients current functioning and then compare it with premorbid functioning.
   - Its onset, duration, progression, aggravating and relieving factors including any associated factors.
   - They should explore for any possible organic causes for his change in behaviour and risks.

5. **Areas of importance to pass the station:**
   - Eliciting details about the patients functioning and the onset, duration and progress of dementia (40%).
   - Explore premorbid functioning and gather information pertaining to reduction in functioning in a patient with Down syndrome and assess current risks (30%).
   - Rule out other causes for the deterioration in functioning (20%).
   - Show advanced listening skills and be empathetic towards mum (10%).

6. **Equipment checklist:**
Not applicable.

Station 148: Learning disability: Collateral history

Theme: Depression in learning disability

1. **Instructions to the candidates:**

   You are doing a special interest session in adult learning disability team. Mrs Jemma Harris is attending your clinic to discuss her 35-year-old son Joshua Harris who suffers from Down syndrome. Joshua has gradually become socially isolated and his appetite has reduced. He gets easily wound-up and irritable and becomes verbally hostile towards his mum.

   Talk to Mrs Harris and gather information about her problems.

2. **Instructions to the role player:**
   - You are Mrs Jemma Harris, 58-year-old mother to Joshua who suffers from Down syndrome. You live with your husband Mark Harris who is 60 years old.
   - Joshua has been socially isolated for the past 6 months. He has stopped going out of the house and has become completely housebound for the last 4 months. He has stopped talking to his friends and has become irritable.
   - You have started to feel scared of Joshua if he is in a bad mood. Last week when you suggested that he should try and go out shopping with Mark, he became very agitated and started hitting his head on the wall. This is the first time you have noticed him in this state.
   - He has low mood, decreased motivation, poor attention and concentration. He has reduced appetite and lost some weight.
   - If the doctor asks, only then provide the following information. Joshua has always been a good lad. He was always very loving, caring, has made friends locally and attends a group every week in Birmingham Town Centre for people with learning difficulties. He has been attending this group for the last 10 years and used to enjoy going there up until 6 months ago.
   - You do not know why he has become socially isolated. There has been no change in the family circumstances, no changes in his routines, recent routine health check-up and blood tests did not reveal any abnormalities. There are no stressors, worries or anxieties that would have triggered this behaviour.
   - He has mentioned once that the family would be better off without him. No previous history of mental illness, self-harm or harm to others.
   - He does not smoke cigarettes, drink alcohol or take illicit drugs.

3. **Construct:**

   This station assesses candidate's ability to gather collateral history from a concerned mother whose son suffers from learning disability.

4. **Expanded construct:**
   - The candidate should use a good mix of open and closed questions.
   - They should demonstrate sensitivity and empathy towards the distressed mother.
   - They should explore precipitating factors, onset, duration, progression of the problem and its impact on the patient and others around the patient.

- They should explore the following causes for his behaviour in addition to others:
  - o Environmental changes
  - o Organic causes
  - o Psychiatric illnesses.
- They should inquire about pre-morbid personality and functioning.
- They should elicit risks to patient and others around him. The candidate may wish to discuss risk management strategies depending on the risk assessment.
- They should discuss formulation but add that assessment is ongoing and would like to assess the patient. The candidates are not expected to make a diagnosis in the station but are expected to ask for relevant symptoms.

5. Areas of importance to pass the station:

- Eliciting collateral information–depth and range of symptoms (40%).
- Exploring possible precipitating factors and premorbid personality (20%).
- Assessment of risk–to self or others (20%).
- Communication (20%).

6. Equipment checklist:

Not applicable.

7. Psychotherapy

Psychotherapy Stations for CASC Examination

1. Introduction:

Assessment and management of mental disorders are based on biopsychosocial approach. One of the most important areas in psychiatric training is to understand the patient experiences in the context of cultural, religious, social and psychological concepts. Understanding mental disorders on the basis of psychological theories helps in deciding the most appropriate psychological treatment. Psychotherapy stations assess these skills. These stations include assessment of the patient's suitability for a particular therapy or explaining a particular therapy is administered and how likely it might work.

Assessment stations:

In the examination situation, many candidates get thrown away by seeing the psychotherapy assessment stations. In fact, they do not even perform the assessments that they do in daily clinical practice. Important thing to remember is that it is very difficult to assess a patient for psychotherapy in 7 minutes or ten minutes. Having said that, the examiners assess the candidates' ability to understand the patient's experience in psychological terms based on certain theories. It is, therefore, important that the candidates are able to demonstrate that they can understand patient's psychological experience. To start with they should be able to pick up patient's cues. Many a times candidates get frustrated when patient does not come out with information. In psychotherapy assessment stations, this in itself may be a cue. Therefore, the question that might be worth asking is whether the patient finds it difficult to share some of the experiences. Also it is worth exploring past experiences with therapists. If a patient doesn't open up the best way is to explore their life situation, work, personal life, relationships, etc. As this goes on, exploring their way of dealing with situations will help the candidates to have a psychological formulation. Even if the candidates do not utter this out in the exam hall examiners will easily pick up.

In addition to understanding patient's experience one should assess the following factors:

(i) Psychological mindedness of the patient.
(ii) Insight into the problem.
(iii) Motivation to change.
(iv) Adequate ego strength.
(v) Ability to tolerate distress and frustration.
(vi) Ability to form and sustain relationships.
(vii) Use of alcohol and drugs to cope with the situation.

A good candidate will touch upon these aspects in assessing the patient.

Explanation Stations:

In explanation stations, candidates should follow the framework. At the same time, they should also be flexible to (a) answer patient's questions and (b) personalize the theories to patient experiences. Many candidates explain the therapy well but personalizing it to the patient helps the patient and the examiner will be able to assess your competency.

To do this, it is important to practise stations with such case histories and try to make a psychological formulation. In these stations drawing a 'five-area' model or a 'Hot-cross bun' model with patient experience will help the candidate to pass the station easily.

Most important thing to remember is that patients want to know some basic information.

- Whether this therapy will help them?
- How it will help and how long it will take them to recover?
- Who will give the therapy?
- Where the therapy will be given?
- How long, how often they have to attend the sessions?
- What is the duration of each session?
- What happens in between the sessions?
- Will it talk about their past?
- Confidentiality issues.
- Will it make them feel worse?
- What to do in a crisis situation?
- Whether they should continue medication?

These questions can easily be answered if the candidates have a set of answers. Even if they find it difficult to explain the principles behind the therapy, they can answer many of the questions and sail through the station.

The principles of confidentiality apply to psychotherapy stations in the same way as our clinical practice. So we can answer the patient by telling that unless there is a risk to self or others all the details discussed in the psychotherapy sessions will be confidential.

Finally, it is important for the candidate to talk about self-help as well as how the family or friends could help the patient. These are very well explained in Royal College of Psychiatrists' patient information leaflets.

Cognitive Distortions in Depression

1. **All or nothing also known as black and white or dichotomous reasoning:** Person sees two extremes and does not see the exceptions or in between possibilities. For example: Either I am a complete success or an utter failure.
2. **Overgeneralisation:** A general conclusion is drawn (usually a negative one) from a few or even a single bad experience. "I could not pass exams this time. So I am a complete failure."
3. **Labelling:** Instead of seeing the situation a person starts giving names to himself. "I'm an idiot".
4. **Discounting the positives:** The person disregards the positive qualities or information. Rather gives his own explanations. "He is praising me to be kind."
5. **Selective abstraction:** Person looks at a little component selectively and concludes about the outcome rather than looking at the context.
6. **Global judgments:** It is similar to selective abstraction. The person looks in to one feature or quality and makes an overall judgment. "He came late to work. This means he is an irresponsible person."
7. **Jumping to conclusions or arbitrary inference:** Jumping into conclusions without looking at the evidence.
8. **Mind reading:** Sometimes people may assume what others would be thinking, feeling or doing without looking for evidence.
9. **Fortune telling:** Person anticipates and predicts negative or worst outcomes in future, often in the absence of facts.
10. **Magnification and minimization:** The person overemphasizes the negative and underemphasizes the positives. "It will be a disaster."
11. **Emotional reasoning:** Person makes conclusions based on the emotional experience or feelings, "I anxious so something bad is going to happen."
12. **Use of moral imperatives:** This is also known as absolute thinking. The person has rigid thinking and makes unreasonable demands on themselves. "I should be like this", "I must always be doing this way."
13. **Mental filter:** The person finds only the negatives and losses and dwell on them. Information that confirms his negative views are seen as proof, while facts that don't fit are seen as rare exceptions and ignored; "I will always lose", "no one cares about me."
14. **Personalisation:** The person erroneously believes that he is the cause of events. "We lost the game because of me."
15. **Blaming:** The opposite of personalization, the reason bad things are happening is because of what the other person is doing or not doing. The person overlooks his own contributions to the problem.

Recommended Reading:

1. Royal College of Psychiatrists' leaflets on different therapies (www.rcpsych.ac.uk).

2. Patient information leaflets from different psychotherapy association websites: e.g., www.acat.me.uk: website for the association of Cognitive Analytical Therapists.

Linked Stations: 149–156

Station 149: Link 1. Assess: Patient's suitability for cognitive behaviour therapy (CBT)
Station 150: Link 2. Discuss: Cognitive behaviour therapy (CBT) with the patient/relative/social worker/student nurse

Station 149: Link 1. Assess: Patient's suitability for cognitive behaviour therapy (CBT)

Theme: Assessment for suitability for CBT

1. **Instructions to the candidates:**
You are a Specialty Registrar in Psychiatry. You are seeing Mr Mankad a 40-year-old gentleman with recurrent depressive disorder. He has recovered partially with venlafaxine XL 150 mg OD. The GP has referred him for cognitive behaviour therapy (CBT).
Talk to the patient and assess his suitability for CBT.

2. **Instructions to the role player:**
   - You are Mr Mankad a 40-year-old man. You live on your own and are not working.
   - You see yourself as a failure. You do not see your friends anymore because you feel that they do not want to spend time with a miserable person like you. You feel worthless.
   - You worked as an electrician until a few years ago. For nobody's fault suddenly there was a power failure at work. All the computers were damaged and this led to loss of all stored information. The company had to reinvest a huge amount to rebuild the database. You attributed this to your fault and resigned the job because of guilt. The managers explained you that it was nobody's fault. But you feel that they were just helping you out of sympathy.
   - You do not see your achievements in the past 10 years, i.e., you designed the whole electrical circuit for this company and was awarded best employee award 5 years ago. You feel that nobody can help you in this situation.

3. **Construct:**
The candidate should demonstrate fluently the assessment of patient's suitability for CBT.

4. **Expanded construct:**
   - Candidate should be able to demonstrate advanced listening skills.
   - Candidate should be able to assess negative cognitions in the patient.
   - Candidate should be able to briefly assess suicide risk.
   - Candidate should be able to rule out alcohol and drug dependence.
   - Candidate should be able to assess personality traits that may interfere with therapy.

5. **Areas of importance to pass the station:**
   - Communication skills (20%).
   - Eliciting negative cognitions or cognitive distortions (70%).
   - Explores suicide risk (10%).
6. **Equipment checklist:**
   Not applicable.

   Tips: Candidates should focus on the cognitive triad in depression, i.e., negative view of the self, negative view of the future and negative view of the world. They should elicit hopelessness, worthlessness and helplessness.

   Demonstrating cognitive distortions in the patient is important to pass this station.

Station 150: Link 2. Discuss: Cognitive behaviour therapy (CBT) with the patient/relative/social worker/student nurse

Theme: Explain cognitive behavioural therapy

1. **Instructions to the candidates:**
   You have assessed Mr Mankad in the previous station. His wife is worried about him. She wants to know more about the proposed psychological treatment. She is a nurse on the Medical ward.

   Talk to her and address her concerns.

   Explain cognitive behaviour therapy.

   Discuss self-help materials in CBT.
2. **Instructions to the role player:**
   - You are Hema Mankad, a nurse in the medical ward. You read about CBT on the internet. You are not sure how this would help your husband. You also heard about some websites as well as self-help books. You are keener in knowing about these as you can help your husband.
   - Open the station with "Doctor why everyone says that it is his thinking. I feel he is suffering from a medical condition and nobody acknowledges this."

   Ask the following questions:
   - **Does CBT mean positive thinking?**
   - **What is a mood diary and how it is maintained?**
   - **What is activity scheduling?**
   - **Does he need medication once talking therapy starts?**
   - **How CBT will help my husband?**
   - **What is the waiting period?**
   - **My husband is a private person and does not want to talk about his childhood.**
   - **Will he be followed up by the psychiatrist?**
   - **Is there any book that can be used as a self-help source of information?**
   - **Is there any website available to learn about CBT?**

3. **Construct:**
The candidate should fluently explain about CBT.

4. **Expanded construct:**
- Candidate should be able to demonstrate advanced communication skills.
- Candidate should be able to quote examples from negative cognitions in the patient.
- Candidate should be able to clarify that CBT is not synonymous with positive thinking.
- Candidate should be able to talk and explain about mood diary, thought-feeling diary, activity scheduling and home work.
- Candidate should be able to explain about the role of self-help in CBT.
- Candidate should be able to aware of self-help websites and books for CBT.

5. **Areas of importance to pass the station:**
- Communication skills (20%).
- Addressing the ideas concerns and expectations (10%).
- Explaining about CBT (40%).
- Talking about self-help resources (30%).

6. **Equipment checklist:**
Not applicable.

Self-Help:
- Commonly prescribed books:
  (i) Mind Over Mood
  (ii) Overcoming Depression
- Commonly prescribed websites:
  (i) Beating the blues: Patients can register on this website through the GP and it is free.
  (ii) Living life to the full.com.
  (iii) Mood gym (Australian website).

Station 151: Link 1. Assess: Patient's suitability for Inter Personal Therapy (IPT)

Station 152: Link 2. Discuss: Inter Personal Therapy (IPT) with a patient

Station 151: Link 1. Assess: Patient's suitability for Inter Personal Therapy (IPT)

Theme: The station tests the ability of a candidate to assess suitability for interpersonal therapy

1. **Instructions to the candidates:**
Mrs Jenny Johnson is a 59-year-old patient, currently living with her dog. She lost her husband 15 months ago. She was treated by her GP with anti-depressants. She is attending your clinic.

- **Assess depressive symptoms.**
- **Assess suitability for interpersonal psychotherapy.**

In the next station, her daughter will meet you to discuss about interpersonal therapy.

2. Instructions to the role player:

- You are Mrs Jenny Johnson, 59 years old. You work as a teacher in the primary school but at present off sick from work due to depression.
- School atmosphere created lot of anxiety in you. You lost your confidence in teaching. You started crying in front of the children. So the head teacher took you again to your GP who gave a sick note to you for 4 weeks.
- You have two children. Your son is 26 years old and daughter is aged 22 years. The son works for a multinational company, lives with his partner and child in London. He keeps in touch with you by phone regularly. Due to work commitments, he could not visit you for the past 3–4 months. Your daughter moved out of home 9 months ago when she got married started working in Wales.
- You were married for 30 years and very close to your husband. Your husband died suddenly due to cardiac arrest, 15 months ago.
- Seven months ago you started feeling very low. You were feeling tired all the time. You were not eating and lost weight. You could not focus on work and started seeing yourself as a failure. Your daughter was worried about you and she took you GP who started you on Fluoxetine 20 mg OD. He also advised you to be off sick.
- But you went to work as you felt that work was 'therapeutic'. You felt that by going back to work you can be focused. Slowly you started eating well and sleeping well. However, you still had phases of low mood. You did not enjoy things as before. At work you were promoted and her responsibilities have increased.
- Open the conversation 'I hate continuing medication'. Ask the doctor 'Am I mentally ill'. If the doctor asks you about suicidal thoughts tell that you want to join your husband, but you would not kill yourself. You do not hear voices or see things.

3. Construct:

The candidate demonstrates knowledge and skills about interpersonal factors playing a role in depression, assess the suitability of patient for interpersonal therapy.

4. Expanded construct:

- Candidate should be able to establish interpersonal contributing factors in depression.
- Candidate should be able to establish potential interpersonal factors for depression in this patient.
- Candidate should be able to elicit patients past experience with psychotherapies.
- Candidate should be able to elicit current risk.
- Candidate should be able to demonstrate advanced listening skills.
- Candidate should be able to engage in a conversation.

5. Areas of importance to pass the station:

- Communication skills (20%).

- Assessing depressive symptoms (20%).
- Understanding interpersonal factors contributing to depression (60%).

6. **Equipment checklist:**
   Not applicable.

Station 152: Link 2. Discuss: Interpersonal Therapy (IPT) with a patient

Theme: The candidate should explain interpersonal therapy to a depressed patient

1. **Instructions to the candidates:**
   You assessed Mrs Johnson in the previous station. Her daughter Shelly Beck is waiting to discuss with you about the proposed treatment plan.
   Explain about interpersonal therapy.
   Address her ideas, concerns and expectations.

2. **Instructions to the role player:**
   Open the station by asking the doctor, "I think my mother needs to find a suitable person, which is the only way she would get better. She still misses my dad".
   Ask the following questions:
   - **What is wrong with my mother?**
   - **Does she need medication once talking therapy starts?**
   - **What type of therapy is proposed?**
   - **How will it help mother?**
   - **How is the therapy given?**
   - **Who will administer the therapy?**
   - **How often mother needs to meet the therapist?**
   - **How long the therapy will go on for?**
   - **How long it takes for mother to recover?**
   - **Mother is a private person and does not want to talk about her childhood.**
   - **Will she be followed up by the psychiatrist?**
   - **Any source of information.**

3. **Construct:**
   Candidate explains the interpersonal therapy in fluent and focused way.

4. **Expanded construct:**
   - Candidate should be able to understand patient/relative's background and understanding of the illness.
   - Candidate should be able to explain the illness based on interpersonal theory.
   - Candidate should be able to explain how interpersonal therapy could help the patient.
   - Candidate should be able to explain other details like where, who, how, how long, how often the therapy is delivered.

5. **Areas of importance to pass the station:**
   - Communication skills (20%).
   - Explaining the interpersonal theory in patient's context (70%).
   - Giving other sources of information (10%).

6. **Equipment checklist:**
   Not applicable:
   Information about IPT
   - IPT is a here and now therapy.
   - It is time-limited and focuses on interpersonal issues, which are understood to be a factor in the genesis and maintenance of depression.
   - IPT views depression as a medical illness.
   - The targets of IPT are symptom resolution, improved interpersonal functioning, and increased social support.
   - Courses of IPT range from 6–20 sessions with provision for maintenance treatment as necessary.
   - *Structure of treatment:* Treatment sessions have three phases: A beginning (1–3 sessions), middle, and end (3 sessions).
   - The patient and therapist work together.

   IPT addresses four major areas:
   - **Grief:** Patient could be going through a normal grief reaction, prolonged grief reaction or pathological grief reaction. The IPT therapist facilitates the grieving process, learning to accept difficult emotions, and replacing lost relationships.
   - **Role dispute:** The patient learns to understand the interpersonal disputes, communication issues, and how to alter communication strategies.
   - **Role transition:** IPT helps with the transition, allowing the client to express concerns and providing strategies and techniques to aid in moving forward.
   - **Interpersonal deficits:** Interpersonal and communication challenges are addressed with a variety of exercises.

   The candidates should learn about Interpersonal triad (Acute interpersonal crisis, Attachment and biopsychosocial/cultural/spiritual vulnerabilities/strengths and inadequate social support). They should also used techniques in IPT, i.e., interpersonal inventories, Interpersonal incidents, Communication analysis, etc.
   Resource: www. interpersonalpsychotherapy.org

Station 153: Link 1. Assess: Suitability for long-term psychotherapy

Station 154: Link 2. Explain: Psychoanalytic therapy to a patient

Station 153: Link 1. Assess: Suitability for long-term psychotherapy

Theme: Assess this patient for suitability for psychodynamic therapy

1. **Instructions to the candidates:**

   You are a CT3 trainee in psychiatry. GP asked you to see Mr Spencer, a 30-year-old man. Mr Spencer has been anxious recently. He works as a plumber and is in a relationship. He has recently moved in with his partner. His partner has expressed her wish to marry him. Mr Spencer continues to work with some difficulties. He has disturbed sleep and reduced appetite. He is not suicidal. He does not misuse alcohol or illicit drugs.

   Assess him.

   Address his ideas, concerns and expectations.

2. **Instructions to the role player:**
   - You are Mr Spencer, a 30-year-old man. You work as a plumber. You met Susan Alexander a 28-year-old woman last year and you both love each other. She wanted to marry you and moved in with you. This made you anxious.
   - You found difficulty in sleeping. Your appetite has gone down. Susan started telling you that already you are a changed person. You are not jovial anymore. You go home late and started avoiding discussions with her. You continue to work with some difficulties. You are not suicidal.
   - You were born in Doncaster. Your father owned a farm and was a very busy person. When you were 7 years old, your mother left your father for another man. Your father never recovered; however, did not marry. Your father never spoke much about relationships but told you not to trust any woman.
   - Your grandmother was telling you stories about how your grandfather left her for another woman.
   - You met Tracy when you were 19 years old. You both developed a deep love. You proposed to marry her. She said 'Yes'. However, within a week she got married to another man. She refused to meet you or discuss with you about any details. This was a big blow to you. You were upset and low for couple of months. You started focusing on your work and enjoying the life.
   - When Susan spoke about marriage you remembered about Tracy 'ditching' you. You are worried that Susan might leave you. This made you anxious. You also remember about your grandmother's story as well as your father's story.
   - To start with talk to the doctor generally, explain about your job, your life and how much you love 'Susan'. When he asks about your future plans, say 'I don't know'.
   - Don't tell the doctor about your worries that Susan might leave you unless he is empathic and listens to you. If he asks the reason ask 'how do you know that she would not do like Tracy?'
   - Don't tell about your parents unless the doctor asks you about this.
   - If the doctor asks for permission to discuss about you with Susan say 'yes'. Otherwise ask whether the doctor will all these to Susan, towards the end of the session.

3. **Construct:**

   Candidate demonstrates skills in assessing a patient's suitability for psychodynamic psychotherapy.

4. **Expanded construct:**

   - Candidate should be able to demonstrate advanced listening skills.
   - Candidate should be able to understand the reasons for patient's anxiety.
   - Candidate should be able to elicit past history of relationship breakdown.
   - Candidate should be able to elicit history of parental separation.
   - Candidate should be able to understand patient's experience in psychodynamic terms.

5. **Areas of importance to pass the station:**

   - Advanced listening skills (20%).
   - Understanding patient's experience (60%).
   - Addressing patient's ideas, concerns and expectations (20%).

6. **Equipment checklist:**

   Not applicable.

Station 154: Link 2. Explain: Psychoanalytic therapy to a patient

Theme: Explain Psychoanalytic psychotherapy

1. **Instructions to the candidates:**

   You have assessed Mr Spencer in the previous station. His partner is eager to discuss with you to discuss the management plan.

   Talk to her and address her ideas, concerns and expectations.

   Explain about psychoanalytic psychotherapy.

2. **Instructions to the role player:**

   - You are Miss Alexander. You are in relationship to Mr Spencer for the past 1 year. You want to marry him. You thought Mr Spencer was also interested, but recently he was feeling low in himself and was found to be anxious all the time.
   - You are worried about him and wanted to know what was wrong with him. You yourself feel at times that you may not be a perfect match to him.
   - You are worried whether Mr Spencer is in another relationship. You asked him about these but he has denied these. You know that deep inside he loves you.

   Ask the following questions to the doctor:

   - **What is wrong with him 'is he depressed'?**
   - **Does he need medication?**
   - **What type of therapy is proposed?**

- **How will it help him?**
- **How is the therapy given?**
- **Who will administer the therapy?**
- **How often he needs to meet the therapist?**
- **How long the therapy will go on for?**
- **How long it takes for him to recover?**
- **He is a private person and does not want to talk about her childhood.**
- **How will you know that he gets benefit with therapy?**
- **Will she be followed up by the psychiatrist?**
- **Any source of information.**

3. **Construct:**
   The candidate should fluently explain about psychotherapy.

4. **Expanded construct:**
   - Candidate should be able to express empathy and shows advanced listening skills.
   - Candidate should be able to explain in simple jargon-free language about the principles of psychodynamic therapy.
   - Candidate should be able to explain the patient's experience in psychodynamic model.
   - Candidate should be able to talk about various terms in simple language: Transference, counter-transference, therapeutic relationship, boundaries, resistance, interpretation, defense mechanisms, etc.

5. **Areas of importance to pass the station:**
   - Advanced communication skills (25%).
   - Explaining psychodynamic theory in the context of the life experiences (50%).
   - Explaining about the details of the therapy, i.e., settings, duration, who, how, how long etc. (25%).

6. **Equipment checklist:**
   Not applicable.

Station 155: Link 1. Assess: Suitability for systemic family therapy

Station 156: Link 2. Explain: Systemic family therapy

Station 155: Link 1. Assess: Suitability for systemic family therapy

Theme: Assessment of behavioural problems in a boy and suitability for systemic family therapy

1. **Instructions to the candidates:**
   Boy's name: Tom Parsons; Age: 6 years

Mother's name: Jennifer Hutchison

You are a CT3 trainee working in a family consultation clinic. You receive a referral to see a boy who has been disruptive to the teaching sessions.

- **Elicit history of present illness from the mother.**
- **Address her ideas concerns and expectations.**

2. **Instructions to the role player:**

Boy's name: Tom Parsons; Age: 6 years

Mother's name: Jennifer Hutchison

- You are Jennifer Hutchison and you have two children aged 12 and 6 years. You live with your boyfriend and two children in a council accommodation.
- You were married for the past 13 years and separated from your husband 1 year ago. You met your current boyfriend and he moved in to live with your family for the past 4 months.
- Three months ago, your boyfriend assaulted your husband in an argument. Since then your husband stopped contacting you or visiting children. For the past 2 months Tom, the younger one has started isolating himself. He started bedwetting on and off. Tom has on occasions been rude to your boyfriend and sworn at him.
- Your boyfriend trying to put certain boundaries in place, e.g., homework, table manners and getting ready for school.
- You started getting reports from school that he is not so keen or attentive in the school anymore. He also started becoming disruptive in the school. Teachers called you for an urgent meeting. You are worried that he might be evicted from school.
- Tom was born by normal delivery, normal milestones of development. Tom had no medical problems and had jabs at appropriate age. Prior to this, he had no problems in school. No bullying in school.
- Start the station by asking "will you give a letter to the school so that Tom stays in school'?
- Ask whether Tom has ADHD.
- If doctor starts telling that his behaviour is because of the home situation, express guilt and ask whether you are the reason for Tom's condition.
- Ask whether tablets could help Tom to be calm and quiet in the school.
- If doctor empathizes with you and approaches the topic sensitively, tell the whole story. Otherwise show your frustration and tell that Tom does not understand life.

3. **Construct:**

The candidate should be in a position to assess the behavioural problems in a 6-year-old child.

4. **Expanded construct:**

- Candidate should be able to approaching the topic sensitively.
- Candidate should be able to use advanced listening skills.
- Candidate should be able to assess the behavioural changes in the boy.
- Candidate should be able to systematically assess the causes of behavioural changes in the child.

- Candidate should be able to address the ideas concerns and expectations of the mother.
- Candidate should be able to explain briefly how the child could be helped.
- Candidate should be able to systematically rule out other causes of behavioural disturbances in a 6-year-old boy.

5. **Areas of importance to pass the station:**
   - Communication skills (20%).
   - Assessing the biopsychosocial causes of behavioural change (60%).
   - Addressing ideas, concerns and expectations (20%).

6. **Equipment checklist:**
   Not applicable.

Station 156: Link 2. Explain: Systemic family therapy

Theme: Candidate should explain about systemic family therapy

1. **Instructions to the candidates:**

   You met Tom's mother in the previous station. Subsequently you assessed Tom. You found him to be getting more and more isolated and depressed. You wanted to meet the family to discuss the option of family therapy. Jennifer Hutchison (Mother) was upset about this and asked her boyfriend to come and meet you.
   - **Explain to him about systemic family therapy.**
   - **Do not take a history.**

2. **Instructions to the role player:**
   - You are Gary Sobers, a 30-year-old man. You are in relationship with Jennifer which actually gave you some direction in life. You are currently jobless and want to get a job so that you can prove yourself as a grown up adult.
   - You like Jennifer's children and try to show affection to them. Jennifer's older son Mathew is friendly with you. But younger one, i.e., Tom isolates himself. You do not know why this should be the case. You are not violent towards Jennifer or her children.
   - You were shocked when Tom's teachers called Jennifer for a meeting at school. You were annoyed and angry when the doctor suggested family therapy.

   You are meeting the doctor and ask the following questions:
   - **Whether the problem will be solved if you leave the family?**
   - **What is wrong with Tom?**
   - **Why the doctor accuses the family to be the cause of Tom's problem?**
   - **What is family therapy?**
   - **Why this therapy will help Tom?**
   - **Should I be attending the session with Jennifer?**
   - **How long the sessions last for?**

- **How many sessions will be conducted?**
- **Who will do the therapy?**
- **Who else will be there?**
- **How it is done?**
- **Will Jennifer be criticised?**
- **What if he does not get better?**
- **What to do if the behaviour gets worse?**

If the doctor is sensitive and empathic then calm down and show interest in the topic.

If the doctor starts giving a lecture then get angry and frustrated. Say that "you do not know how much I love these kids. How can you say that I am the cause of Tom's problems?"

3. **Construct:**
Candidate should be in a position to explain fluently about family therapy.

4. **Expanded construct:**
- Candidate should be able to empathise with the parent.
- Candidate should be able to open the topic sensitively and explain the term 'identified patient'.
- Candidate should be able to explain how changes in family circumstances could lead to changes in the behaviour.
- Candidate should be able to explain the process of family therapy.
- Candidate should be able to explain how it will help Tom.
- Candidate should be able to explain how it will help the family.
- Candidate should be able to explain how Tom will be helped–monitoring, counselling etc.

5. **Areas of importance to pass the station:**
- Communication skills (20%).
- Demonstrated knowledge and explains about family therapy in a focused and fluent way (60%).
- Explains other support systems that will be offered to the child and family (20%).

6. **Equipment checklist:**
Not applicable.

Key Information about systemic family therapy:
- Many a times behavioural problems in a child could be a manifestation of problems that are going on within the family. The child is the 'identified patient'.
- Systemic family therapy is a common form of family therapy.
- In family therapy, the therapist or team of therapists work with the family as a unit which is a group of people living together and care for each other.
- Offering family therapy does not mean that family is the cause. Ideally people involved in family functioning should aim to attend sessions. Gary should, therefore, try to attend.
- The therapy aims to encourage families to think of alternate means of communicating within families, to avoid confrontations and solve matters amicably.

- The family therapists try to help family members find constructive ways to help each other.
- They do not only work in the families but they also do individual and group work. They work with children as well as adults with wide range of issues.
- According to systems theory, each family is made up of systems and subsystems. Each system or subsystem could affect the other.
- Read about circular communication, linear communication, etc.
- The family therapy sessions last up to 6 months. They will take place in the clinic settings.
- Each session could last for 1–2 hours. There will usually be fortnightly or monthly sessions depending on your needs and availability.
- Process: One therapist will be sitting and discussing the issues with the family in the meeting room and a group of therapists will be observing from the other room through a one-sided mirror. After about 90 minutes there will be a break. The therapist will bring other therapists into the room who will explain their observations and communication styles. The session is non-judgmental and non-critical and it aims to improve the communication patterns. This in turn helps to replace the dysfunctional pattern of behaviour with a more adaptive behaviour.
- It is evidence-based therapy for not only depression, but also for other disorders like eating disorder.

Single Stations: 157–161

Station 157: Discuss cognitive analytic therapy (CAT) with a patient

Theme: Explain cognitive analytic therapy

1. **Instructions to the candidates:**

   You are a CT3 trainee in psychiatry. The GP referred Miss Monica Bender, a 24-year-old patient. Miss Bender has difficulties at work as well as in relationship. She was self-harming by cutting herself. She was diagnosed as borderline personality disorder. She is keen to change for the better.

   Explain about cognitive analytic therapy.

   Address her ideas, concerns and expectations.

2. **Instructions to the role player:**

   - You are Miss Monica Bender, a 24-year-old female, working in a superstore. You have difficulty facing people. You get annoyed easily when people ask explanations. You had tough time at customer services. You think about leaving the job. But this is the 12th job in the past 2 years. You find difficult to hold on to a job.
   - Same thing happens in relationships. You can't trust people. You have chronic feelings of emptiness and boredom. You self-harm to get relief. For the past 2 months you have been thinking of how to change this life.
   - You discussed about this with the GP who referred you to the psychiatrist. You were diagnosed as borderline personality disorder. Today you are going to meet the psychiatrist to learn about CAT.

Ask the following questions to the doctor:

- **What is borderline personality?**
- **Do I need medication?**
- **What type of therapy is proposed?**
- **How will it help me?**
- **Will it help me to have a stable family life?**
- **How is the therapy given?**
- **Who will administer the therapy?**
- **How often I need to meet the therapist?**
- **How long the therapy will go on for?**
- **How will I know that I am getting better?**
- **Will I be followed up by the psychiatrist?**
- **Source of information.**

3. **Construct:**
   Candidate fluently explains about cognitive analytic therapy to the patient.
4. **Expanded construct:**
   - Candidate should be able to empathise with the patient experience.
   - Candidate should be able to explain about the principles of cognitive analytic therapy in focussed and fluent way.
   - Candidate should be able to give explanations with examples from patient's life situation.
   - Candidate should be able to explain about the duration, course of therapy and about who will give therapy, etc.
   - Candidate should be able to address patient's ideas, concerns and expectations.
   - Candidate should be able to demonstrate advanced communication skills.
5. **Areas of importance to pass the station:**
   - Communication skills (20%).
   - Explaining CAT (60%).
   - Addresses patient's ideas concerns and expectations (20%).
6. **Equipment checklist:**
   Not applicable.

Information on Cognitive Analytic Therapy (CAT)

- CAT is a talking therapy. It is focussed and time limited. It combines the principles of CBT and psychoanalytic psychotherapy.
- Principle behind CAT: As we grow up, we develop certain coping skills. CAT focuses on these repeating patterns as a way of coping with emotional difficulties.
- Maladaptive procedures and harmful relationship roles will be identified and the therapist and patient will work on recognising these patterns.
- After the initial assessment sessions, the therapist writes a reformulation letter to the patient, which is the working hypothesis for the therapy. It helps promote change.
- It is a collaborative work between a therapist and patient.

- Usually the sessions are held weekly and each session lasts for 50–60 minutes. A course of therapy can be from 16–24 sessions.
- Between 1 and 5 follow-up sessions are offered after the end of regular therapy. This can be negotiated with the therapist.
- The important feature of CAT is that the ending is identified in the initial sessions.
- CAT is used with a wide variety of problems, such as, relationship difficulties, self-harm, substance misuse and eating disorders.
- Patients will be given homework tasks from time to time to encourage recognising and revising maladaptive procedures.

Station 158: Explain: Systematic desensitization with the patient/relative/carer

Theme: Management of agoraphobia by systematic desensitisation

1. **Instructions to the candidates:**

   Patient's name: Sally Saunders; Age 35 years.

   You are a senior registrar working in a community mental health team (CMHT). Today, you are reviewing Ms Saunders at her home along with the care coordinator. Sally has not left the house for the past 3 years. She was an efficient administrator and wants to go back to work and live independently. She tried medication, but was not getting better. Hence, the psychologist proposed psychological treatment for her.

   - **Explain the systematic desensitisation.**
   - **Address her ideas concerns and expectations.**

2. **Instructions to the role player:**

   - You are Sally Saunders who is a 35-year-old and you live with your husband and 3-year-old son Mathew.
   - Your problems started 3 years ago. On day one when you went to the gym you felt sick. You had a panic attack and came back home. You tried to go to gym on couple of occasions, however, you were getting more panic attacks. You felt like collapsing. You discontinued attending the gym.
   - You started avoiding public places. When you went back to work you felt confused and dizzy. You could not focus on work. You started sweating and shaking. You asked for a week's leave and came home. Since then you never left home. You do everything at home and look after Mathew.
   - Your GP prescribed you with medication which did not help. You slept too much and started gaining weight. So you stopped all the medication 3 months ago.
   - You were upset that you couldn't even drop Mathew to nursery. Soon Mathew will be starting his preschool and you want to take him to school daily. You also want to earn more and place Mathew in a private school.
   - You start by asking the doctor "Will I ever be going out of my home?"
   - If the doctor is reassuring too much say "You are talking like my husband, I do not think that I can go out and enjoy this life".
   - If the doctor puts too much stress on "psychological" ask "Do you mean that it is all in my mind?"

   You ask the following questions:

   - **What is wrong with me?**

- **What type of therapy is proposed?**
- **How will it help me?**
- **How is the therapy given?**
- **Who will administer the therapy?**
- **How often will I need to meet the therapist?**
- **Will the therapist come to my home?**
- **How long it takes for me to recover?**
- **Will my child be taken away from me?**
- **Will I be followed up by the psychiatrist?**
- **Any source of information.**

3. **Construct:**
Candidate should be able to explain the management of agoraphobia in a fluent and focused way.

4. **Expanded construct:**
- Candidate should be able to demonstrate advanced communication skills.
- Candidate should be able to explain the behavioural model of Agoraphobia.
- Candidate should be able to explain the role of Psycho education, Medication and Psychological therapies.
- Candidate should be able to avoid giving a lecture.
- Candidate should be able to give examples from patient's story and explain the management principles.
- Candidate should be able to explain systematic desensitisation clearly.
- Candidate should be able to explain the role of family.
- Candidate should be able to explain prognosis in realistic terms and avoid false reassurance.

5. **Areas of importance to pass the station:**
- Advanced communication skills (30%).
- Psycho-education (20%).
- Explaining psychological management of agoraphobia (40%).
- Explains prognosis and long-term management (10%).

6. **Equipment checklist:**
Not applicable.

Systematic desensitisation for agoraphobia: Key points

Understanding the illness in terms of behavioural models is important.

Principles behind systematic desensitisation: When someone has an irrational fear of going out, the usual reaction is to avoid going out and staying in door. Avoidance reduces anxiety and reinforces the avoidance behaviour. Thus the cycle continues. The goal of systematic desensitisation is to help you overcome the avoidance behaviour by learning relaxation techniques and gradually practise going out of the home.

Stages or steps of systematic desensitisation:

(a) Learning to relax. This could be in the form of deep breathing, progressive muscle relaxation or visualisation.

(b) Constructing a hierarchy of anxiety arousing situation.
(c) Presenting phobic situations either by imagination or in real life situation while the patient learns to inhibit the anxiety by relaxation.

The advantage of this approach is that you don't have to do everything at once. You take one small step at a time.

If for some reason the task is more difficult than you anticipated rather than avoiding it, discussing with the therapist and revising the list would be beneficial.

How it is done in the CMHT setting: The patient learns relaxation techniques and sets hierarchy with the help of therapist.

Usually the community support worker (CSW) will work with the patient in the stage of exposure. The number of sessions could range from 10 to as many as required. They are usually weekly sessions. Each session lasts for 30–40 minutes. The patient performs a task with the help of the community support worker. As anxiety increases, the patient should start relaxing, being in the situation. Once the anxiety is under control, the patient moves to the next stage in the hierarchy.

Unknowingly and unintentionally, family can play a big part in the maintenance of symptoms. Family can help the patient in this the treatment process by learning the steps. The illness could have relapses hence, patient should continue to apply the principles of psychological treatment after achieving the goals.

Station 159: Explain: Dialectic behaviour therapy (DBT)

Theme: Explain dialectical behaviour therapy (DBT) to your patient/carer

1. **Instructions to the candidates:**

   You are a CT3 trainee in psychiatry, currently working with complex needs services. Earlier the consultant had assessed Ms Emma Thomas a 35-year-old female patient. She has been self-harming since the age of 14 years. She was also suicidal on couple of occasions. She was diagnosed as suffering from Borderline Personality Disorder.

   The consultant has asked you to explain her about dialectical behaviour therapy.

   Address her ideas, concerns and expectations.

2. **Instructions to the role player:**
   - You prefer to be called Emma. You had a difficult past. You started harming yourself at the age of 12 years. You wanted to get better and understand more about dialectic behaviour therapy.

   You ask the following questions to the doctor:
   - **What is Dialectical Behaviour Therapy (DBT)?**
   - **What are the indications of DBT?**
   - **How will DBT help me?**
   - **I do not prefer groups. Can I get individual sessions?**
   - **Can I contact the therapist in between sessions?**
   - **What happens if I feel desperate and self-harm during therapy?**
   - **How long the therapy will go on?**
   - **Does it preach Buddhism?**
   - **Is there any resource available to know more about DBT?**

3. **Construct:**

   Candidate should be able to explain about DBT fluently avoiding jargons.

4. **Expanded construct:**
   - Candidate should be able to demonstrating advanced listening skills.
   - Candidate should be able to explain the therapy using examples from patient's history, without offending the patient.
   - Candidate should be able to explain about the principles of DBT.
   - Candidate should be able to tell about the key components of DBT.
   - Candidate should be able to clarify 'boundaries' used in DBT.
5. **Areas of importance to pass the station:**
   - Communication skills (30%).
   - Explaining about DBT in simple terms (70%).
6. **Equipment checklist:**
   Not applicable.

   Information on dialectic behaviour therapy:
   - Dialectical behaviour therapy (DBT) combines principles of CBT and Buddhism principle called mindfulness.
   - DBT is effective for people who self-harm, e.g., people with borderline personality disorder, patients with self-destructive behaviour, such as eating disorders and substance abuse.
   - It helps patient to learn about tolerating the distress, understand and regulate emotions and improve relationships with others.
   - DBT helps a person identify their strengths and builds on them so that the person can feel better about themselves and their life.
   - It is a collaborative therapy. Overall, the therapy could go on from 6 months to one and half years.
   - DBT consists of individual therapy, group therapy as well as telephonic contact with the therapist in between the sessions.
   - DBT teaches skills to people and these are taught as modules. Usually these are 2 hours long sessions and focus on the following: Mindfulness, interpersonal skills, distress tolerance, skills and emotional regulation.
   - Once a person attends skills groups he/she is asked to complete homework assignments, to role-play new ways of interacting with others, and to practice skills that are learnt.
   - The therapist validates patient's feelings without necessarily agreeing to it.
   - If the patient self-harms in between the sessions contact with therapist is discouraged and patient is advised to seek medical help.
   - Information and self-help resource: www. dbtselfhelp.com.

Station 160: Explain: Exposure and response prevention to a patient who suffers from obsessive compulsive disorder (OCD)

Theme: The candidate explains the behavioural management of OCD to the patient

1. **Instructions to the candidates:**

   Patient's name: Thomson Casey; Age 36

   Thomson Casey is a 36-year-old patient referred to you by her GP. Thomson was diagnosed with OCD 2 years ago. He continues to take fluoxetine 60 mg a day which has helped him to control the obsessions to some extent. Thomson had obsessions about contamination. He used to wash his hands more than 100 times a day. Now it has come down to 25 times a day. He wants to learn about exposure and response prevention. Hence, the consultant asked you to review her in the outpatient clinic.

- **Explain exposure and response prevention.**
- **Candidate is not expected to explain CBT for OCD.**
- **Address patient's ideas concerns and expectations.**

2. **Instructions to the role player:**
   - You are Thomson Casey who works as a lecturer in the University of Bedfordshire. You teach Physics to the university students. You suffer from OCD, mainly having the fear of contamination. You had the fear of contamination for long time, which became worse over the past 2–3 years.
   - Your younger son was born 3 years ago. Following this your wife developed infection in the hospital. She was treated with antibiotics. Your son also had pneumonia and was in intensive care for 10–15 days. The ward staff asked you to wash your hands and clean with alcoholic gel before and after seeing the child. This restarted your habit of washing hands and it went beyond your control.
   - You were spending hours and hours washing hands. You avoid shaking hands with your colleagues or students. You discussed about this with the head of the department. The Head of the Department referred you to the counsellor who in turn referred you to the psychiatrist.

   You ask the doctor the following questions:
   - **What is the proposed treatment?**
   - **What is the rationale?**
   - **Is it effective?**
   - **How it is done?**
   - **Who will administer the therapy?**
   - **How long and how often I need to meet the therapist?**
   - **Will I be cured?**
   - **Can I stop the medication?**
3. **Construct:**
   Candidate should explain the technique of exposure and response prevention, clearly and avoiding jargons.
4. **Expanded construct:**
   - Candidate should be able to demonstrate advanced communication skills.
   - Candidate should be able to explain the technique of exposure and response prevention, clearly and avoiding jargons using patient symptoms as examples.
   - Candidate should be able to empathic and address patient's concerns.
   - Candidate should be able to explain the role of family in helping the patient recovery.
5. **Areas of importance to pass the station:**
   - Advanced communication skills (20%).
   - Explaining exposure and response (60%).
   - Addressing patient concerns (20%).

6. **Equipment checklist:**
Not applicable.

Information about exposure and response prevention:

Exposure and response prevention (ERP) is a behavioural treatment technique for treating OCD and is very effective in treating ritualistic behaviour.

Principles behind the therapy: Obsessional thoughts create anxiety in a patient suffering from OCD. He carries out compulsive rituals to get relief from anxiety temporarily. This reinforces the person to carry out the compulsive rituals in response to obsessions.

In exposure and response prevention, therapist will help the patient to understand this cycle.

The patients are taught relaxation techniques as well. Once the patient is ready for the treatment, they are exposed to situations which trigger their obsessive thoughts. They are taught to resist/not to carry out compulsive acts. Initially this may intensify the anxiety, but over a period of time patients learn to deal with obsessional thoughts with less anxiety.

For example, people who have obsessions about contamination are instructed to hold something dirty in their hands and then not wash their hands for some hours.

Usually the sessions are carried out on weekly basis and the course of sessions will be around 20.

The combination of medication and ERP is more effective.

Station 161: Assess: Patient not engaging in therapy and wants to talk to you

Theme: Assess the patient who is not willing to follow-up with psychotherapy sessions

1. **Instructions to the candidates:**

You are assessing a 42-year-old female who was referred to you by your GP. She was started on fluoxetine 20 mg by her GP about 6 months ago for depressive symptoms. She did not respond well. Hence, the GP referred her to the Improving Access to Psychological Therapies (IAPT) services. She attended three sessions with the psychologist. She did not want to continue her sessions with the psychologist.

- **Assess the reason as to why the patient did not want to continue with psychotherapy sessions.**
- **Address patient's ideas, concerns and expectations.**

2. **Instructions to the role player:**

- You are Christina Brookes, a 42-year-old.
- You lost your job 2 years ago. You were divorced 1 year ago. You live with your 14-year-old son.
- For the past 9 months, you have been feeling low in yourself. You don't want to get up and do things. But you force yourself so that Victor could get ready and go to school. You do not feel hungry. You have lost a stone in the last 2 months.
- Your GP prescribed fluoxetine and this did not help. In the end, GP referred you for psychological treatment. You attended three sessions. You do not want to continue the sessions. Hence, GP referred you to the psychiatrist.

When the psychiatrist asks questions you can easily disclose the above details. Show a bit of reluctance if he asks personal questions without being sensitive.

- The following details can be disclosed only if the psychiatrist asks you. If you get a feeling that the psychiatrist is judgmental show your frustration "why all the men behave in the same way?"

- Your father was very strict. Your mother was very kind to you, but she could not talk to your father. "It was like living in a Barrack". You left home at the age of 18 years. You still call your mother on and off and talk to her. You avoid your father as much as possible. He is still the 'same'.
- You got married 15 years ago. You have not been working for the past 2 years. Your husband was also not bothered. He was always telling "don't worry, things will be fine". You felt that he was very insensitive. He was running a successful business and was least bothered about your job.
- You felt that he was like your father. You both fell apart and separated. All these play in your mind and create hatred towards men. You went to psychotherapy sessions where the psychologist was telling you not to worry too much.
- He started giving you homework, treating you as a child. You did not like him telling you to do things. These reminded you of your father. So stopped attending the sessions.
- **Tell the candidate "I will be fine if I get a job". "All I need is a job to recover".**
- **If the candidate insists on therapy ask whether he would refer you to some other therapist so that you can have your therapy.**
- **If the candidate agrees thank him.**
- **If the candidate disagrees show that you are annoyed. But if he/she gives a valid reason agree for further sessions.**

3. **Construct:**
Candidate should demonstrate skills and elicit transference issues.

4. **Expanded construct:**
   - Candidate should be able to empathise with the patient and show advanced communication skills.
   - Candidate should be able to validate patient experience without colluding.
   - Candidate should be able to sensitively probe transference issues.
   - Candidate should be able to explain the reason to continue therapy.
   - Candidate should be able to gently suggest raising transference issues with the therapist and discuss further.

5. **Areas of importance to pass the station:**
   - Advanced communication skills (30%).
   - Candidate focuses on transference issues and elicits appropriate reasons (50%).
   - Explaining to the patient about the need to continue therapy and discuss issues with therapist (20%).
   - Colluding with the patient and agreeing for change of therapist will lead to failure in the station.

6. **Equipment checklist:**
Not applicable.

Further Reading

- References and useful reading list is provided as a separate section due to the format of stations and content. This list is not exhaustive, however, we believe that the following references are the most useful for preparation and revision of CASC.

Communication Skills

- Kurtz S.M., Silverman J. and Draper J. (2005) *Teaching and learning communication skills in medicine,* 2nd edn. Oxford: Radcliffe Publishing.
- Morrison J. (2014) *The First interview,* 4th edn. New York, NY, United States: Guilford Publications.
- Neighbour R. and Reade P. (1987) *The inner consultation: How to develop an effective and intuitive consulting style*. Dordrecht: MTP Press.
- Silverman J., Kurtz S., Draper J., Deveugele M. and Suchman A.L. (2013) *Skills for communicating with patients,* 3rd edn. London: Radcliffe Publishing.
- Tate P. and Tate E. (2014) *The doctor's communication handbook,* 6th edn. Oxford, U.K.: Radcliffe Publishing.
- Woollard J. and Jenkinson J. (2016) *Core skills for the CASC*. United Kingdom: RCPsych Publications.

Diagnosis and Classification

- Association, A.P. (2013) *Desk reference to the diagnostic criteria from DSM-5*, 5th edn. Washington, DC: American Psychiatric Publishing.
- LLC S.P. (2015) *Dsm-5 pocket guide (speedy study guides)*. United States: Dot Edu.
- Organization W.H. (1994) *Pocket guide to ICD-10 classification of mental and Behavioural disorders: WITH glossary and diagnostic criteria for research DCR-10*. Edited by John E. Cooper. Edinburgh: Churchill Livingstone.

Cognitive Assessment

- Hodges J.R. (2007) *Cognitive assessment for clinicians,* 2nd edn. New York: Oxford University Press.

Psychopathology

- Casey P.R., Brendan and Kelly B. (2007) *Fish's clinical psychopathology: Signs and symptoms in psychiatry*, 3rd edn. London: Royal College of Psychiatrists.
- Oyebode F. (2014) *Sims' symptoms in the mind: An introduction to descriptive psychopathology*, 5th edn. Edinburgh, United Kingdom: Saunders (W.B.) Co.

Physical Health Examination

- Britton R. and Danielson, E. (2013) *Macleod's clinical examination: With STUDENT CONSULT online access*. Edited by Graham Douglas, Fiona Nicol and Colin Robertson, 13th edn. Edinburgh, United Kingdom: Churchill Livingstone Elsevier.
- Hampton J.R. (2013) *The ECG made easy*. 8th edn. Edinburgh: Churchill Livingstone/Elsevier.

Useful General and Core Psychiatry Books

- Committee J.F. (ed.) (2016) *British National Formulary (BNF): No. 72*. London, United Kingdom: Pharmaceutical Press.
- Cowen P., Harrison P.J. and Burns T. (2012) *Shorter Oxford textbook of psychiatry,* 6th edn. Oxford: Oxford University Press.
- IVONNE P. (2014) *Kaplan and Sadock's synopsis of psychiatry: Behavioral science/Clinical Psychiatry*. Lippincott Williams and Wilkins.
- Puri B.K., Hall, A. and Ho R. (2013) *Revision notes in psychiatry,* 3rd edn. Boca Raton, FL: CRC Press/Taylor and Francis Group.
- Semple D. and Smyth R. (eds.) (2013) *Oxford handbook of psychiatry*, 3rd edn. Oxford: Oxford University Press.
- Stahl S.M. and Muntner N. (2013) *Stahl's essential Psychopharmacology: Neuroscientific basis and practical applications*, 4th edn. Cambridge: Cambridge University Press.
- Taylor D., Paton C. and Kapur S. (2015) *The Maudsley prescribing guidelines in psychiatry*. Hoboken NJ, United States: John Wiley and Sons.

Useful Website:

Guidelines

https://www.nice.org.uk/guidance/conditions-and-diseases/mental-health-and-behavioural-conditions

Leaflets

http://www.rcpsych.ac.uk/healthadvice/atozindex.aspx

Useful information for discussion with patients; has information on diagnosis, management in simple and jargon free manner

https://www.rethink.org/home
http://www.mind.org.uk/